I R Brent

Atlas of Endourology

Atlas of Endourology

Kurt Amplatz, M.D.
Professor and Chief
Cardiovascular and Interventional Radiology Section
Department of Radiology
University of Minnesota Medical School
Minneapolis, Minnesota

Paul H. Lange, M.D.
Professor and Vice Chairman
Department of Urologic Surgery
University of Minnesota Medical School
Chief of Urology
Minneapolis Veterans Administration Medical Center
Minneapolis, Minnesota

YEAR BOOK MEDICAL PUBLISHERS, INC.
Chicago • London

Library of Congress Cataloging-in-Publication Data
Main entry under title:

Atlas of endourology.

   Includes bibliographies and index.
   1. Nephrostomy—Atlases. 2. Kidneys—Calculi—
Surgery—Atlases. 3. Ureters—Surgery—Atlases.
4. Urology—Atlases. I. Amplatz, Kurt, 1924–
II. Lange, Paul, 1941–   . [DNLM: 1. Urinary Tract—
surgery—atlases. 2. Urography—methods—atlases.
3. Urology—methods—atlases. WJ 17 A862]
RD575.A77   1986   617′.46   85-26352
ISBN 0-8151-0160-0

1 2 3 4 5 6 7 8 9 0 Y C 90, 89, 88, 87, 86

Sponsoring Editor: James D. Ryan, Jr.
Manager, Copyediting Services: Frances M. Perveiler
Copyeditor: Deborah Thorp
Production Project Manager: Etta Worthington
Proofroom Supervisor: Shirley E. Taylor

This work is dedicated to Carol (K.A.), my best friend; and to Lucy, my wife (P.L.).

CONTRIBUTORS

Kurt Amplatz, M.D.
Professor and Chief
Cardiovascular and Interventional Radiology Section
Department of Radiology
University of Minnesota Medical School
Minneapolis, Minnesota

Demetrius H. Bagley, M.D.
Associate Professor of Urology and Radiology
Thomas Jefferson Medical College
Attending Urologist and Radiologist
Thomas Jefferson University
Philadelphia, Pennsylvania

Wilfrido Castañeda-Zuñiga, M.D.
Professor, Cardiovascular and Interventional Radiology Section
University of Minnesota Medical School
Attending Radiologist
University of Minnesota Hospitals and Medical School
Minneapolis, Minnesota

Carol C. Coleman, M.D.
Assistant Professor
Department of Radiology
University of Minnesota
Attending Radiologist
Ramsey Clinic and University of Minnesota Hospitals
Minneapolis, Minnesota

Betty Dale, R.N., B.S.N.
Head Nurse
Urologic Surgery
University of Minnesota Medical School
Supervisor of Nurses
University of Minnesota Hospitals and Medical School
Minneapolis, Minnesota

Ricardo Gonzalez, M.D.
Professor, Department of Urologic Surgery
Head, Pediatric Urologic Surgery
Attending Urologist
University of Minnesota Medical School
Minneapolis, Minnesota

John C. Hulbert, M.D.
Assistant Professor
Department of Urologic Surgery
Attending Urologist
University of Minnesota Medical School
Minneapolis, Minnesota

David W. Hunter, M.D.
Assistant Professor
Cardiovascular and Interventional Radiology Section
Department of Radiology
Attending Radiologist
University of Minnesota Medical School
Minneapolis, Minnesota

Paul H. Lange, M.D.
Professor and Vice Chairman
Department of Urologic Surgery
University of Minnesota Medical School
Chief of Urology
Minneapolis Veterans Administration Medical Center
Minneapolis, Minnesota

Pratap K. Reddy, M.D.
Assistant Professor
Department of Urologic Surgery
University of Minnesota Medical School
Attending Urologist
University of Minnesota Hospitals and Medical School
Minneapolis, Minnesota

Joseph W. Segura, M.D.
Department of Urology
Mayo Clinic
Rochester, Minnesota

Antony T. Young, M.D.
Assistant Professor, Department of Radiology
Attending Radiologist
Christchurch Hospital
Christchurch, New Zealand

FOREWORD

This atlas is directed to the practicing urologist and radiologist, instructing them, in practical step-by-step fashion, in the performance of the many endourologic procedures.

Not surprisingly, the book begins with a chapter by Kurt Amplatz on radiation protection. It is incumbent on the prospective endourologist, and not only those who are radiologists, to protect self and patient from excessive radiation exposure.

This atlas then takes the reader systematically through endourological procedures under the guidance of a good mix of urologist and radiologist authors. There are many discussions elsewhere of how to do a percutaneous nephrostomy, but here, the subject has been divided logically into five chapters for a more thorough review: indications, renal anatomy, positioning and draping of the patient, opacification of the collecting system, and creation of the definitive puncture. Here, as throughout the book, the various available techniques, including those especially suited to children and patients with stones, are presented so that the reader understands what options are available in various cases. Equally important, each step of a procedure is illustrated, thus simplifying the text and facilitating review.

Gadgetry is an integral part of endourology, and the reader becomes familiar with the many different drainage tubes and stents now on the market. One is taught to insert them correctly and, if mishaps occur, how to reestablish drainage. The reader also is taught to use rigid and flexible nephroscopes and their numerous accessories.

Minute attention is given to the details of removing renal calculi, from selecting the proper puncture site through tract dilatation to stone extraction by various fluoroscopic and endoscopic techniques. Even with the introduction of the ex-

tracorporeal lithotriptor, mastery of these techniques is important, as 20%–30% of renal stones are not suitable for destruction from the outside.

Every urologist will encounter complications, and Paul Lange has outlined a practical approach to managing them. Naturally, problems are best avoided, but since this is not always possible, one must be prepared.

I am pleased to see that endourology of the ureter is well represented in this atlas, especially now that new equipment is making the ureter more accessible to closed, controlled manipulation. I also note with pleasure the consideration given to recent approaches to upper-tract pathology in John Hulbert's chapter on intrarenal surgery.

It is in new areas such as endourology that workers most need a special environment. Many of the procedures described in this atlas were pioneered or developed at the University of Minnesota, where two physicians have been especially helpful. The urologists have been strongly encouraged by Elwin Fraley, whose skepticism about the perfection of each seeming triumph stimulated further refinement. In the radiology department, Kurt Amplatz turned many dreams into reality, conceptualizing and making many new instruments needed to do the job. At Minnesota, a combination of exceptionally innovative people and a stimulating environment has been immensely productive. Its most recent accomplishment is the atlas you now hold.

ARTHUR D. SMITH, M.D.
Chairman, Division of Urology
Long Island Jewish Hospital
Hillside Medical Center
New Hyde Park, New York

PREFACE

In 1979, we proposed the term "endourology" in response to the new and dramatic applications of percutaneous nephrostomy and the assimilation of many other techniques of interventional radiology to the field of urologic surgery and uroradiology.[1] In the broadest sense, endourology refers to the discipline that involves closed intervention to any part of the urinary tract for visualization and manipulation. However, over the years, endourology most often has been used to refer to any procedure done through a percutaneous approach to the kidney and upper collecting system, and also to retrograde ureteroscopy. This is the definition of endourology that applies in this book.

The recent explosion of interest in endourology is the result of many factors, including the development of reliable methods to achieve percutaneous access, the invention and manufacture of instruments designed to work effectively through these percutaneous tracts, and the creation of methods to successfully manage many urologic problems through the percutaneous approach. Yet, perhaps the greatest factor in this rapid evolution was the development of cooperative teams composed of urologic surgeons and interventional radiologists. This team approach began in 1977 at the University of Minnesota and evolved a most creative and productive environment, because each specialty contributed a unique blend of insights and skills.

Many books on endourology are now available or will be soon. Generally, these works give a didactic approach to the subject. This atlas is not intended to repeat these efforts, but rather offers a pictorial description of the major technical maneuvers of this field. Furthermore, emphasis is placed on actual photographs, particularly of endoscopic findings, since verbal descriptions are often inadequate.

The authors hope the material presented here is uniquely useful both to physicians who are beginning endourology and to those with some prior experience. This work evolved through the efforts of many people. We would particularly like to thank Cook Inc. and the 3M Foundation, St. Paul, Minn., for their financial support.

KURT AMPLATZ, M.D.
PAUL H. LANGE, M.D.

1. Smith A.D., Lange P.H., Fraley E.E.: Application of percutaneous nephrostomy. *J. Urol.* 121:382, 1979.

ACKNOWLEDGMENTS

We would like to express our sincere thanks to Bill Cook, President of Cook Incorporated, who provided financial support.

We acknowledge with gratitude the work of the pioneers in endourology here at the University of Minnesota: Dr. Robert Miller, Dr. Ralph Clayman, and Dr. Arthur Smith.

Thanks are also expressed to the Chairman of the Department of Urology, Dr. Elwin Fraley, and the Chairman of the Department of Radiology, Dr. Eugene Gedgaudas, who made it possible for us to advance this new field so rapidly.

CONTENTS

CHAPTER 1

Radiation Protection

Kurt Amplatz, M.D.

Because of the long fluoroscopy time and type of x-ray equipment used in endourologic procedures, a prohibitive x-ray exposure may result to the operator. It is therefore of paramount importance that the urologist be aware of this hazard and acquaint himself with the basic principles of radiation protection. These principles should be well known to radiologists as well.

X-rays are a form of electromagnetic radiation similar to light, but with a much shorter wavelength and higher energy. X-rays are part of the large spectrum of ionizing radiation; they have three unique properties that are the basis for their diagnostic and therapeutic use.

1. X-rays penetrate matter and are absorbed differentially, which results in the radiographic image.

2. Because of their high energy, x-rays are able to knock out electrons from atoms, producing ions (charged particles). This ion production has profound biologic effects, which constitute the basis for radiation therapy and also radiation damage.

3. While passing through matter, x-rays produce new so-called scattered (secondary) x-rays, which expose and endanger the operator.

This secondary radiation is emitted from the patient in all directions (Fig 1–1). The operator, therefore, will be exposed to this secondary or scattered radiation and ions will be produced in his body that may cause biologic defects, particu-

larly if exposure occurs over a long period of time. The safe level of x-ray exposure to operating personnel is not known, but it should be kept at a minimum. State and government guidelines have been developed that give the maximum permissible x-ray exposure limits to occupationally ex-

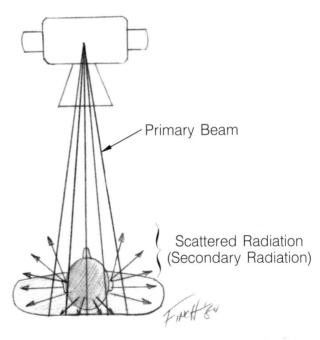

Fig 1–1. Diagrammatic representation of the production of secondary radiation (scattered radiation). The body exposed by the primary x-ray beam becomes the source of new x-rays which radiate in all directions from the patient (*arrows*).

posed personnel. To determine the x-ray exposure of personnel, the radiation has to be monitored and measured. There are no legal limits for the exposure of the patient.

Radiation dose is measured by the roentgen unit (R), which is the ionization produced in 1 cu cm of air. Since this measurement determines the amount of ion produced, it reflects also the biologic effect of x-rays. For dose measurement the milliroentgen (mR) is commonly used, which is $1/1,000$ of a roentgen. Another unit is the rem (roentgen equivalent—man), which is identical to the roentgen in the range of diagnostic radiation. Radiation safety measurements are commonly expressed as rems rather than roentgens.

For the measurement of the shorter wavelengths, as in γ-radiation, it is common to use the rad (radiation absorbed dose). Consequently, in radiation therapy, doses are usually expressed in rads.

For all practical purposes all three units (R, rem, and rad) are interchangeable in the diagnostic range of x-ray radiation.

RADIATION MONITORS

By law, all personnel working with x-ray and γ-radiation are required to wear a radiation monitor to determine the radiation exposure.

The simplest device is the so-called film badge (Fig 1–2,A), which is a radiographic film that is hermetically sealed and mounted in a plastic frame. One film badge should be worn underneath a protective lead apron to monitor the x-ray exposure to the body and another at the level of the collar outside the apron to record radiation exposure to the head and neck (in particular, the thyroid gland).

The exposure to the operator's hands is particularly high with endourologic procedures. Ring dosimeters can be worn beneath surgical gloves (Fig

1–2,B). They are so-called thermoluminescent dosimeters (TLD) using lithium fluoride as a phosphor. If heated to 200 C, the irradiated lithium fluoride gives off light and the amount of emitted light is proportional to the amount of x-ray exposure, thus, the term "thermoluminescent dosimeter." These are more expensive than film badges but can be reused; TLDs are also available as wrist dosimeters.

The film badges are mailed monthly to a responsible company that develops the films and reads radiation exposure of TLDs. A computer printout of the monthly and yearly radiation dose is mailed to the radiation safety officer of the institution, who supervises accumulative radiation exposure of personnel. These records are kept indefinitely.

Radiation safety regulations vary from state to state but they are usually patterned according to the regulations of the National Council on Radiation Protection and Measurements (NCRP) or the Occupational Safety and Health Administration (OSHA).

OSHA RECOMMENDATIONS

The yearly limit of radiation to occupationally exposed personnel should not exceed: 5 rems to head and neck; 5 rems to total body, bloodforming organs, and gonads; and 75 rems to the extremities (Fig 1–3). Maximal permissible dose to the extremities is much more liberal because the long bones contain primarily fatty, non–blood-forming bone marrow. However, because of the red bone marrow in the skull bones and the radiosensitivity of the lens of the eye and, particularly, the thyroid gland, exposure limits to head and neck are the same as to the gonads, namely, 5 rems/year. The gonads and body are covered by a protective lead apron, but head and neck are not. Therefore, legal limits of radiation exposure are most commonly exceeded because of excessive radiation exposure to the head and neck.

RADIATION HAZARD WITH ENDOUROLOGIC PROCEDURES

In diagnostic radiology there are two basic different arrangements of the x-ray tube and image intensifier:

1. X-ray tube below the patient.
2. X-ray tube above the patient (Figs 1–4,A and B).

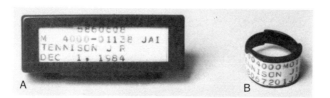

Fig 1–2. **A,** close-up view of film badge, which is least-expensive, simplest radiation monitor. It contains a hermetically sealed photographic film. The degree of blackening on the developed film is the measure of the exposure levels. **B,** close-up view of a ring containing a thermoluminescent phosphor (lithium fluoride); thermoluminescent dosimeters are also available in other configurations.

Yearly Limit of
Occupationally Exposed Personnel– OSHA

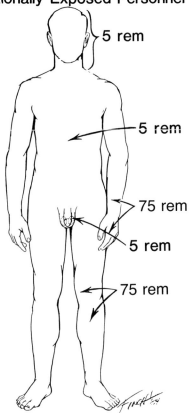

5 rem

5 rem

75 rem

5 rem

75 rem

Fig 1–3. Diagram demonstrating yearly limit of radiation exposure to occupationally exposed personnel. For head and neck, total body, and gonads, yearly limits are identical.

Because of the much lower radiation exposure to the operator the under-table tube mounting (as in Fig 1–4,B) is standard in diagnostic radiology. In urologic procedures the tube is mounted above the table (as in Fig 1–4,A) because a 40-in. distance is required to take radiographs, a necessity in urology.

Figures 1–4,A and B demonstrate the strikingly different scatter radiation and radiation hazard with each type of equipment. Isodose measurements were made using a 5 × 5 in. field 2 MA and 100 KVP. As can be seen, the level of exposure to the body of the operator is less than half in Figure 1–4,B as compared with Figure 1–4,A. Furthermore, the head and neck of the operator are completely protected by the image intensifier in Figure 1–4,B. On the other hand, in Figure 1–4,A, the operator's eyes and thyroid gland receive about 500 mR/hour! In about 15 hours of fluoroscopy time, the operator would exceed the yearly dose limit of permissible radiation to head and neck. Considering the fact that endourologic procedures may require one hour or longer of fluoroscopy time, only very few patients can be examined safely.

Why this dramatic difference in radiation exposure?

1. In the arrangement in Figure 1–4,B, the image intensifier absorbs virtually all secondary radiation. The observer cannot see the irradiated field and, consequently, no secondary rays can strike his eyes. This is, however, only true for an operator of standard height and with the image intensifier close to the patient (Fig 1–5,A). With the over-the-table tube mounting (Fig 1–5,B), the head and neck of the small or tall operator are exposed. The tall person, however, receives less secondary radiation because of greater distance from the source (inverse square law).

2. With the under-the-table tube arrangement, much less secondary radiation exits from the body.

As x-rays pass through the body, the beam is markedly attenuated by absorption (Fig 1–6,A and B). Of course, it is this differential absorption of the x-ray beam that forms the radiographic image. If the entry dose is 100%, the exit dose is only about 1% to 2%. If the operator, for example, inadvertently places his hand in the primary beam (as seen in Fig 1–6,A), it receives only 1% of the

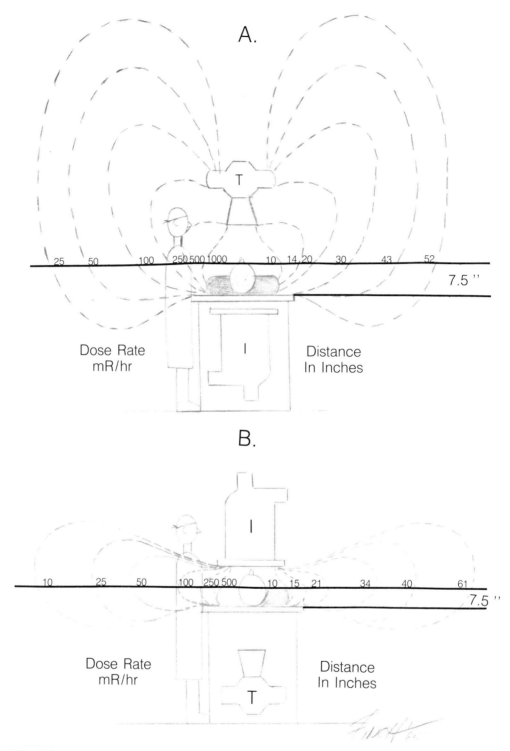

Fig 1–4. **A,** isodose measurement made on urologic equipment with the x-ray tube mounted above the table (2 ma, 100 KVP, 5 × 5 inch field). An operator standing close to the table receives 0.5 roentgens (R) (500 milliroentgens [mR]) per hour. **B,** isodose measurements made on a standard fluoroscopic unit with the x-ray tube beneath the table. Isodose curves are flat due to the protection by the image intensifier. Operator's head and neck receive virtually no radiation (1 to 2 mR/hour). Arrangement in **A** represents a radiation hazard in endourologic procedures.

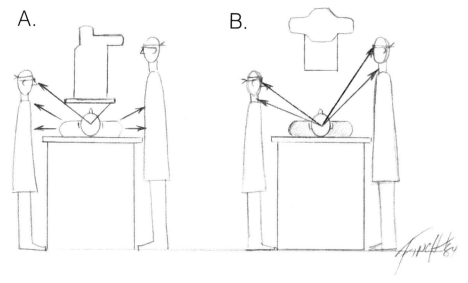

Fig 1–5. **A,** diagrammatic demonstration of difference between radiation exposure of head and neck of a tall and small person. Small person may receive a considerable amount of exposure to head and neck, in spite of the under-the-table tube arrangement. **B,** with x-ray tube mounted above the table, small and tall persons are exposed to scattered radiation.

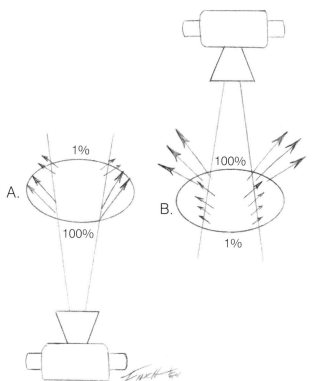

Fig 1–6. **A,** diagram demonstrating the absorption of x-rays passing through the body with the x-ray tube beneath the patient. Entry dose is 100%; exit dose is only 1% to 2%. Consequently, much more scatter is produced at the entry site and is largely absorbed by the body. (The amount of scatter produced is indicated by the length of the arrows.) **B,** diagram demonstrating production of secondary radiation with the x-ray tube mounted above the patient. The relatively unattenuated beam produces a large amount of scatter, which is only attenuated by the body to a minor degree. (The amount of scatter is indicated by the length of the arrows.)

entrance dose. The operator's hand using standard urologic equipment (as in Fig 1–6,B) receives 100% of the dose. Due to this rapid attenuation of the primary x-ray beam while passing to the body, the formation of scatter is much greater at the entry site than the exit site. Furthermore, secondary radiation is also absorbed (attenuated) by the body as is the primary radiation. The patient's body is therefore an efficient filter for the secondary beam, providing protection to the operator.

PRINCIPLES OF DECREASING RADIATION EXPOSURE TO PERSONNEL

Protection by Proper Coning

All fluoroscopic units are equipped with a coning device, which allows the operator to limit the radiated field size to the area of interest. Field size, therefore, should always be as small as possible, since this improves not only image quality but also dramatically decreases x-ray exposure to the patient and operator. By decreasing a 4-in. field to 3 in., the secondary radiation is reduced by 80% (Fig 1–7).[1]

Protection by Limiting Fluoroscopy Time

X-ray exposure of patient and operator is linearly related to fluoroscopy time. Consequently, fluoroscopy time should be as short as possible. This is accomplished by activating the fluoroscopic switch only while the operator is observing. Fluoroscopy time can also be saved by freezing the image on the monitor with a videodisc recorder or by the use of pulsed fluoroscopy.

Protection by Distance

Ionizing radiation decreases in intensity with the square root of the distance. This so-called inverse square law is a simple and effective means of radiation protection, particularly of personnel not involved in the procedure. X-ray technicians and anesthetists should be as far distant as possible from the patient. On the other hand, the operator himself should stand as close as possible to the image intensifier, which provides almost 100% radiation protection for head and neck.

Protection by Radiation Barriers

Radiation barriers are an effective and inexpensive means to reduce radiation exposure. Lead or lead glass is most commonly used as shields, gloves, aprons, etc. A 0.5-mm lead equivalent absorbs 90% of the radiation in the 75-KVP range and 75% at the 100-KVP level.

RECOMMENDATIONS FOR PROTECTION AND FOR DECREASING X-RAY EXPOSURE DURING ENDOUROLOGIC PROCEDURES:

1. Careful dose measurements should be made by a qualified radiation physicist prior to the operation of the radiographic equipment.
2. X-ray equipment should only be operated by trained, professional personnel under the supervision of a qualified radiologist.
3. All operating personnel should wear x-ray monitoring badges and protective aprons.
4. A lead apron is made of leaded rubber encased in fabric. Since the lead aprons may become brittle and crack with time, they should be radiographed at yearly intervals. Aprons with cracks should be discarded.
5. The best protection could be obtained by a thick lead apron. Because of weight, a compromise has to be made, which is to use a 0.5-mm lead equivalent. Lead aprons of less lead content are lighter but not recommended, since they absorb secondary radiation inefficiently.

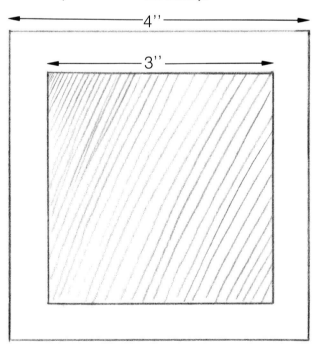

Fig 1–7. Diagram demonstrating the effect of coning on the production of scatter. If the 4 × 4-in. field size is reduced to 3 × 3 in. (shaded area) the amount of secondary radiation is reduced by 80%.

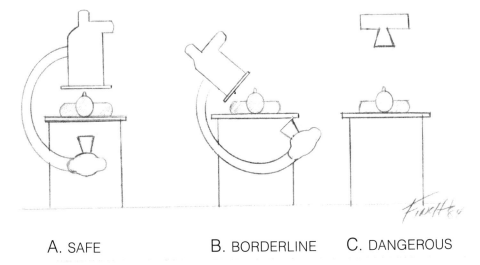

A. SAFE   B. BORDERLINE   C. DANGEROUS

Fig 1–8. Diagram demonstrating the radiation hazard of various x-ray tube/image intensifier mountings. **A,** image intensifier straight above the patient causes no excessive radiation to the operator's head and neck. **B,** with the image intensifier oblique, as with a tilted C-arm, the operator receives a considerable amount of radiation to the head and neck and legal limits may be exceeded. **C,** x-ray tube mounted above the patient constitutes a radiation hazard to the operator's head and neck. To stay within legal limits, a radiation helmet may be required.

6. Lead aprons are only protective in the direction of the x-ray beam and, consequently, the operator has to face the source of radiation, which is the patient. Personnel not facing the patient are to wear "wraparound" aprons, which protect front and back of the body. The disadvantage of "wraparound" aprons is increased weight.

7. In addition to wearing lead aprons, portable lead radiation shields can be used, which provide additional protection.

8. X-ray exposure to operating personnel is to be carefully monitored; state and government safety guidelines cannot be exceeded.

9. Exposure to head and neck is monitored by a collar badge on the outside of the lead apron. Exposure to total body and gonads is determined by a radiation monitor worn beneath the protective apron.

10. The over-the-table tube arrangement as used in urology is dangerous, unless additional special protective barriers are used; otherwise, the number of patients that can safely be examined is about 30 per year.

11. The amount of secondary radiation produced with the under-the-table tube arrangement is much less and is, therefore, the preferred tube mounting.

12. With tube mountings such as C- and U-arms in the oblique position, the image intensifier may no longer protect the operator's head and neck, and radiation limits may also be exceeded.

13. The under-the-table tube arrangement with the image intensifier above the patient is considered safe. The C-arm arrangement (with the C-arm tilted) is "borderline" in terms of safety, and the over-the-table tube arrangement is considered a radiation hazard (Fig 1–8).

14. The field size should always be as small as possible.

15. The operator's hands should never be placed in the direct x-ray beam.

16. A plastic handle should be used for puncture (see Chapter 6).

17. The fluoroscopic switch should be used intermittently only during observation. A videodisc recorder can further decrease radiation dose.

18. Protection of the thyroid gland by a thyroid shield is advisable (Fig 1–9). Thyroid shields should be worn routinely, like lead aprons. Some lead aprons have an attached thyroid shield.

19. The operator's eyes can be protected by lead

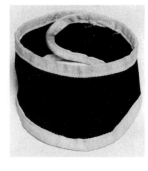

Fig 1–9. Close-up view of a thyroid shield made of 0.5-mm lead equivalent. It is an effective means of reducing radiation exposure to the thyroid, which is very radiosensitive.

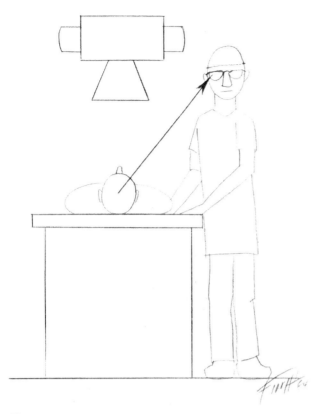

Fig 1–10. Diagram demonstrating an operator with protective lead eyeglasses observing television monitor during fluoroscopy. Since he is not looking in the direction of the source of scattered radiation *(arrow)*, his eyes are not protected.

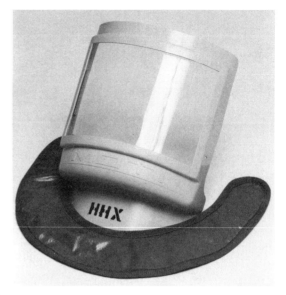

Fig 1–12. Close-up view of a protective radiation helmet, which protects the entire head and neck.

glasses. Lead glasses are only protective if the face is turned in the direction of the x-ray beam. The operator's eyes are not protected while viewing a television monitor during fluoroscopy (Fig 1–10).

20. To provide effective protection of the eyes, glasses with side flaps have to be worn (Fig 1–11).

21. Even with thyroid shields and protective lead glasses, the legal permissible x-ray exposure limit to head and neck may be exceeded unless a radiation helmet is worn (Fig 1–12). Such protec-

tive helmets are rather cumbersome, but may be the only protective solution for equipment with over-the-table tube mounting.

22. A simple, effective means to decrease secondary radiation exposure to the operator is the application of two pieces of lead apron directly on the patient's flanks (Fig 1–13). The lead flaps are taped on the patient in such a way that they do not interfere with fluoroscopic observation. Contrary to fixed protective shields, there is no interference with manipulation. Secondary radiation to the operator is decreased considerably (Figs 1–14,A and B).

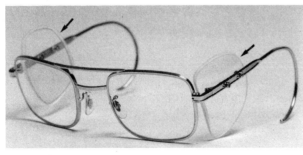

Fig 1–11. Close-up view of protective eyeglasses providing adequate shielding of lateral scatter by side flaps *(arrows)*.

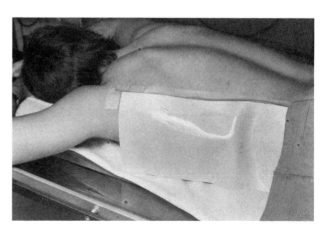

Fig 1–13. Photograph showing patient prior to stone removal. Lead flaps have been taped to both flanks. Oblique fluoroscopy was carried out to make sure that there was no interference with oblique fluoroscopic observation. The significant reduction of scatter radiation is demonstrated in Figures 1–14, A and B.

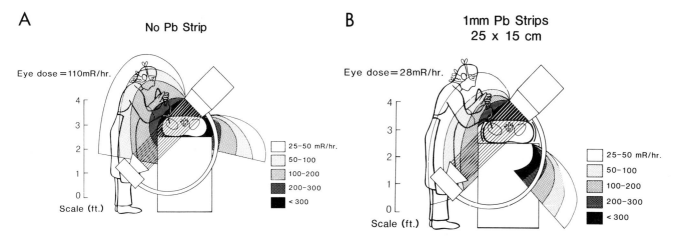

Fig 1–14. Comparison of scatter isodose measurements with the C-arm in oblique position. **A,** no lead side flaps. **B,** additional lead flaps attached to both flanks of the patient. The dose to the operator's head and neck is markedly reduced.

CHAPTER 2

Percutaneous Nephrostomy: Indications and Preparations

Paul H. Lange, M.D.

INDICATIONS

The major indication for percutaneous nephrostomy is obstruction. This obstruction should be sufficient to merit surgical intervention, which may be a subjective judgment, but usually involves a dilated upper collecting system sufficient for symptoms or for the impairment of kidney function. In this context one should attempt to determine if kidney function is potentially salvageable, since placing a tube into a kidney that is "not worth saving" may only introduce pyonephrosis, ultimately requiring nephrectomy. This fear, however, should not inhibit intervention in equivocal cases; often, a tube left in a kidney that is subsequently discovered to be nonsalvageable can be safely removed after instillation of antibiotics prior to actual removal.

A second indication for primary percutaneous nephrostomy is infected urine in a collecting system that does not allow sufficient natural drainage; percutaneous nephrostomy effects drainage of the urine. It can also be used as the first step in an endourological procedure, such as percutaneous nephrolithotomy or ureteral stinting.

Percutaneous nephrostomy can also be used purely as a diagnostic maneuver, either for anatomical delineation (e.g., antegrade pyelography) or for assessment of function (e.g., a Whitaker test; see Chapter 11). Here the procedure may entail only the temporary insertion of a thin needle. However, percutaneous puncture should be utilized with extreme caution in those situations in which the possibility of transitional cell carcinoma of the upper collecting system exists, since this tumor has a propensity to seed wounds and, at least theoretically, extravasation of urine may invite retroperitoneal tumor growth. (For the same reason percutaneous puncture should not be done in patients with active renal tuberculosis.) Finally, in rare circumstances primary percutaneous nephrostomy is used purely to divert urine in the presence of a urinary fistula. One should know, however, that without coexisting obstruction, the urinary flow may not be totally diverted.

CONTRAINDICATIONS

The contraindications to percutaneous nephrostomy are all relative. The most serious contraindication is the existence of an uncorrected or uncorrectable coagulation disorder. Less serious contraindications include those rare conditions in which visualization becomes impossible, such as an extreme case of kyphoscoliosis or in cases of massive obesity. Another relative contraindication is a history of serious reaction to contrast media. When appropriate, the procedure can still be done using carbon dioxide exclusively (see Chapter 6). Of course, another contraindication is the presence of terminal cancer, when the alleviation of pain or the possibility of palliative treatment is not a consideration.

PREPARATION

The patient preparation begins with informed consent. The patient should realize that this is an interventional procedure and should understand the various complications, including failure to gain access, perinephric abscess, bleeding, and even emergency surgery. Some assessment of kidney function should be made of the pertinent kidney. This may require only an intravenous pyelogram or renography. There should also be some confirmation of upper tract dilation, in most cases by ultrasonography. A simple x-ray of the kidney is probably also desirable to rule out the possibility of other unappreciated defects, such as stones. Preoperative preparation includes serum electrolytes, BUN, and creatinine determinations, as well as urinalysis, urine culture, hemoglobin measurement, complete blood cell count, and coagulation studies. Although these procedures are often performed under local anesthesia, an ECG and chest roentgenogram are usually appropriate, also. It is important to correct the abnormalities when possible, such as coagulation disorders, severe azotemia, and hyperkalemia.

Whenever possible, food and drink should be withheld for at least 12 hours, even though the procedure is performed under local anesthesia. A sterile urine is desirable, although in less optimal circumstances the patient should be given coverage with appropriate antibiotics or at least with broad-spectrum antibiotics. In most cases a urethral catheter should be placed.

CHAPTER 3

Percutaneous Nephrostomy: Renal Anatomy

Carol C. Coleman, M.D.

One of the most neglected aspects of percutaneous renal and ureteral stone removal is that of anatomy. Everyone is too excited about jumping in and performing the procedure without a thoughtful analysis of the situation. Because of this grave error, many a failure and complication have occurred.

It is of paramount importance that the radiologist as well as the urologist understand the anatomy associated with stone removal. It is the purpose of this chapter to teach and familiarize the reader with this anatomy, so as to prevent potential complications, to maximize successes, and minimize failures.

POSITION

The human kidneys are paired, retroperitoneal organs; one kidney lies on either side of the vertebral column between the twelfth thoracic and second to third lumbar vertebrae. The renal axis parallels the psoas muscle and lordotic curvature of the lumbar spine, so that the upper pole is medial and posterior to the lower pole (Figs 3–1 and 3–2). The lateral edge of the kidney is also positioned posterior to the medial edge, placing the medially positioned renal hilum more anterior to the lateral convex border of the kidney, i.e., the kidney is tilted about 30 degrees posterior to the coronal plane of the body (Fig 3–3).

RETROPERITONEAL RELATIONSHIPS

The retroperitoneal space is bordered by the posterior parietal peritoneum anteriorly and by the transversalis fascia posteriorly. It ranges from the pelvic brim inferiorly to the diaphragm superiorly. The structures within the retroperitoneum include (1) the adrenal glands, kidneys, and ureter; (2) the descending, transverse, and ascending portions of the duodenum and pancreas; (3) the great vessels and branches; and (4) the ascending and descending colon.[1] The extraperitoneal region is distinctly outlined by quite noticeable fascial planes. As described by Meyers[1] there are three individual extraperitoneal compartments: (1) the anterior pararenal space containing the ascending and descending colon, the duodenal loop, and the pancreas; (2) the perirenal space containing the adrenals, kidneys, and proximal ureters; and (3) the posterior pararenal space, composed of fat (Fig 3–4). Each space can produce characteristic roentgenographic findings when involved with fluid or gas. The reader is referred to Meyers' excellent descriptions for more detailed analysis.[1]

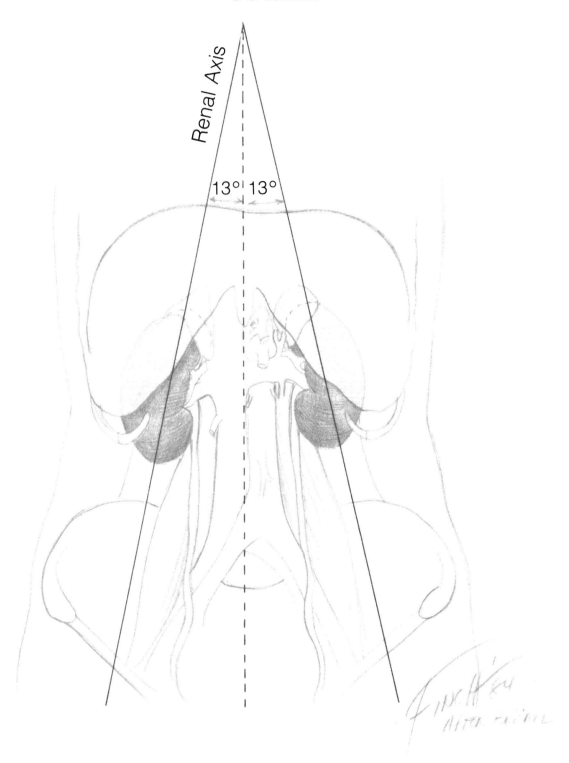

Fig 3–1.   Anterior view of the abdomen. The kidneys follow the course of the psoas muscles. As a result their axis tilts approximately 13 degrees from the vertical, placing the upper pole more medial to the lower pole.

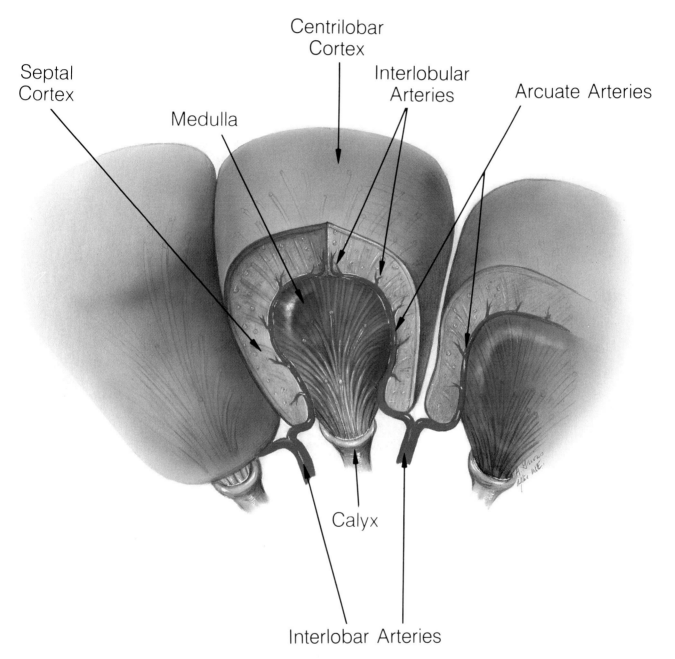

Septal
Cortex

Centrilobar
Cortex

Medulla

Interlobular
Arteries

Arcuate Arteries

Calyx

Interlobar Arteries

Plate 1. Early in the embryo there is a one-to-one relationship of the calyx and papilla. The cortex of the renunculus surrounds the papilla on three sides. The interlobar artery supplies arcuate arteries to adjacent lobes.

ANTERIOR VIEW

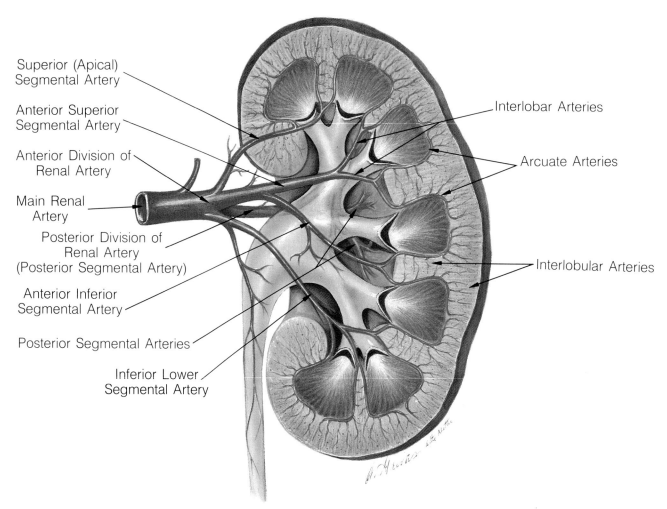

Superior (Apical)
Segmental Artery

Anterior Superior
Segmental Artery

Anterior Division of
Renal Artery

Main Renal
Artery

Posterior Division of
Renal Artery
(Posterior Segmental Artery)

Anterior Inferior
Segmental Artery

Posterior Segmental Arteries

Inferior Lower
Segmental Artery

Interlobar Arteries

Arcuate Arteries

Interlobular Arteries

Plate 2. Anterior view of an example of a patient with a single renal artery: The renal artery divides into anterior and posterior divisions. There are then four anterior segmental arteries and one posterior segmental artery. These subdivide into interlobar, arcuate, and interlobular branches.

POSTERIOR VIEW

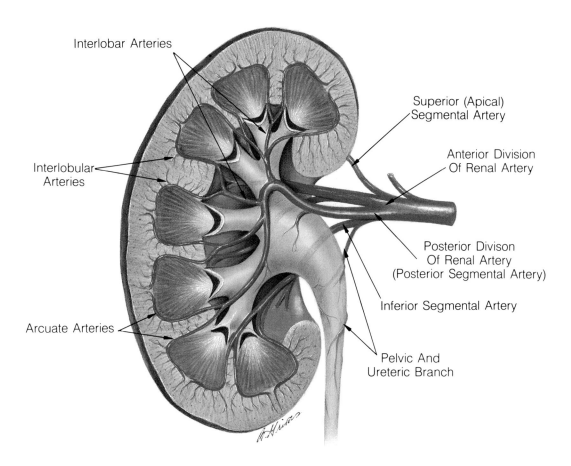

Interlobar Arteries

Interlobular Arteries

Arcuate Arteries

Superior (Apical) Segmental Artery

Anterior Division Of Renal Artery

Posterior Divison Of Renal Artery (Posterior Segmental Artery)

Inferior Segmental Artery

Pelvic And Ureteric Branch

Plate 3. Posterior view of the kidney: The posterior segmental artery usually crosses over the upper pelvis or proximal upper pole infundibulum and then divides to supply blood to the posterior aspect of the kidney. Note that the interlobar arteries may cross the infundibulum near the calyx. Laceration of one of these larger arteries could potentially cause uncontrolled bleeding.

SAGITTAL VIEW

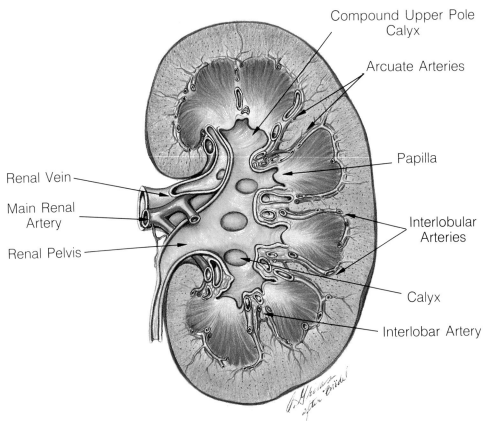

Plate 4. Sagittal section through the kidney: This view again demonstrates the close relationship between the interlobar and proximal arcuate arteries with the infundibula and calyces. The smaller interlobular arteries are the least likely to cause significant bleeding.

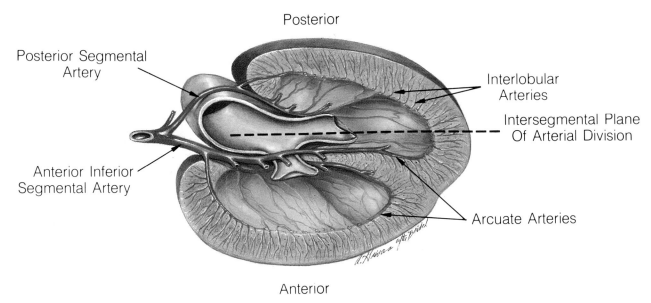

Plate 5. Cross-section of the midpolar region: Here an anterior segmental artery is supplying the anterior surface of the posterior calyx. The division between the anterior and posterior segmental arteries bisects the posterior calyx and its papillae. A puncture into an infundibulum could lacerate an interlobar artery and cause uncontrolled bleeding.

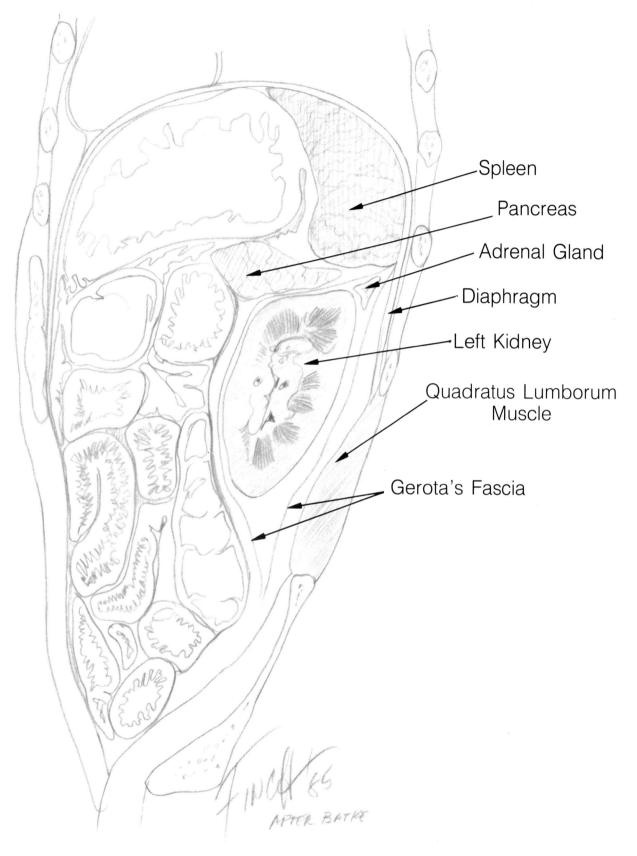

Spleen

Pancreas

Adrenal Gland

Diaphragm

Left Kidney

Quadratus Lumborum Muscle

Gerota's Fascia

Fig 3–2. Lateral view of the abdomen. The kidneys lie next to the psoas muscles also in the anteroposterior direction and follow the lumbar curvature of the spine. The upper pole, therefore, is posterior to the lower pole.

POSTERIOR

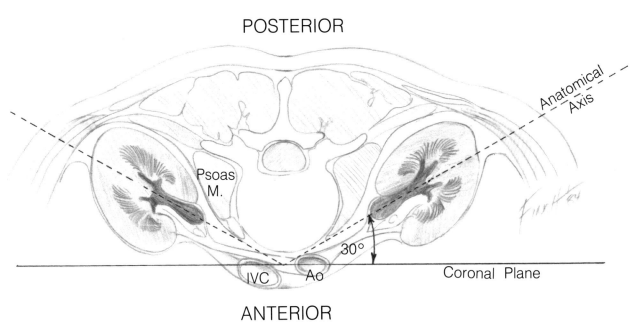

ANTERIOR

Fig 3–3. Cross-section of the abdomen through the level of the kidneys. The anatomical axis of the kidneys is tilted approximately 30 degrees posterior to the coronal plane of the body.

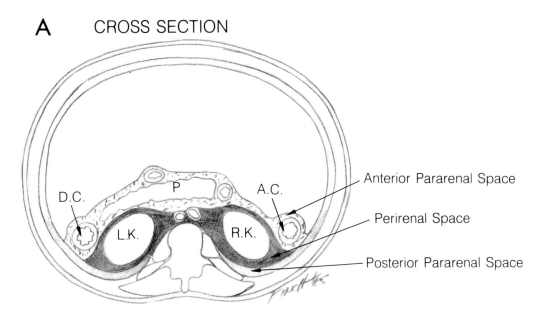

A CROSS SECTION

D.C.

P

A.C.

L.K.

R.K.

Anterior Pararenal Space

Perirenal Space

Posterior Pararenal Space

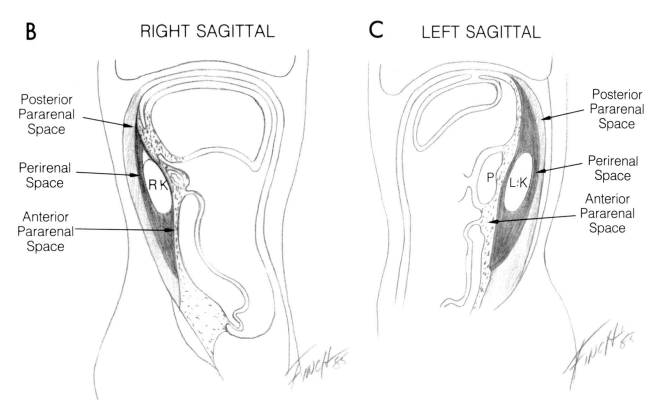

B RIGHT SAGITTAL

Posterior Pararenal Space

Perirenal Space

Anterior Pararenal Space

R K

C LEFT SAGITTAL

Posterior Pararenal Space

Perirenal Space

Anterior Pararenal Space

P L.K.

Fig 3–4. Cross-section of the body through the level of the kidneys **(A)** and right sagittal **(B)** and left sagittal **(C)** views of the kidney. The anterior pararenal space includes the extraperitoneal portions of the alimentary tract, the ascending and descending colon, the duodenal loop, and the pancreas. The perirenal space contains the adrenals, kidneys, and proximal ureters. The posterior pararenal space contains no organs but is composed of fat. P indicates pancreas; LK, left kidney; RK, right kidney; AC, ascending colon; and DC, descending colon.

The surface of the kidney is closely covered by a fibrous renal capsule. However, the capsule is not adherent to the kidney. Each kidney is surrounded by perirenal fat, which extends into the renal sinus. The fat is enveloped by posterior and anterior layers of renal fascia (Gerota's fascia). Laterally, these two layers of fascia fuse behind the ascending and descending colon to form the lateroconal fascia. The lateroconal fascia continues around the flank to blend with the peritoneal reflection, forming the paracolic gutter (Fig 3–5). Medially, the posterior fascial layer fuses with the psoas or quadratus lumborum fascia. The anterior renal fascia blends into the dense connective tissue surrounding the aorta and inferior vena cava in the root of the mesentery and also behind the pancreas and duodenum. Inferiorly, Gerota's fascia fuses around the ureter, but this is a weak fusion. Superiorly, the two layers firmly fuse above the adrenal glands and to the diaphragmatic fascia.[1] These relationships are particularly important in analyzing perinephric and paranephric fluid collections.

The musculature posterior and medial to the kidney consists of the erector spinae muscle oc-

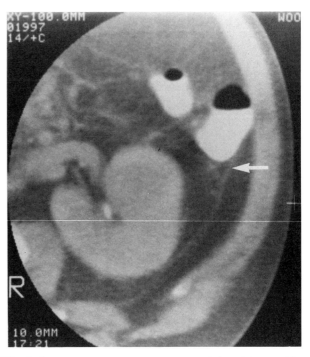

Fig 3–5. Computed tomographic scan of the abdomen. The lateral conal fascia *(arrow)* blends with the peritoneal reflection, forming the paracolic gutter.

MUSCLES AND FASCIAE OF THE BACK

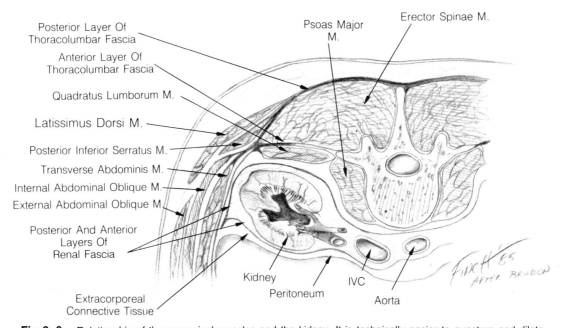

Fig 3–6. Relationship of the paraspinal muscles and the kidney. It is technically easier to puncture and dilate lateral to the erector spinae muscle. There is also less pain associated with the more lateral puncture.

cupying the vertebrocostal groove of the back and the quadratus lumborum muscle adjacent to the posterior paranephric space. Posterior laterally are the latissimus dorsi, posterior inferior serratus, external oblique, internal oblique, and transversus abdominis muscles and their related fascia (Fig 3–6). The thoracolumbar fascia and renal capsule commonly give resistance to the puncturing needle or dilating catheter during percutaneous nephrostomies and tract dilations.

RELATIONSHIP TO PLEURA AND RIBS

Posteriorly, the 12th rib crosses the kidney at a 45-degree angle such that one third or more of the kidney lies above and is beneath the last two ribs (Fig 3–7). This is more pronounced on the left because of the lack of inferior hepatic displacement. However, this can be modified by the position and variable length of the 12th rib. On the left the lower half of the kidney usually extends below the pleural reflection, whereas on the right about two thirds of the kidney extends below. These rela-

tionships are important when considering supracostal or infracostal approaches.

The diaphragm is attached to the 12th rib and arcuate ligament. The reflection of the posterior costal pleura to the diaphragm is along a horizontal line starting at the lateral surface of the 12th thoracic vertebra on the same level or a little below the origin of the 12th rib, and passes obliquely downward and laterally[2] (see Fig 3–7). At the axillary line it lies under the tenth rib. The 12th rib crosses the pleural reflection 4 cm from the rib's proximal edge. Therefore, the proximal 4 cm of the rib lies above the level of the pleura, whereas the distal portion lies below it. Irrespective of the length of the 12th rib, or its absence, the lower line of the pleural reflection remains the same. It is therefore important to know whether the last palpable rib is the 11th or the 12th. One can determine the number of paired ribs by counting downward from above.

The two major problems associated with supracostal punctures are pneumothoraces and hydrothoraces. Within the reflection of the pleura are the pleural reserve sinuses, which are invaded by

POSTERIOR VIEW OF VISCERA IN SITU

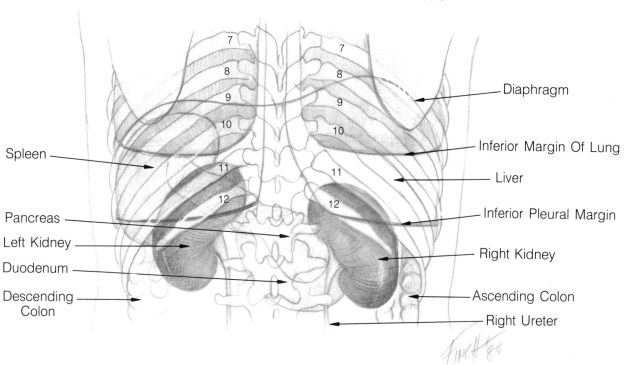

Fig 3–7. Posterior view of the viscera in situ. The upper one third to one half of the kidneys are covered by the ribs and, therefore, by the pleura. The inferior posterior pleural reflection runs along a horizontal line from the 12th rib medially and passes slightly obliquely downward as it goes laterally. At the axillary line it is positioned under the tenth rib. Medially, the pleura can be below the 12th rib.

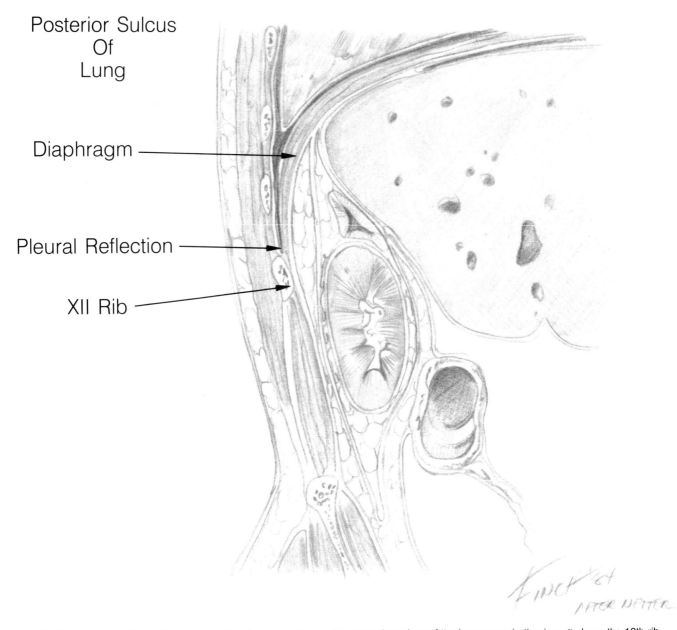

Posterior Sulcus
Of
Lung

Diaphragm ——————

Pleural Reflection ——————

XII Rib ——————

Fig 3–8.   Lateral view of the lower chest and upper abdomen. The posterior sulcus of the lung on expiration is well above the 12th rib in most patients. It is important, therefore, when planning a supracostal puncture to perform fluoroscopy of the lung in the lateral position to determine the depth of inspiration or expiration needed to avoid puncturing the lung.

the lung margins only on deep inspiration (Fig 3–8). During expiration the pleural leaves of the recesses are approximated. Therefore, unless otherwise planned, when puncturing the kidney one must be aware of the pleural reflections and puncture below the 12th rib. For planned high punctures, usually midpole or upper-pole punctures, lateral fluoroscopy should be used to determine the amount of expiration required to keep the lung above the 11th rib to avoid its puncture and, therefore, to avoid a pneumothorax. The hydrothorax in supracostal punctures comes from irri-

gation fluid dissecting along the nephrostomy tract into the chest. It can be prevented by keeping the Teflon sheath or cystoscopic sheath in place during the stone removal, whether the tract is new or old. (Even though a tract may be two weeks of age, pleural adhesions have most likely not formed, and there remains a potential tract into the chest cavity.)

When puncturing near the 11th or 12th ribs, rubbing of the sheath or tube against the inferior margin could cause pain from irritation from the intercostal nerve or significant bleeding from lac-

A

ANTERIOR

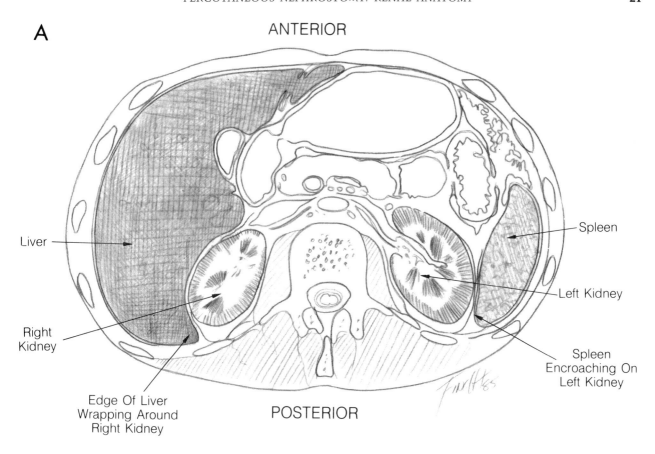

Liver

Right
Kidney

Edge Of Liver
Wrapping Around
Right Kidney

POSTERIOR

Spleen

Left Kidney

Spleen
Encroaching On
Left Kidney

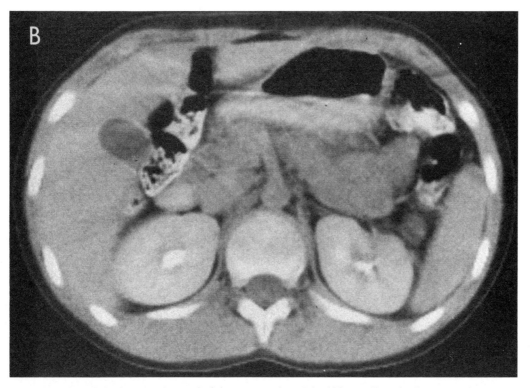

Fig 3–9. A, cross-section of the body at the level of the upper poles of the kidneys. Here the liver and spleen are in their larger dimensions, sometimes abutting along the posterior lateral margin of the kidneys leaving only a small space for entrance of the puncturing needle. **B,** computed tomographic scan demonstrating the same relationships seen in **A.**

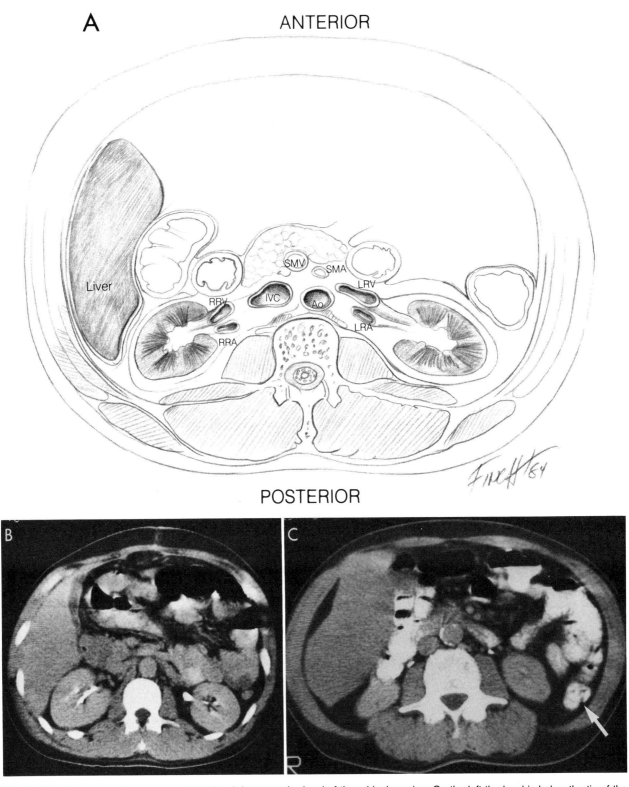

Fig 3–10. A, cross-section lower down in the abdomen at the level of the midpole region. On the left the level is below the tip of the spleen; the descending colon is nearby, but not encroaching on the kidney. On the right the liver has receded laterally, giving a little more room for a lateral puncture if needed. RRV indicates right renal vein; RRA, right renal artery; IVC, inferior vena cava; AO, aorta; SMV, superior mesenteric vein; SMA, superior mesenteric artery; LRV, left renal vein; and LRA, left renal artery. **B,** computed tomographic (CT) scan demonstrating the same relationships in **A. C,** CT cut in the abdomen through the lower poles of the kidneys. The colon or, as in this case, the small bowel *(arrow)* can be positioned posteriorly and medially compromising again the space for a safe puncture. Here, puncturing the small bowel, which is an intraperitoneal structure, could cause a serious complication. The ascending and descending colon are in the retroperitoneal space; therefore, a perforation of these organs is more contained.

eration of the intercostal artery. Also, if the drainage tube rubs the periosteum of the superior aspect of the 12th rib it can also cause significant pain. Therefore, the best site for puncturing is exactly between the 11th and 12th ribs or at least 1 cm below the 12th rib. A more in-depth discussion on supracostal punctures is contained in Chapter 17.

RELATIONSHIPS TO ADJACENT ORGANS AND STRUCTURES

The important adjacent anatomical structures in renal stone removal are the diaphragm and pleura, liver, spleen, and the right and left colon. These particular organs are important because of the potential for perforation by the puncturing needle and dilators. The diaphragm and pleura have already been discussed.

Depending on the level of puncture, various adjacent organs pose a problem. High in the abdomen (upper pole of the kidney) the liver and spleen are quite medial (Fig 3–9), therefore giving little room for error. As one punctures lower, the liver and spleen regress laterally; however, the right and left colon begin to appear (Fig 3–10), still forcing the puncture medially but not to the extent that occurs in the upper pole. We have found that puncturing just adjacent to the lateral border of the paraspinal muscles gives a consistently safe route of entry into the renal collecting system (Fig 3–11).

In the patient with hepatosplenomegaly a CT examination should be performed to determine the relationships between the kidney and adjacent organs before the percutaneous nephrostomy is performed (Fig 3–12).

LOBAR ANATOMY

Embryologically, most fetal kidneys have 14 lobes (renunculi): seven anterior and seven posterior. Deep surface clefts delineate the margins of the lobes. Caliceal development at this time corresponds to the pattern of lobar clefts. Each lobe has one calyx, one papilla, and surrounding cortex on its base (centrilobar cortex) and sides (septal cortex) (Plate 1). Following the 28th week of ges-

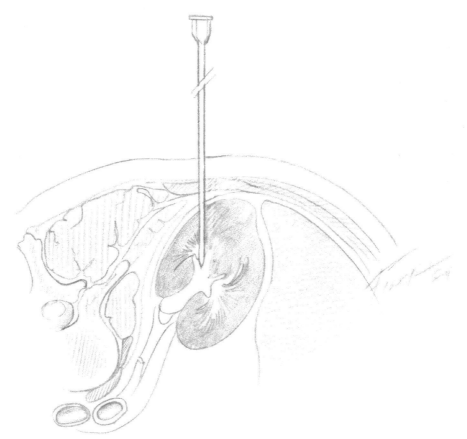

Fig 3–11. Usual skin entrance site of the puncturing needle is adjacent to the lateral edge of the paraspinal muscles. The exact site will be influenced by the position of the underlying calices and the pole entering.

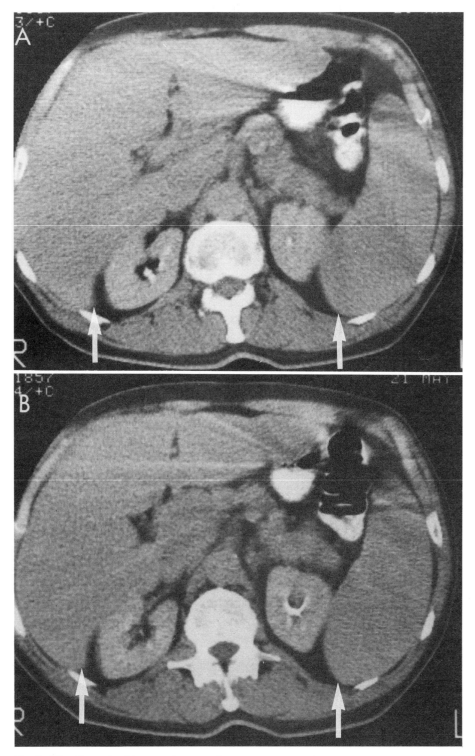

Fig 3–12. Example of hepatosplenomegaly seen on computed tomographic scan. Upper pole **(A)** and lower upper pole **(B)** regions of the kidneys are encroached upon by both the liver and spleen *(arrows)*. The left kidney is displaced medially and anteriorly by the enlarged spleen. An upper pole puncture in this case is inadvisable.

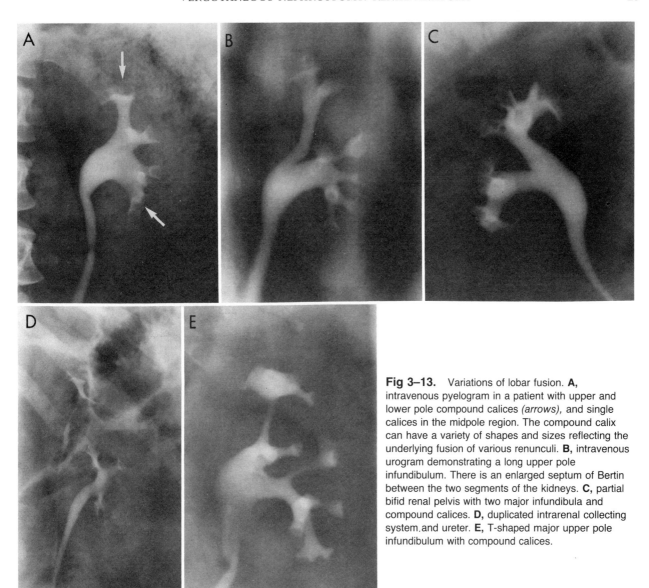

Fig 3–13. Variations of lobar fusion. **A,** intravenous pyelogram in a patient with upper and lower pole compound calices *(arrows),* and single calices in the midpole region. The compound calix can have a variety of shapes and sizes reflecting the underlying fusion of various renunculi. **B,** intravenous urogram demonstrating a long upper pole infundibulum. There is an enlarged septum of Bertin between the two segments of the kidneys. **C,** partial bifid renal pelvis with two major infundibula and compound calices. **D,** duplicated intrarenal collecting system and ureter. **E,** T-shaped major upper pole infundibulum with compound calices.

tation, varying degrees of assimilation of the independent lobes occur. A reduction in the number of calyces, papillae, and surface lobar clefts follows. There is a greater degree of fusion of the calices than the papillae, resulting in a lesser number of calyces than papillae by the time of birth. In the adult kidney there is an average of 8.7 calyces and 10.7 papillae.[3, 4] The process of fusion results in the compound calyx, usually in the upper and lower lobes, into which two, three, or more papillae drain. The calyx therefore loses its one-to-one relationship with an individual lobe and may drain multiple adjacent lobes (Fig 3–13).

Another result of fusion can be the disappearance of the septal cortex. When the fusion is complete, the septal cortex is completely lost and the medullary portions of adjacent lobes abut each other directly (Fig 3–14). When lobar fusion does not occur the septal cortex remains extending into the renal sinus to the level of the papilla. One septal cortex fuses with the adjacent septal cortex (septa of Bertin). Therefore, in this case the relationship of a single calyx to a single papilla is preserved. Fusion between the anterior and posterior lobes in the interpolar region is rare, and in the midregion of the kidney single calyces are frequently found. In the upper and lower poles there is usually fusion of anterior lobes to posterior lobes with compound calyces and papillae commonly seen. Intermediate degrees of fusion also

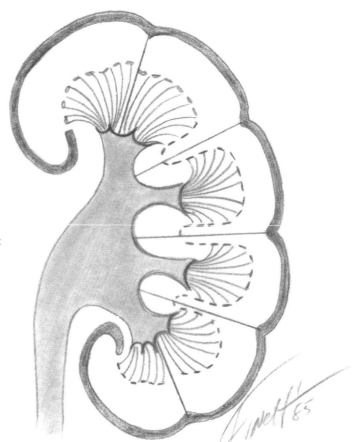

Fig 3–14. Schematic representation of a kidney after fusion of the renal lobes. In the upper and lower poles, the fusion has been complete with loss of the intervening cortex. In the midpole region fusion has not occurred and there is one papilla per calix and fusion of the septal cortex of adjacent lobes (septa of Bertin). Dashed line demarcates cortex from papillae, i.e., the corticomedullary junction.

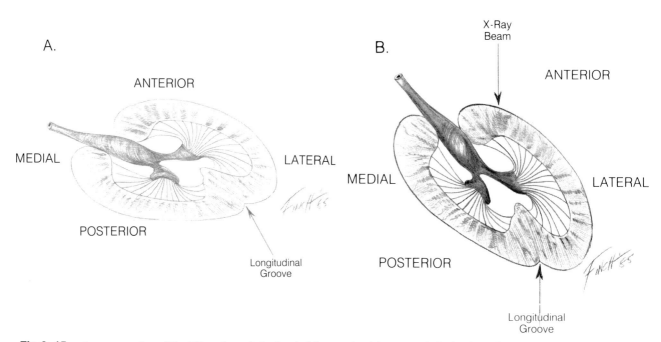

Fig 3–15. **A,** cross-section of the kidney through the level of the renal pelvis as a pathologist views the kidney. The hilum is anterior and medial and the longitudinal groove (plane between the anterior and posterior aspects of the kidney) is posterior and lateral. This places the anterior calices more lateral and the posterior calices more medial in position. **B,** same cross-section seen in **A,** but tilted as positioned in the body. This brings the anterior calices into an even more lateral position and the posterior calices more medial.

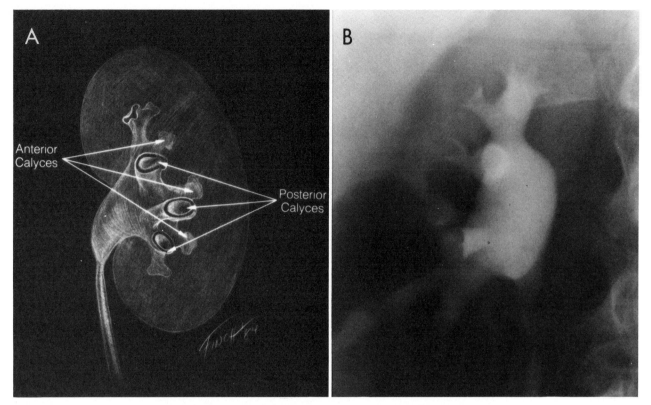

Fig 3–16. **A,** posterior view of the collecting system as seen at fluoroscopy. The calices seen en face are the posterior calices and those seen tangentially are the anterior calices. **B,** intravenous pyelogram with the posterior calices seen en face and the anterior calices tangentially.

occur. In these cases the septal cortex persists between the lobes to varying depths[3–5] (see Fig 3–13).

Offsetting the lobar pattern is the hilus opening on the anterior surface of the kidney near its medial border. The resultant effect is that relative to the main renal coronal plane, the longitudinal plane between the two groups of lobes is on the posterior lateral surface of the kidney. This places the anterior papillae more laterally and the posterior papillae more medially relative to one another (Fig 3–15,A). This is more often seen in the mid-polar region. Compound calyces tend to be more in the midline of the kidney without anterior and posterior positioning.

The posterior angulation of the kidney parallel to the psoas muscle further accentuates the lateral position of any anterior calyx and the medial position of any posterior calyx (Fig 3–15,B). The result is that the posterior calyces are seen en face or end-on, and the anterior calyces are seen tangentially (Fig 3–16,A and B). The midcalyces generally are paired and arranged in two rows on either side of a line that divides the kidney longitudinally into anterior and posterior halves. The anterior calyces are irregularly arranged about

70 degrees anterior to the frontal plane of the kidney.[6, 7] The posterior calyces are more regular in position and lie about 20 degrees posterior to their frontal plane (Figs 3–17 and 3–18). However, a word of warning: there is great variability in the positioning of the calyces and occasionally just the opposite occurs. Therefore, before puncturing the calyx use lateral fluoroscopy or oblique views from an intravenous or retrograde pyelogram to determine which calyx or calyces are posterior and which are anterior.

ARTERIAL ANATOMY

Brödel was the first to recognize the segmental distribution of the renal artery.[8] However, it was Graves, in 1954,[9] whose excellent work described the constant pattern of intrarenal arterial distribution, which usually divides the renal parenchyma into specific anatomical segments.[10] The renal artery divides into anterior and posterior divisions. The anterior division is the direct continuation of the main renal artery and divides into three or four branches. The posterior division continues without significant further branching.

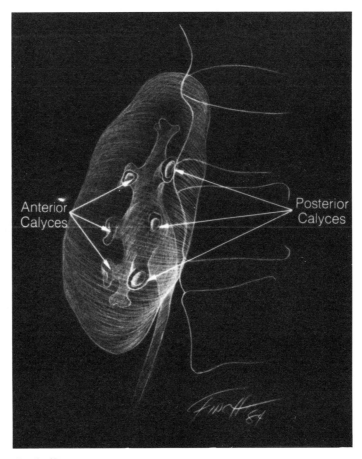

Fig 3–17. Lateral view of the kidney. The nonfused calices tend to be arranged in anterior and posterior rows. Oblique fluoroscopy can demonstrate the position of the calices in question.

From the two main divisions there are five arterial segments in the human kidney that are constant (Plates 2 through 4). There are four anterior segmental arteries—apical, upper, middle, and lower—and one posterior segmental artery.[9] These segmental arteries are end arteries without communication between them. The segmental arteries divide into eight to 12 interlobar arteries that become arcuate arteries, generally on entering the renal parenchyma at the corticomedullary junction. They are usually paired, one to each adjacent papilla. Therefore, each papilla is supplied from at least two interlobar arteries (see Plate 1). The arcuates run in the corticomedullary junction, giving off perpendicular interlobular arteries supplying the cortex. The size of the individual segments is variable; therefore, the frontier between them varies from kidney to kidney.[11, 12] In addition tongues of tissue from one segment project into another, creating an irregular intersegmental line (Fig 3–19). The planes between the segments have no constant or predictable relationship to any re-

sidual fetal lobulation seen on the surface of the kidney.[12, 13]

The anterior segmental arteries supply the anterior and posterior surface of the anterior row of calyces. They extend onto the posterior renal surface and provide vascular supply to the anterior surface of the posterior row of calyces.[6, 10, 14] The posterior segmental artery crosses the posterior aspect of the upper pelvis or proximal upper infundibulum and supplies the posterior aspect of the posterior row of calyces (Fig 3–20). However, the size of the posterior segmental artery is highly variable.

In greater than 50% of the kidneys the posterior segmental artery is confined to the middle or upper half of the posterior renal surface without extending to the midcoronal plane or convex lateral border. In this group the posterior segmental artery vascularizes only the posterior parenchyma of the posterior row of calyces (Plate 5). In 30% of the population, the posterior segmental artery reaches the lateral border of the kidney or beyond

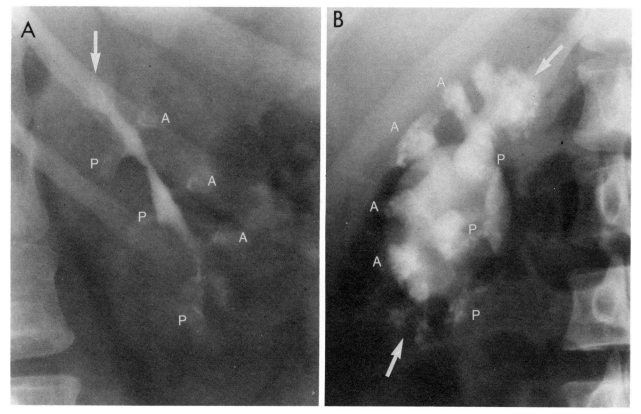

Fig 3–18. **A,** lateral view of the kidney from an intravenous pyelogram demonstrating the anterior and posterior rows of the calices. Superiormost upper pole calix is in midline *(arrow)*. A indicates anterior; P, posterior. **B,** patient with a medullary sponge kidney and multiple renal tubular stones. The collecting system is dilated from a ureteropelvic junction obstruction. The lateral view of the kidney nicely demonstrates the anterior and posterior rows of calices and the midline position of the compound calices in upper and lower poles *(arrows).* A indicates anterior; P, posterior.

RENAL VASCULAR SEGMENTS

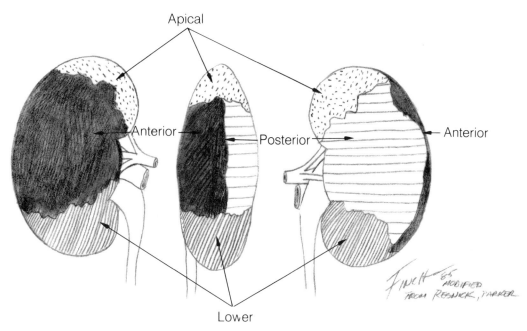

Fig 3–19. Diagram of the intersegmental lines in a kidney: The apical and lower segmental arteries supply the polar regions of the kidney, often both anteriorly and posteriorly. The parenchyma between these two poles is supplied by the remaining three segmental vessels, the anterior aspect by the upper and middle segmental arteries, and the posterior surface by the posterior segmental artery. The junction between the anterior and posterior segments is usually on the posterior surface of the kidney. Irregular tongues of tissue may extend from one segment into another. These intersegmental lines can be only determined at surgery with selective injection of a dye into the segmental arteries.

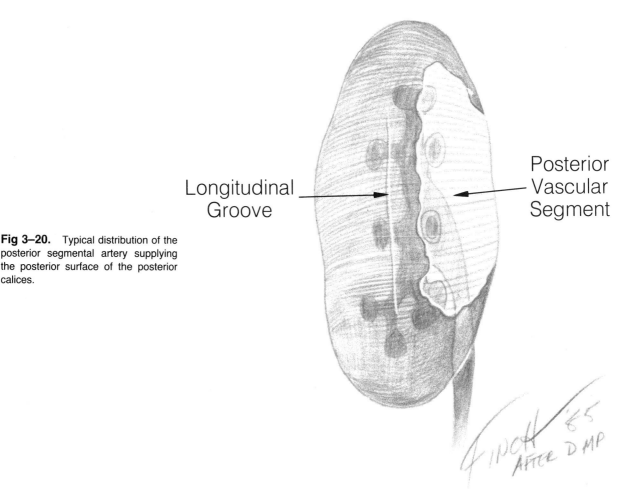

Longitudinal Groove

Posterior Vascular Segment

Fig 3–20. Typical distribution of the posterior segmental artery supplying the posterior surface of the posterior calices.

to meet the adjacent anterior segmental artery in the midcoronal plane. Here the posterior segmental artery assumes more of the vascular supply of the posterior row of calyces. It is only in the rare kidney that the posterior segmental artery supplies the entire anterior surface of the posterior row of calyces.[10]

It is obviously important that any puncture and subsequent dilation tract should avoid transsection of any major artery. The major segmental arteries lie in a relatively deep plane within the kidney, running close to the infundibula within the hilar area. By the time their branches have reached the more peripheral level of the calyces they have become considerably smaller. Once the cortical medullary junction has been reached (beyond the territory of the major collecting system) the vessels are quite small in caliber. Therefore, the puncture site chosen should be made as far peripherally as possible. Ideally the puncture should enter the calyx end-on rather than side-on, avoiding the interlobar arteries, which can cross the infundibula.

POSITIONING

The problem now is how to put all this information to good use. Once the entry site into the collecting system has been determined, the patient and fluoroscope must be positioned correctly to facilitate the easiest and safest puncture possible.

Generally, because of the smaller vessels involved, the posterior calyx is entered end-on. In order to do this, the affected side is raised from the tabletop. For example, in the patient with the kidney at a posterior oblique angle of 30° and the posterior calyx at an angle of 20° posterior to the frontal plane of the kidney, the affected side would have to be raised 30° to 40° (Fig 3–21) to see the posterior calyx on end. This will vary from patient to patient and can be determined fluoroscopically.

The skin entrance site is important because of the surrounding organs that might be punctured. The safest route is just adjacent to the paraspinal muscles. If one goes too far laterally, then the liver, spleen, or colon might be punctured.

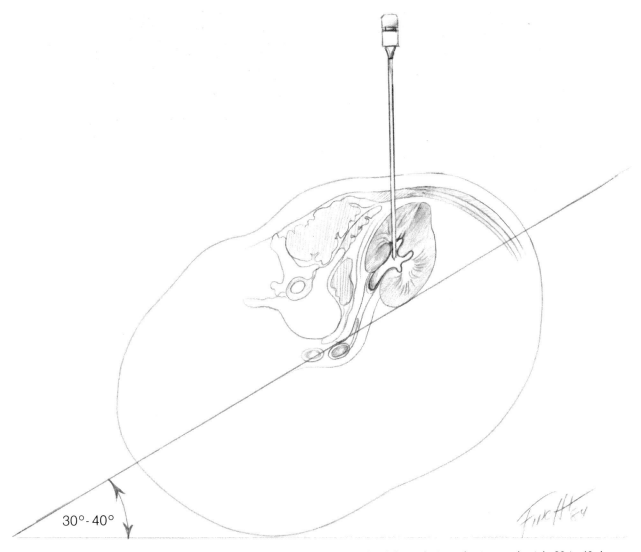

Fig 3–21. To puncture the posterior calix end-on, usually the affected side of the patient is raised approximately 30 to 40 degrees. Alternatively, the fluoroscope could be moved to line up the calix with the puncturing needle.

SUMMARY

In selecting a puncture site for stone removal it is important to know the individual patient's calyceal anatomy and the location of the stone or stones; to understand the renal arterial distribution, in order to stay away from the larger arteries; and to know the relationships of adjacent organs, to avoid puncturing them. Without this knowledge, catastrophic complications, as well as failed or difficult stone removals, can occur.

REFERENCES

1. Meyers M.: The extraperitoneal spaces: Normal and pathologic anatomy, in *Dynamic Radiology of the Abdomen Normal and Pathologic Anatomy.* New York, Springer-Verlag, 1976, pp. 113–194.
2. McVay C.: Abdominal cavity and contents, in *Surgical Anatomy*, ed. 6. Philadelphia, W.B. Saunders Co., 1984, chap. 15, pp. 585–777.
3. Davidson A.J.: Renal anatomy, in *Radiologic Diagnosis of Renal Parenchymal Disease.* Philadelphia, W.B. Saunders Co., 1977, pp. 17–35.
4. Hodson J.: The lobar structure of the kidney. *Br. J. Urol.* 1972;44:246–261.
5. Hodson J.C.: The renal parenchyma and its blood supply. *Curr. Probl. Diagn. Radiol.* 1978;7:1–32.
6. Spirnak J.P., Resnick M.I.: Anatrophic nephrolithotomy. *Urol. Clin. North Am.* 1983;10:665–675.
7. Kaye K.W., Goldberg M.E.: Applied anatomy of the kidney and ureter. *Urol. Clin. North Am.* 1982;9:3–13.

8. Brödel M.: The intrinsic blood vessels of the kidney and their significance in nephrotomy. *Johns Hopkins Hosp. Bull.* 1901;12:10–15.

9. Graves F.T.: The anatomy of the intrarenal arteries and its application to segmental resections of the kidneys. *Br. J. Surg.* 1954;42:132–139.

10. Resnick M.I., Parker M.D. (eds.): Intrarenal anatomy, in *Surgical Anatomy of the Kidney.* Mt. Kisco, N.Y., Futura Publishing Co., 1982, chap. 2, pp. 17–34.

11. Graves F.T.: The vascular anatomy and the principles of intra-renal access, in Wickham J.E. (ed.): *Intra-renal Surgery.* New York, Churchill Livingstone, 1984, pp. 1–29.

12. Boyce W.H.: Anatrophic nephrotomy, in Wickham J.E. (ed.): *Intra-renal Surgery.* New York, Churchill Livingstone, 1984, pp. 154–165.

13. Sykes D.: The correlation between renal vascularization and lobulation of the kidney. *Br. J. Urol.* 1964;36:549–555.

14. Graves F.T.: *The Arterial Anatomy of the Kidney: The Basis of Surgical Technique.* Bristol, England, Wright, 1971.

CHAPTER 4

Percutaneous Nephrostomy: Patient Positioning and Draping

Carol C. Coleman, M.D.

POSITIONING

Positioning of the patient is important for the care of the patient as well as for the puncture and tract establishment.

The arms are placed above the head for both accessibility to the intravenous line and for keeping the ipsilateral arm out of the way during the stone removal. The head is turned to the side for unobstructed breathing.

For the puncture, the body is usually placed in a prone oblique position with the involved side elevated 30 to 40 degrees using wedge pillows (Fig 4–1). This enables a vertically held needle to puncture the calyx end-on. If a C-arm is used, the fluoroscope can be angled instead of the patient. During actual stone removal the patient is placed completely prone for easier access to the tract by the urologist or radiologist, and for easier collection of irrigating fluid. If the patient is oblique during the stone removal, the irrigant may flow to the opposite side of the table from the fluid collection pocket.

The legs are positioned so as to assure accessibility to the ureteral and Foley catheters. Occasionally it is necessary to reposition the ureteral catheter. Time is saved by having it easily accessible and untaped from the leg. The ureteral catheter should be connected to the contrast medium source before draping (Fig 4–2). The bladder retention catheter is connected to a dependent drainage bag at the side of the table. It must be emptied periodically.

If general anesthesia is used, chest rolls are placed to facilitate breathing. Pads are placed under the elbows, knees, and feet to prevent ulnar nerve palsy and ischemic pressure points.

For young patients the gonads are shielded by a lead shield. In addition, a lead strip is taped to the involved lateral flank area to aid in decreasing the

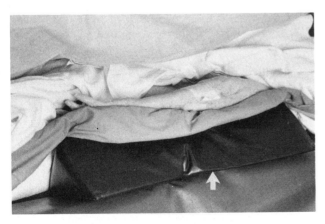

Fig 4–1. A plastic-covered foam rubber wedge *(arrow)* is used to elevate the patient's side (where stone is located) to 30 to 40 degrees.

scattered radiation reaching the fluoroscopist (see Chapter 1) (Fig 4–3).

For right-sided stones, we work on the right side of the patient; for left-sided stones we work on the left. With some fluoroscopic units, the left-sided stones may require that the patient's head be placed at the "foot end" of the table. The body is placed on the table in such a fashion that the kidneys and bladder can be seen fluoroscopically.

DRAPING

Draping is extremely important for the control of the irrigation fluid and for the protection of the radiographic equipment.

A vinyl waterproof drape is placed directly on the tabletop to stop any seepage of flushing solution and blood through the table or over the tabletop edge. Two cloth sheets are placed on top of the vinyl drape to absorb the patient's perspiration. After preparing the patient's back, any of several types of drapes can be used, either with an aperture or without an aperture. We find that the 3M

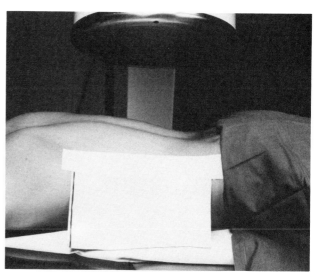

Fig 4–3. Strip of lead taped to patient's flank provides protection for the radiologist and urologist against scattered radiation.

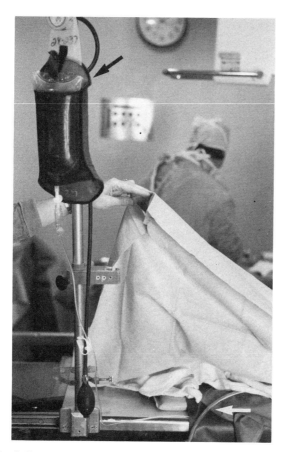

Fig 4–2. Pressurized bag of 30% solution of contrast medium *(black arrow)* connected to the patient's ureteral catheter. Foley catheter placed to dependent drainage *(white arrow).*

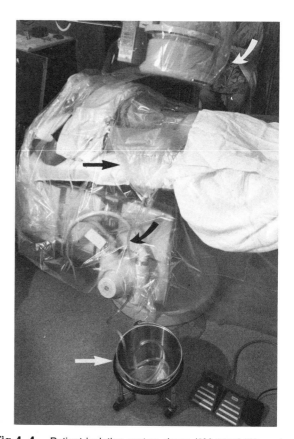

Fig 4–4. Patient isolation system drape (3M 1017). There is a generous adhesive area, allowing for a large latitude of puncture sites without potential repositioning of the drape. In this system there is a funneled side pocket *(straight black arrow).* The pocket is connected to clear plastic drainage tubing *(curved black arrow)* placed to dependent drainage in a bucket *(straight white arrow).* The fluoroscopic tube is covered with a fluoroscopic drape (3M 1012) *(curved white arrow).*

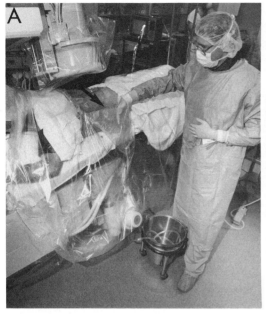
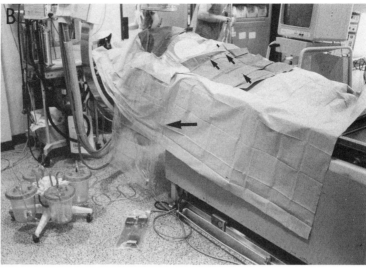

Fig 4–5. **A,** funneled side pocket of the 3M system *(arrow).* **B,** large fluid collection bag of the barrier nephroscopy sheet *(black arrow).* In this system, the pocket is much larger and more efficient in collecting irrigation fluid. There are also multiple flaps with perforations *(small black arrows)* to hold the equipment needed for stone removal.

1017 patient isolation system drape (3M Corp., St. Paul, Minn.) or the barrier nephroscopy sheet (Surgikos, Arlington, Texas) is quite useful. These drapes have a large, clear adhesive area with no aperture (Fig 4–4). The puncture can be made anywhere within the prepared area. With incorrectly placed aperture drapes, repositioning is required, which decreases the adhesive properties. The drapes have large side pockets for fluid collections (Fig 4–5). The drainage tube at the bottom of the pocket can be connected to suction or to dependent drainage. It is of paramount importance to make sure that there is a uniform seal of the adhesive section of the drape to the skin. Incomplete adhesion of the drape allows fluid to seep onto the tabletop and floor and into the radiographic equipment. If two persons hold the drape taut during its placement and smooth it out while applying it to the skin, air pockets and gaps should be prevented. If the procedure is a follow-up case, then an aperture drape such as the 3M 1090 femoral angiography drape can be used if use of irrigation fluid is not anticipated; or the 3M 1017 patient isolation system drape and barrier nephroscopy sheet can be used as an aperture drape by simply cutting a hole within the adhesive area.

If a leak under the drape occurs, a small 3M 1092 minor procedure aperture drape is applied over the tubes after the skin has been appropriately dried. This usually will seal the leak, but the added drape may interfere with the operator's functioning.

The foot pedal and x-ray tube have to be draped separately. The image intensifier is draped to prevent potential contamination of equipment (Fig 4–6).

An ultrasonic lithotriptor has its own suction port to remove irrigation fluid and fragments (Fig 4–7). The fragments are collected in a sieve (Fig 4–8); therefore, the flushing fluid does not have to be strained manually for stones.

An alternative closed fluid collecting system is the nephrostomy cannula or the Rutner adapter (both from Cook Urological, Spencer, Ind.). The nephrostomy cannula is a 34 F size that is introduced over a 28 F dilator. It has a side port that connects to the drainage tubing and a gasket that provides a seal (Fig 4–9) for the scope. The Rutner adapter fits on top of the Teflon sheath from the standard Amplatz renal dilator set (Cook Inc., Bloomington, Ind.) (Fig 4–10). One size fits the 24 and 26 F sheaths and a larger size the 28 and 30 F sheaths. It also has a side port for draining the irrigation fluid. Although we have preferred the open fluid system, the Rutner technique makes draping much simpler.

The setup for each patient and each individual's radiographic suite has to be adapted according to the particular situation. The foregoing are only guidelines and suggestions that have proved valuable to us (Fig 4–11).

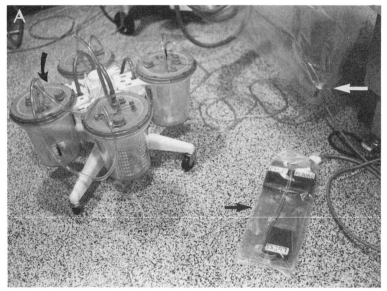

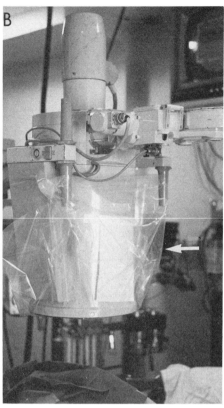

Fig 4–6. **A,** draped foot-switch *(black arrow).* Note suction system and tubing *(curved black arrow)* with four collection containers for removal of the irrigating fluid from the drainage pocket *(white arrow).* **B,** fluoroscopic drape *(arrow).* If possible, the controls of the tower should be covered in case the radiologist wishes to move the tower himself or herself during the procedure.

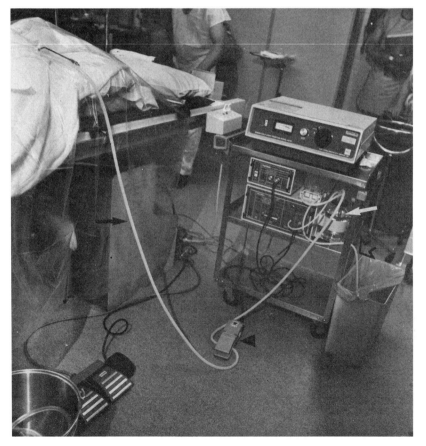

Fig 4–7. Ultrasonic lithotriptor unit. Tubing from the ultrasonic lithotriptor *(black arrow)* connects to a suction bottle *(white arrow),* which removes the irrigation fluid and filters it at the same time. The efferent fluid from the suction bottle passes through another drainage tube into a bucket *(open black arrow).* Foot-switch for the ultrasonic lithotriptor *(arrowhead)* controls both the suction and lithotripsy.

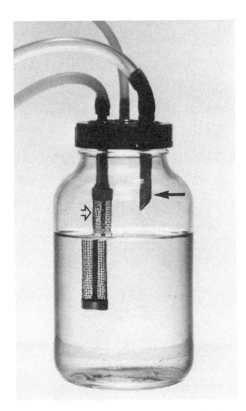

Fig 4–8. Suction bottle from the ultrasonic lithotriptor with its filtering device. The irrigation fluid enters the bottle through a beveled metal tube *(black arrow)* and leaves through the sieve *(open arrow)*. The sieve prevents the stone fragments from leaving the suction bottle, thus containing all the fragments within the bottle.

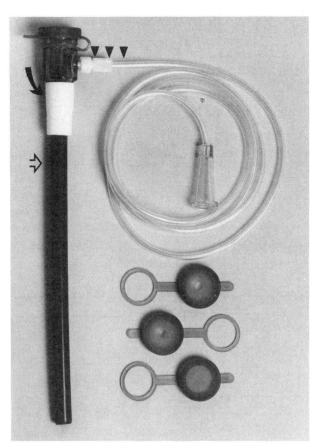

Fig 4–10. Rutner adapter. The adapter *(curved arrow)* fits onto an Amplatz Teflon sheath *(open arrow)*. Tubing for drainage is connected to the side port *(arrowheads)*. The set comes with various-sized gaskets to adapt to the different types of cystoscopes.

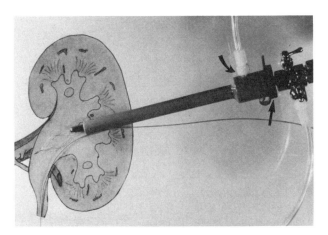

Fig 4–9. Nephroscopy cannula. The urologic scopes are introduced through a tight-fitting diaphragm *(straight arrow)* into the cannula. The side port *(curved arrow)* is connected to a drainage tube for collection of the irrigating fluid.

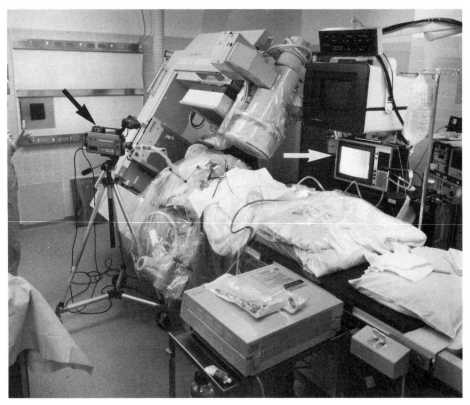

Fig 4–11. Fluoroscopic room with patient positioned. The urologist can use a camera *(black arrow)* and television system *(white arrow)* for viewing and manipulating the scopes.

CHAPTER **5**

Percutaneous Nephrostomy: Opacification of Collecting System

Antony T. Young, M.D.

THE NECESSITY FOR OPACIFICATION OF THE COLLECTING SYSTEM

It is necessary to opacify the collecting system prior to nephrostomy puncture because it is only after the introduction of contrast material that the pelvicalyceal system is visible on the fluoroscopic monitor. Percutaneous nephrostomy should be performed under fluoroscopic control because fluoroscopy is the only modality that provides real-time imaging with sufficient resolution to clearly determine the relationships to the collecting system of the needles, wires, and catheters used during nephrostomy placement. Contrast material, therefore, defines the collecting system, allowing an accurate assessment of the unique anatomy of a particular kidney, presents a target for puncture, and confirms suitable position of the nephrostomy instruments.

Exceptions

In the presence of a dilated pelvicalyceal system, "single-stick" punctures into an appropriate calyx are possible with ultrasound guidance. However, contrast is usually injected after the passage of the initial fine needle in order to confirm suitable location in the collecting system.

The presence of a calculus, usually of the staghorn type, within the calyx or infundibulum targeted for puncture may in itself act as a contrast material, obviating the need for further contrast. However, the injection of contrast medium can identify acalculous areas and distend the collecting system, facilitating puncture (Fig 5–1).

CHOICE OF CONTRAST AGENT

Positive Contrast

Conventional iodinated contrast is the most widely used means of opacifying the collecting system. The chemical composition of the contrast agents is of little consequence when used in the urinary tract. They are ionic in solution and, in the usual 60% concentrations, are also hyperosmolar and hyperbaric compared with urine.

Techniques
Iodinated contrast material may be delivered to the kidney by a retrograde ureteral catheter, intravenously, by direct fine-needle puncture of the renal pelvis, or by reflux from a urinary conduit.

39

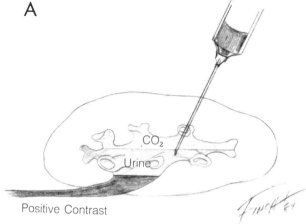

A

Positive Contrast

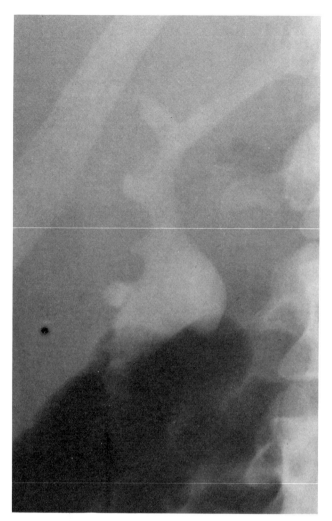

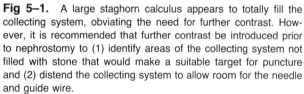

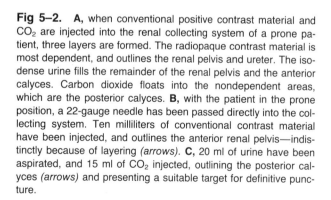

Fig 5–1. A large staghorn calculus appears to totally fill the collecting system, obviating the need for further contrast. However, it is recommended that further contrast be introduced prior to nephrostomy to (1) identify areas of the collecting system not filled with stone that would make a suitable target for puncture and (2) distend the collecting system to allow room for the needle and guide wire.

Fig 5–2. **A,** when conventional positive contrast material and CO_2 are injected into the renal collecting system of a prone patient, three layers are formed. The radiopaque contrast material is most dependent, and outlines the renal pelvis and ureter. The isodense urine fills the remainder of the renal pelvis and the anterior calyces. Carbon dioxide floats into the nondependent areas, which are the posterior calyces. **B,** with the patient in the prone position, a 22-gauge needle has been passed directly into the collecting system. Ten milliliters of conventional contrast material have been injected, and outlines the anterior renal pelvis—indistinctly because of layering *(arrows).* **C,** 20 ml of urine have been aspirated, and 15 ml of CO_2 injected, outlining the posterior calyces *(arrows)* and presenting a suitable target for definitive puncture.

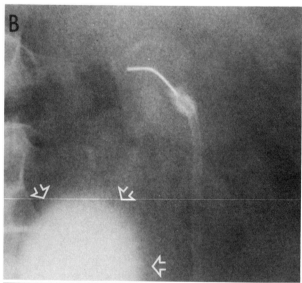

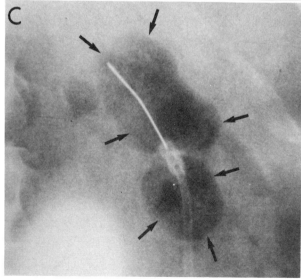

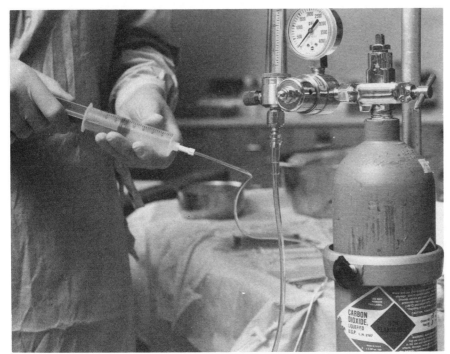

Fig 5–3. A disposable plastic syringe is filled with CO_2 using a sterile connecting tube attached to a cylinder of medical grade CO_2, which is fitted with a pressure-reducing valve and a flow meter.

Advantages

Positive contrast material results in a high degree of contrast, which is easy to see on the fluoroscopic monitor.

The intravenous route provides satisfactory opacification in many situations without causing trauma to the kidney.

Disadvantages

Being hyperbaric, the density of conventional radiographic contrast material is greater than urine, which results in layering of the contrast into the dependent portions of the collecting system (the renal pelvis and anterior calyces in the prone patient). This is mainly a problem with dilated systems, in which posterior calyces may be impossible to visualize (Fig 5–2).

The intravenous administration of contrast carries the potential for allergic reactions and nephrotoxicity.

If positive contrast material extravasates from the collecting system, it has a relatively long half-life and may obscure detail of the collecting system and compromise the procedure.

Radiopaque calculi, particularly when small, may be obscured by relatively low concentrations of positive contrast material.

Negative Contrast

Negative contrast agents include carbon dioxide (CO_2) and nitrous oxide (N_2O), both soluble gases with a documented high margin of safety, even when inadvertently injected intravascularly. The gas is introduced into the collecting system either through a retrograde ureteral catheter or by antegrade fine-needle puncture of the kidney.

Technique

Medical-grade CO_2 is used. The cylinder is attached to a pressure-reducing valve and a flow meter and, using a sterile connecting tube, a plastic syringe is easily filled with gas (Fig 5–3). A stopcock may be used to close the nozzle of the CO_2-filled syringe.

Advantages

- The density of the negative contrast agents is less than urine; this allows initial filling of nondependent portions of the collecting system, which in the prone patient are the posterior calyces (see Fig 5–2,C).
- The presence of gas in the collecting system results in improved visibility of calculi.
- When extravasated, the gas has a very short half-life, and clears faster than iodinated contrast material.
- There have been no documented allergic or toxic reactions.

Disadvantages

- The intravenous route cannot be used.
- The degree of contrast produced by negative

agents is less than with positive contrast agents; therefore, details of the collecting system are more difficult to see.

• Bowel gas overlying the collecting system may be confusing.

CONSIDERATIONS WHEN CHOOSING A METHOD FOR CONTRAST INTRODUCTION

When choosing a method for the introduction of contrast material into the collecting system, consideration should be given to the following factors:

The Indications for Nephrostomy

Complex endourologic procedures require careful planning of the access route and highly accurate puncture of the pelvicalyceal system. The ability to control the degree of distension of the collecting system and to vary the type of contrast material used, along with the avoidance of extravasation, are significant factors in determining the ultimate success of the procedure. Retrograde ureteral catheterization is, therefore, the method of first choice for contrast introduction prior to complex procedures, such as stone removal.

Degree of Dilatation of the Pelvicalyceal System

A distended collecting system provides an easy target for the "blind" insertion of a fine needle, through which contrast can then be injected. Conversely, a nondistended, "spidery" collecting system may be very difficult to puncture, requiring multiple attempts. In such a situation, consideration should be given to the retrograde or intravenous route of contrast administration.

The Presence of Upper Urinary Tract Obstruction

In the presence of high-grade upper urinary tract obstruction, the retrograde technique cannot be used. Intravenous contrast administration is likely to result in delayed opacification. Preinjecting the contrast material one to six hours prior to the procedure may result in satisfactory visualization. However, this is unpredictable, and the usual technique chosen in this situation is fine-needle puncture under ultrasound or fluoroscopic guidance.

Renal Function

When there is impaired renal function, the administration of intravenous contrast usually results in poor opacification of the pelvicalyceal system, and may be contraindicated, particularly in the presence of diabetes or multiple myeloma. Retrograde techniques, opacification by reflux, or fine-needle puncture are therefore used.

RETROGRADE OPACIFICATION

Indications

This is the technique of choice for opacification of the collecting system for nephrostomy prior to complex endourologic procedures.

Advantages

• The degree of distension of the collecting system is controllable. Distension facilitates the initial needle puncture (Fig 5–4).
• The degree of opacification may be varied. Contrast can be introduced or removed in order to determine the position of small calculi. Both positive and negative contrast agents may be chosen.
• Extravasation does not occur prior to the definitive nephrostomy puncture, so the puncture target is clearly visible.
• During percutaneous urinary stone removal, the presence of the retrograde ureteral catheter inhibits the passage of stones down the ureter.
• The retrograde catheter can be utilized for flushing techniques during stone removal.
• In rare situations it is advantageous to pass a guide wire up the ureteral catheter and bring it out of the nephrostomy tract to facilitate dilation and ensure intraluminal location of the nephrostomy catheter.

Limitations

• Retrograde ureteral catheterization requires cystoscopy. This represents an additional procedure.
• Overdistension of the collecting system is possible with the pressurized infusion of contrast. This may cause considerable patient discomfort, and, rarely, rupture of the collecting system.
• The technique cannot be used when there is complete upper urinary tract obstruction.

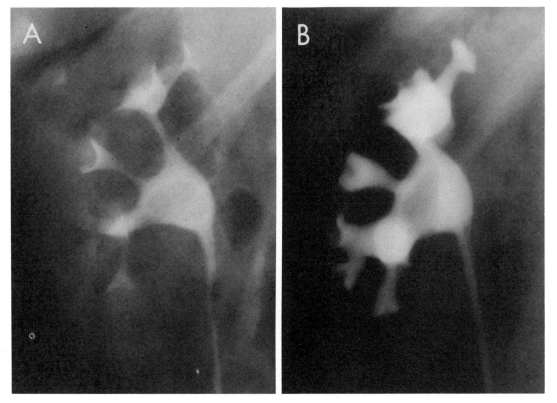

Fig 5–4. Advantages of retrograde opacification. **A,** 10-minute film from the intravenous pyelogram demonstrates a large renal pelvic stone. The calyces and infundibula are "spidery," presenting a difficult target for puncture. **B,** retrograde opacification distends the calyces and infundibula, providing for easier delineation of anatomical relationships, and allowing more successful puncture.

Technique

Cystoscopy is performed using a flexible or a rigid cystoscope. An angiographic guide wire is passed up the ureter and over this a ureteral catheter, 5 to 8 F in size with a single end-hole, is inserted so that its tip lies at the ureteropelvic junction. This is connected to a pressure infusion bag containing 60% iodinated contrast diluted with normal saline, one part contrast to two parts saline (Fig 5–5). The rate of infusion is adjusted for sufficient opacification and distension for the puncture. Negative contrast agent may be easily injected through a side port in the infusion tubing. It is recommended that the infusion be terminated just before puncture, to avoid troublesome extravasation of contrast should the puncture be unsatisfactory.

OPACIFICATION BY REFLUX

Indications

The pelvicalyceal system can be opacified by retrograde reflux of contrast up the ureter in patients with ileal or colonic urinary conduits without obstruction to the upper urinary tract (Fig 5–6). This is a good technique when use of intravenous contrast either is contraindicated or produces inadequate opacification.

Technique

A Foley catheter is placed in the urinary conduit, the balloon inflated with saline, and gentle traction applied to the Foley catheter to "snug"

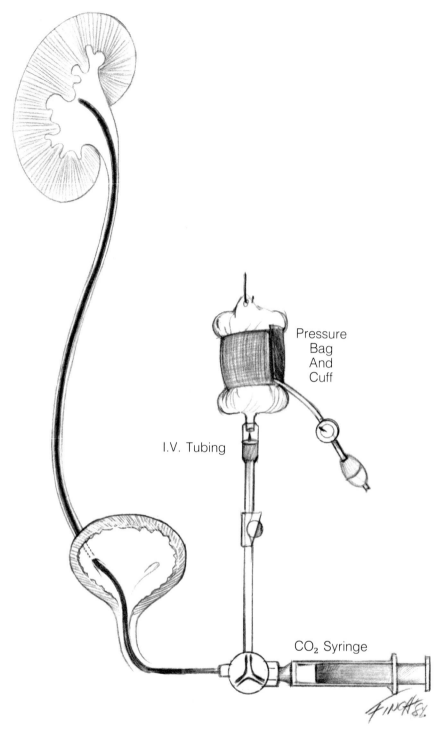

Fig 5–5.   Pressurized infusion bag contains 20% iodinated contrast material. Infusion rate is adjusted to produce satisfactory opacification and distension of the renal collecting system without causing undue patient discomfort. A three-way stopcock allows introduction of CO_2 as a contrast agent or for flushing of ureteral calculi.

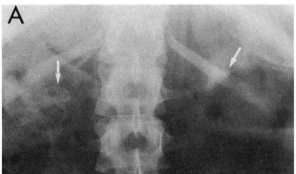

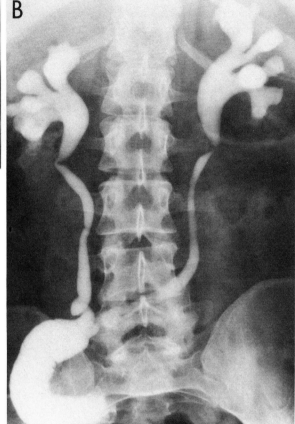

Fig 5–6. **A,** scout film demonstrates bilateral renal pelvic calculi in patient with ileal conduit. **B,** infusion of contrast into the conduit using a Foley catheter results in excellent visualization of the collecting systems, prior to nephrostomy puncture.

the balloon against the internal aspect of the stoma. The patient is placed in the prone-oblique position for the nephrostomy, and diluted contrast is run into the Foley catheter, either using the same pressure infusion system as in the retrograde technique or with a 60-cc syringe. Overdistension of the conduit is avoided by intermittent fluoroscopy.

Advantages

• It is simple and atraumatic.

Disadvantages

• The technique is messy due to the inevitable leak around the Foley balloon.
• In theory, there is an increased risk of sepsis due to the high incidence of infected urine in conduits. However, this has not been a significant problem with the use of prophylactic antibiotics.
• The degree of opacification and distension of the collecting system is unpredictable.

INTRAVENOUS ADMINISTRATION OF CONTRAST

Indications

The pelvicalyceal system is opacified by the intravenous injection of iodinated contrast when there is no gross dilatation, when there is adequate renal function, and when retrograde ureteral catheterization is either not successful or not required, as in nephrostomy for drainage.

Contraindications

A documented previous allergic reaction to intravenous contrast material and renal impairment (particularly when secondary to diabetes mellitus or multiple myeloma) are relative contraindications.

Technique

Fifty to 100 ml of iodinated contrast agent is injected intravenously immediately before nephrostomy puncture. Satisfactory visualization occurs in five to ten minutes. An abdominal compression device may be used to increase distension of the pelvicalyceal system, and so facilitate puncture. In the presence of upper urinary tract obstruction, preinjecting the contrast three to six hours prior to nephrostomy puncture frequently results in satisfactory visualization. Intravenous opacification may be followed either by definitive nephrostomy or by fluoroscopically guided fine-needle puncture, to allow introduction of additional contrast and distension of the pelvicalyceal system prior to definitive puncture.

Limitations

- The degree of distension is difficult to control, and accurate puncture is more difficult than the retrograde method of opacification.
- Once contrast is injected, there is continuous filtration of contrast material for several hours. Therefore, small radiopaque stones may be obscured throughout the remainder of the procedure.
- Even when injected intravenously, the filtered contrast material is denser than the urine already in the collecting system, and may layer with gravity in the dependent portions. Therefore, posterior calyces are sometimes not visualized in the dilated system. Rolling the patient several times may mix the contrast and resolve the problem.

FINE-NEEDLE PUNCTURE

There is general acceptance of the safety of fine-needle puncture (using 21- to 23-gauge needles) into all of the abdominal organs. Even when major blood vessels and bowel loops are traversed by such a needle, the incidence of complications is minimal. Once the needle is in such a collecting system, contrast is injected; this is followed by the definitive nephrostomy puncture.

Indications

This technique is used in the absence of a retrograde ureteral catheter, in the presence of ureteral obstruction, and when intravenous opacification is either contraindicated or suboptimal.

Techniques

The fine-needle puncture may be guided by fluoroscopy alone or with the addition of real-time ultrasound.

FINE-NEEDLE PUNCTURE GUIDED BY FLUOROSCOPY

Punctures are made from a directly posterior approach. This allows easy orientation with respect to the skeletal structures.

The position of the renal collecting system may be inferred by (1) fluoroscopic recognition of the

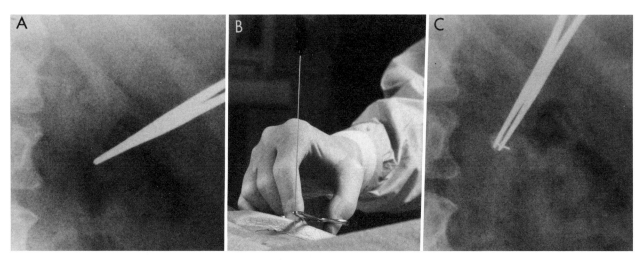

Fig 5–7. Fine-needle puncture guided by fluoroscopy. **A,** hemostat marks the site of initial puncture, immediately lateral to the transverse process of L-2. **B,** the needle is passed in the direction of the primary x-ray beam down onto the kidney. A hemostat keeps the operators hands away from the primary beam. **C,** "Down-the-barrel" imaging projects the needle as a dot. The needle is inserted to a depth of 6 to 10 cm.

renal outline, (2) reference to a previous intravenous pyelogram, (3) the administration of intravenous contrast, or (4) the assumption that the renal pelvis lies immediately lateral to the tips of the transverse processes of the L-1 and L-2 vertebrae.

Reference to a previous sectional image (ultrasound, computed tomographic scan, magnetic resonance imaging) provides a useful guide to the required depth of needle puncture. This is usually between 6 and 12 cm, depending on the size of the patient.

Advantages

- Adequate volumes of contrast can be injected, and the degree of distension of the collecting system can be controlled.
- Both positive and negative contrast agents can be introduced.
- In an obstructed system, the technique is more rapid than waiting for intravenous opacification.

Disadvantages

- Multiple unsuccessful needle passes may result in extravasation of contrast from the collecting system at a subsequent successful puncture. This may compromise the definitive nephrostomy.
- The technique causes more discomfort to the patient than intravenous contrast administration.
- "Spidery" nonobstructed collecting systems may be impossible to puncture despite multiple passes of the "skinny" needle.

Technique

The patient is placed in a prone position, the skin is prepared, and the puncture site is chosen using fluoroscopic guidance of a sterile radiopaque pointer (Fig 5–7,A). The skin is infiltrated with 1% lidocaine solution, a small dermatotomy is made, and then, during quiet respiration, a 22-gauge needle is advanced in the direction of the x-ray beam down onto the kidney (Fig 5–7,B and C). The direction of the needle is checked fluoroscopically every 1 cm or so and readjusted as necessary. A recently developed split handle (Cook Inc., Bloomington, Ind.) can be used to hold the needle. This allows continuous fluoroscopic monitoring during needle insertion, without irradiation of the operator's hands (Fig 5–8). Because a beveled needle tends to deviate in a direction opposite the bevel, it may be "steered" onto a target by judicious rotation (Fig 5–9). The position of the bevel is marked on the hub of the needle.

As the needle enters the kidney there is often a "popping" sensation as the renal capsule is crossed. There is then a characteristic movement of the needle with respiration (Fig 5–10). The needle is advanced a further 2 to 4 cm. Usually there is a second vague popping sensation as the renal pelvis is entered. The stylet is then removed and a connecting tube and syringe attached to the needle hub. Gentle suction is applied, and the needle is slowly withdrawn until urine is aspirated. Once there is free flow of urine, a sample may be taken for Gram stain, and culture if indicated; this is followed by an injection of contrast to opacify the collecting system prior to the definitive nephrostomy (Fig 5–11).

In the presence of upper urinary tract obstruction, and particularly if there is a possibility of infected urine, care should be taken to avoid overdistension of the collecting system for fear of precipitating septicemia. Minimizing the volume of contrast used and injecting an equal volume of contrast to that of the urine aspirated are wise precautions. The use of CO_2 allows initial visualization of the posterior calyces without the requirement of large volumes of contrast material.

If urine is not aspirated, repeated punctures are made, altering the aim slightly each time. Not puncturing deeply enough is a common cause of failure, particularly in obese patients. Lateral fluoroscopy provides a useful indication of the depth of the needle. The renal pelvis lies at approximately the same depth as the middle of the vertebral bodies.

Failure to aspirate urine on multiple passes may indicate a collecting system filled with debris, e.g., clot or fungus balls. A careful injection of contrast in such a situation may outline the collecting system and prove suitable location of the needle in the absence of urine aspirate (Fig 5–12).

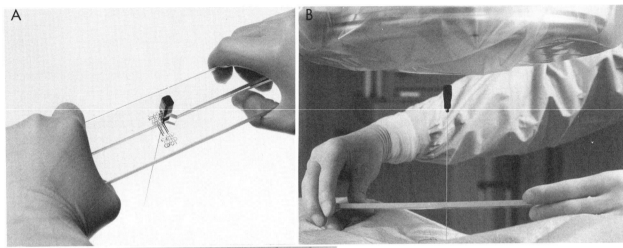

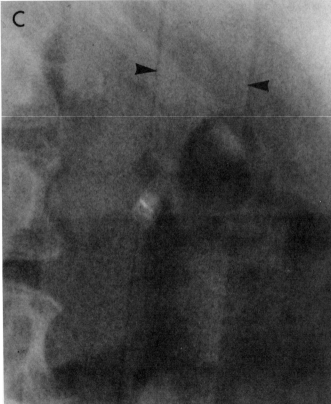

Fig 5–8. Amplatz radiolucent needle holder. **A,** radiolucent needle holder has been developed that allows highly accurate passage of an 18- to 23-gauge needle onto the kidney, in the direction of the primary beam, while keeping the operator's hands away from the primary radiation. **B,** by squeezing the shaft of the needle in the "split" handle, accurate puncture is performed during fluoroscopy. **C,** needle is projected as a dot over the intended site of puncture. Radiolucent handle is faintly visible *(arrows).*

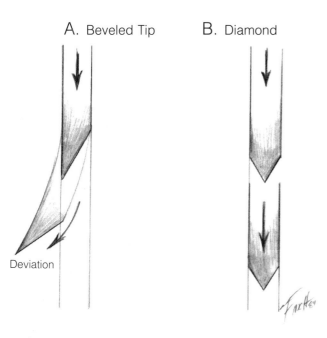

A. Beveled Tip   B. Diamond

Deviation

Fig 5–9. A beveled needle tends to deviate in a direction away from the bevel. This affords some control of the direction of the needle tip by judicious rotation of the hub. A diamond-tipped needle runs a straight course, and is therefore more suitable for definitive nephrostomy.

Fig 5–10. Once the tip of the needle lies within the kidney, there is a characteristic movement of the needle with respiration. Advancement of the needle a further 2 to 4 cm will pierce the collecting system.

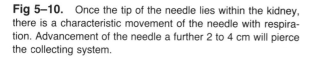

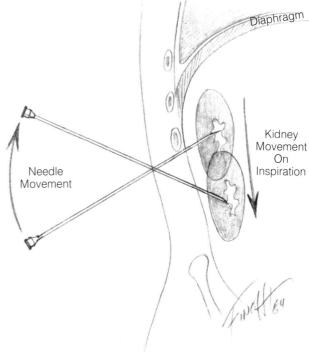

Diaphragm

Needle
Movement

Kidney
Movement
On
Inspiration

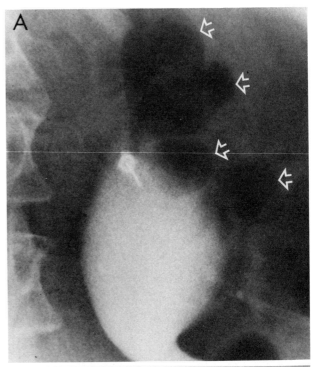

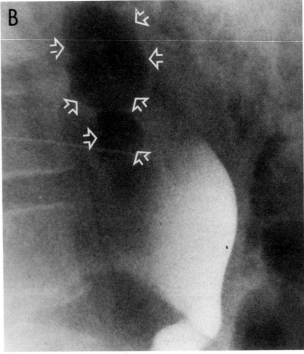

Fig 5–11. Injection of contrast material. **A,** once urine is aspirated from the Chiba needle, 10 to 20 ml of positive contrast is injected. This is followed by the withdrawal of 15 to 30 ml of urine, in order to decompress the system. Ten to 20 cc of CO_2 is then injected in order to outline the posterior calyces *(arrows)*. **B,** a steep oblique view shows the needle in the renal pelvis. Positive contrast outlines the anterior part of the renal pelvis and ureter. The gas-filled posterior calyces are well demonstrated *(arrows)*.

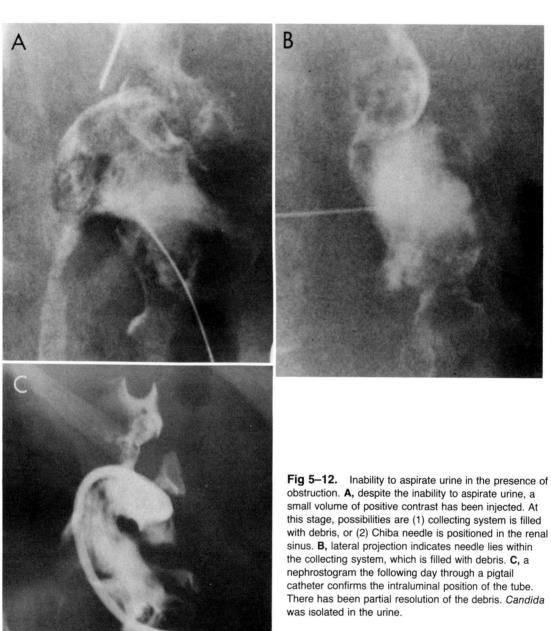

Fig 5–12. Inability to aspirate urine in the presence of obstruction. **A,** despite the inability to aspirate urine, a small volume of positive contrast has been injected. At this stage, possibilities are (1) collecting system is filled with debris, or (2) Chiba needle is positioned in the renal sinus. **B,** lateral projection indicates needle lies within the collecting system, which is filled with debris. **C,** a nephrostogram the following day through a pigtail catheter confirms the intraluminal position of the tube. There has been partial resolution of the debris. *Candida* was isolated in the urine.

FINE-NEEDLE PUNCTURE GUIDED BY REAL-TIME ULTRASOUND

Ultrasound-guided fine-needle puncture is usually performed from a posterolateral approach, in the same way as the definitive nephrostomy puncture. However, the true posterior approach may also be used, as in fine-needle puncture guided by fluoroscopy.

Advantages

- The fluid-filled collecting system, particularly when dilated, may be directly visualized without the need for contrast agents.
- The depth of the required tract to the kidney may be accurately measured.
- The abdominal organs adjacent to the kidney are usually easily recognizable on the ultrasound monitor and, therefore, a safe access route may be ensured.
- There is no radiation exposure to the operator's hands.

Limitations

- Gross obesity severely limits visualization.
- Nondilated, "spidery" collecting systems may be difficult or impossible to puncture, as in the fluoroscopically guided technique.

- The transducers of the commonly available machines cannot be sterilized. Sterile sleeves or gloves may therefore be used, but are often awkward to handle.

Techniques

Real-time ultrasound provides the capability of observing the actual progress of the needle into the kidney. The tip of the needle is often seen as an echogenic focus, and this may be made more obvious by "jiggling" the hub of the needle (Fig 5–13). Three basic techniques are available for directing the fine needle.

- Needle holders are available that attach to the transducer, and these guide the needle along the plane of the beam of sound onto the target, which is under constant observation on the ultrasound monitor (Fig 5–14). While these holders are undoubtedly successful, most operators find them clumsy to use, with difficulties in maintenance of sterility.
- The passage of the needle may be observed on the monitor with equal success without the use of a needle guide, by holding the transducer steady and then manually aiming the needle down the plane of the sound wave to the required depth (Fig 5–15).
- "Memory-guess," however, is the most popular method for guiding the fine-needle puncture

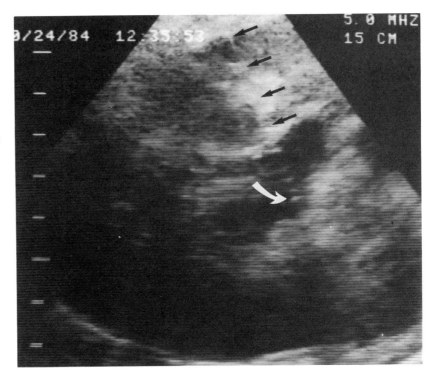

Fig 5–13. Visualization of Chiba needle on ultrasound. A static frame from a portable real-time ultrasound unit demonstrates the path of the needle through the renal parenchyma *(black arrows)* into a prominent extrarenal pelvis. The tip of the needle is identified as an echogenic focus *(curved white)*; this was made more obvious by jiggling the hub of the needle.

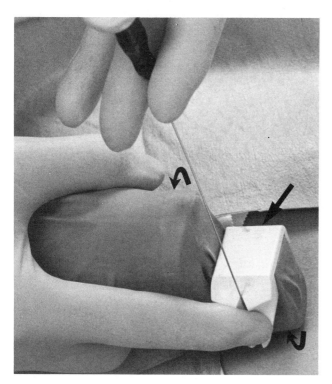

Fig 5–14. Use of ultrasound needle guide. A sterile needle holder *(straight arrow)* is clipped onto the transducer, which is enclosed in a sterile sleeve *(curved arrows)*. The needle is inserted through a slot at the side of the guide, and passes into the kidney within the plane of the sector of sound. Progress of the needle into the kidney may therefore be observed on the ultrasound monitor.

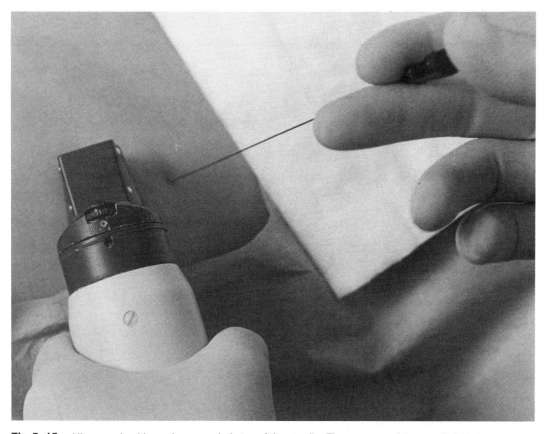

Fig 5–15. Ultrasound guidance by manual aiming of the needle. The passage of the needle into the collecting system may be observed on the ultrasound monitor by directing the needle in the plane of the sector of sound.

with ultrasound. In this technique, the real-time ultrasound unit is used to assess the direction and depth of a potential tract down to the renal pelvis. This is committed to memory (Fig 5–16), the ultrasound unit is put aside, and the needle is then "blindly" passed in the memorized direction to the predetermined depth.

The stylet is then removed and the needle withdrawn until urine is aspirated. Contrast medium is injected, as in the technique guided by fluoroscopy, for fluoroscopic confirmation of successful puncture and opacification of the pelvicalyceal system.

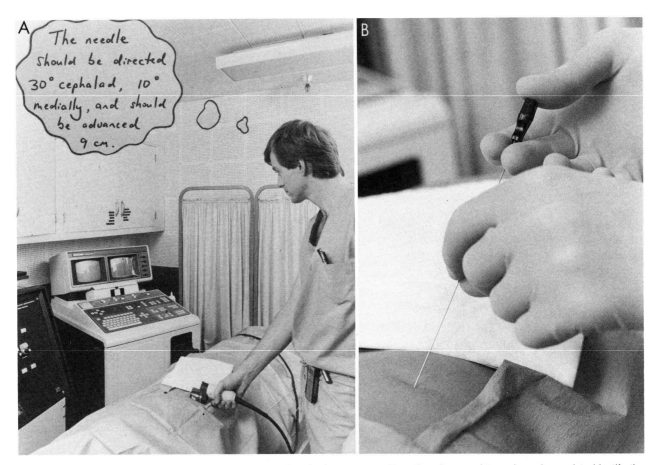

Fig 5–16. "Memory-guess" technique. **A,** with the patient in the prone position, the ultrasound transducer is used to identify the position and depth of the renal pelvis. This is committed to memory. **B,** the Chiba needle is passed in the memorized direction to the predetermined depth.

CHAPTER 6

Percutaneous Nephrostomy: Puncture Techniques

Antony T. Young, M.D.

EVALUATION OF THE ANATOMY

An accurate evaluation of the anatomy of the pelvicalyceal system and its pathology is a prerequisite for successful radiologic-urologic interventions in the upper urinary tract. This is particularly true for the more complex procedures, such as stone extraction, but also applies to simple nephrostomy for drainage.

For drainage, it is usually sufficient to identify a posterior calyx for access. For interventions in the ureter, for example, the antegrade placement of a ureteral stent, consideration should be given to providing access in a way that minimizes the angle between the nephrostomy sheath and the ureter, to reduce the likelihood of troublesome buckling of catheters and guide wires in the renal pelvis. In such a situation, our preference is for a middle- or upper-pole puncture, when possible. For stone extraction, access must be planned in a way that allows appropriate instruments to reach the stone.

Poor attention to this first step may prejudice the whole procedure, and require a de novo nephrostomy puncture.

Identifying a Posterior Calyx

In general terms, a nephrostomy puncture should be made into the periphery of the pelvical-yceal system in order to minimize the risk of laceration of segmental and interlobar arteries, which occupy a more central location. The preferred approach is into a posterior calyx (Fig 6–1). Reasons include the following:

1. Access through an anterior calyx results in a more difficult angle between the nephrostomy tract and the calyceal infundibulum, impeding the passage of not only rigid instruments and dilators, but also of flexible scopes and catheters.

2. The length of the tract through the renal parenchyma is minimized, thus reducing the risk of significant trauma to intrarenal vessels.

3. Posterior calyces are usually more medial than anterior calyces. A more medial nephrostomy tract reduces the chance of violation of organs in lateral relationship to the kidney (spleen, liver, colon).

Posterior calyces are identified by the following methods:

Parallax

This requires radiographic imaging from two or more directions. This is best achieved with a C-arm fluoroscopy unit, which may be rotated axially or in a cephalad-caudad direction. Alternatively, particularly when a conventional radiographic-fluoroscopic table is used, the patient may be rotated axially. Continuous fluoroscopy during these movements of the machine or the patient most clearly demonstrates the relative motion of the calyces with one another, distinguishing anterior from posterior. By rotating the patient or image intensifier, structures closer to the image intensifier show more shift than deeper structures. Since the patient is lying prone, posterior calyces show more shift than anterior calyces, which allows their identification. Biplane units may be used to similar effect.

Negative Contrast Agents

Small volumes of carbon dioxide (CO_2) or nitrous oxide (N_2O) injected into the collecting system float into nondependent calyces. When a patient is positioned prone, these are the posterior calyces. The limited visibility of the gas-filled posterior calyces may be enhanced by rotating the fluoroscope or the patient, as in the parallax technique, providing a relative motion between these calyces and the remainder of the collecting system, which is filled with positive contrast (Fig 6–2).

PLANNING THE ROUTE

Once the optimal entry point into the pelvicalyceal system is chosen (see Chapter 15) attention is directed to the soft tissue tract from the skin down to this point.

When possible, the kidney should be approached from below the 12th rib, to reduce the risk of chest complications. For calyces lying above the 12th rib, and these are usually in the upper-pole group, cephalad angulation of the needle is required. This may result in an unfavorable angle between the nephrostomy tract and the infundibulum, which impedes the passage of instruments from the upper calyx into the renal pelvis or ureter. Depending on the indication for the nephrostomy, our preference is either to consider choosing a different calyx for puncture or to proceed to an intercostal approach (see Chapter 15).

The nephrostomy needle is passed from a posterolateral direction, at an angle of 20° to 30° from

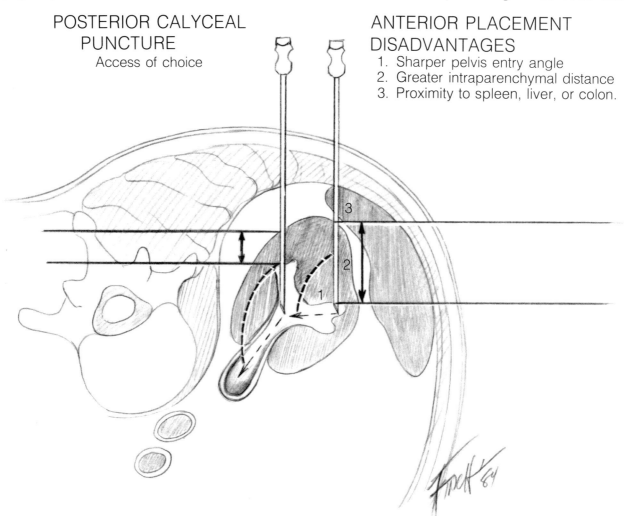

POSTERIOR CALYCEAL
PUNCTURE
Access of choice

ANTERIOR PLACEMENT
DISADVANTAGES
1. Sharper pelvis entry angle
2. Greater intraparenchymal distance
3. Proximity to spleen, liver, or colon.

Fig 6–1. Disadvantages of entry into the collecting system via an anterior calyx.

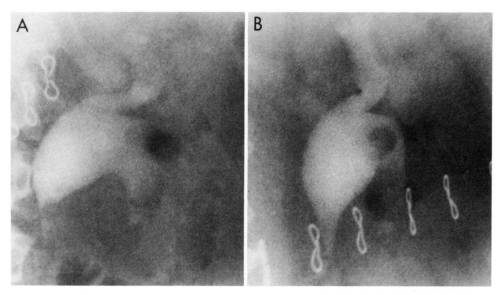

Fig 6–2. Identifying a posterior calyx by carbon dioxide (CO_2) injection. **A,** a small bubble of CO_2 is present within a posterior calyx of the middle-pole group (the patient is in a prone position). Surgical clips are noted in the anterior abdominal wall. **B,** with the patient's right side elevated, approximately 30 degrees, it is seen that the gas-filled calyx has moved toward the left relative to the remainder of the visualized collecting system, confirming that it is indeed a posterior calyx. (The surgical clips in the anterior abdominal wall have moved well toward the right.)

the sagittal plane. A direct posterior approach (in the sagittal plane) passes through the thick paraspinal muscles, and results in a position for the subsequent nephrostomy tube that is uncomfortable for the patient. A puncture directed more than 30 degrees from the sagittal plane increases the chance of piercing organs situated lateral to the kidney, including the colon, spleen, and liver (Fig 6–3). The presence of splenomegaly, megacolon, and, perhaps, hepatomegaly requires particular care, and the use of real-time ultrasound or computed tomography (CT) should be considered to ensure a safe soft tissue tract.

It should be appreciated that because the upper pole of the kidney lies medial to the lower pole, upper-pole punctures should pierce the skin more medially than punctures to the lower pole, to keep within the 30° safety limit (see Chapter 3).

PATIENT POSITION

The position of the patient on the table depends on the type of fluoroscopy unit available and the general condition of the patient. When a nonangulating, "conventional" fluoroscopy unit is used, the optimal position for a patient undergoing nephrostomy placement is semiprone, with the side of interest elevated 20 to 30 degrees on a foam wedge. The nephrostomy puncture may then be made in a vertical direction, and this allows "down-the-barrel" imaging for accurate puncture.

Once the puncture has been successfully achieved, the foam wedge may be removed and the opposite side of the patient elevated 30 to 45 degrees, so as to minimize radiation to the operator's hands, during the manipulation of guide wires and catheters (Fig 6–4).

There is more flexibility in patient position when a C-arm unit is available. Usual choices are semiprone, as outlined above, or true prone. The C-arm is rotated over the needle to allow "down-the-barrel" puncture, and then swung away to provide parallax imaging and also to protect the operator's hands during subsequent manipulations (Fig 6–5). Acutely ill patients, or the very old are often unable to lie in the prone or semiprone position. Punctures are possible, however, with the patient lying in the lateral position with the affected side uppermost, or even in the supine-oblique position with the affected side elevated 60° (Fig 6–6). In the latter position, the needle is passed in a horizontal direction. A C-arm allows highly accurate punctures even in these suboptimal conditions.

EQUIPMENT FOR NEPHROSTOMY PUNCTURE

Nephrostomy Needle

Nephrostomy needles in general use comprise a diamond-tipped stylet and a blunt outer cannula

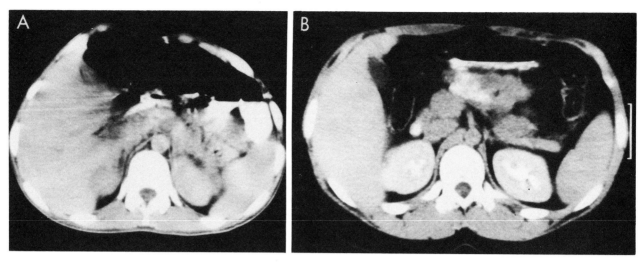

Fig 6–3. Lateral relationships to the kidney. Computed tomographic scans from two different patients demonstrate that **(A)** the spleen and **(B)** the liver may be at risk during nephrostomy, particularly during approaches to the upper pole.

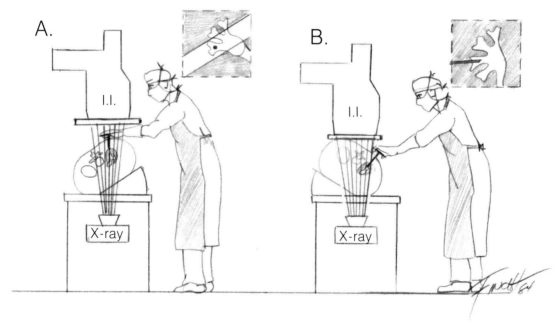

Fig 6–4. Patient position for nephrostomy, with nonangulating fluoroscopy unit. **A,** during nephrostomy the patient is placed semi-prone, with the ipsilateral side elevated 30 degrees on a sponge. This allows "down-the-barrel" imaging during needle insertion. **B,** during subsequent manipulations, the contralateral side is then elevated 30 to 50 degrees, in order to display the nephrostomy tract in profile, and to keep the operator's hands away from the primary beam.

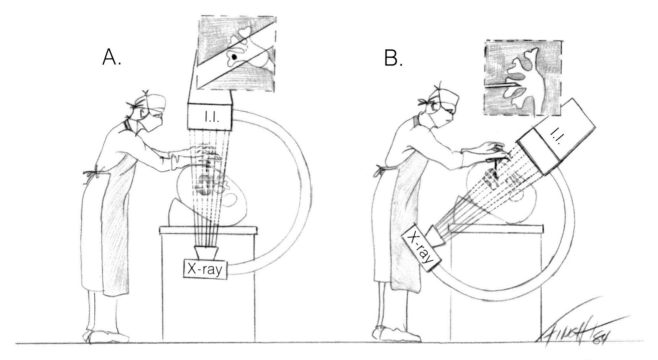

Fig 6–5. Patient position for nephrostomy using C-arm fluoroscopy. **A,** the patient is positioned prone or semiprone, with the C-arm rotated over the needle to allow "down-the-barrel" imaging. **B,** for subsequent manipulations, and for "parallax imaging" the C-arm is swung away, protecting the operator's hands.

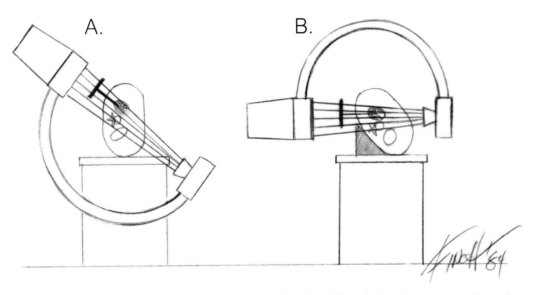

Fig 6–6. Less favorable positions for nephrostomy. In the acutely ill or immobile patient, nephrostomy may be performed with the patient in the lateral **(A)** or supine-oblique position **(B).** Accurate puncture is still possible using the C-arm.

(Fig 6–7). The hub of the assembly is radiolucent. The diamond tip ensures a straight course of the needle, whereas a bevel would tend to deviate the tip of the needle away from the side of the bevel, as with the "skinny" needle (see Fig 6–7). The blunt cannula requires the presence of the inner stylet, properly seated, in order to be advanced. However, once the cannula is within the collecting system it is less likely than a beveled needle to be partly outside the collecting system, and it is also less likely to puncture the anterior wall of the entered calyx. The radiolucent hub allows "down-the-barrel" fluoroscopy without obscuring a small target.

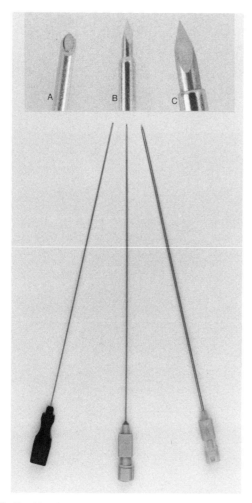

Fig 6–7. Needles commonly used during nephrostomy. **A,** 22-gauge Chiba needle has a beveled tip and therefore runs in a slightly curved course. However, this allows the needle to be "steered" by a rotation of the hub. **B,** 21-gauge "single-stick" needle has a diamond tip stylet, which passes through a blunt outer cannula. This accepts the stiff 0.018-in. mandril guide wire. **C,** standard 18-gauge nephrostomy needle: the rigidity of this needle, and the diamond-tipped stylet allow highly accurate puncture routinely. All of these needles have a radiolucent hub.

Nephrostomy needles are available in different sizes. The standard nephrostomy needle is 18 gauge; this is a rigid needle that is easy to redirect and runs a straight course. These allow direct passage of an 0.038-in. angiographic guide wire, which is the standard working wire for interventional procedures in the upper urinary tract. However, 18-gauge needles are potentially traumatic, and false passes should be avoided. In situations in which highly accurate punctures are not possible (for example, angulated punctures, when only a standard radiographic-fluoroscopic unit is available), consideration should be given to the use of the less-traumatic 21-gauge needles. These needles are finer and therefore more flexible, making straight and accurate puncture more difficult. In addition, they allow passage of only a fine 0.020-in. guide wire, which may be difficult to see fluoroscopically (particularly in the presence of contrast material), and which is insufficiently robust to safely guide catheters or dilators. However, a stiff 0.018-in. guide wire and a tapered dilator have been specially developed; these allow passage of an 0.038-in. guide wire (see "Single-Stick Systems").

A sheathed needle may also be used. This comprises an 18-gauge diamond-tipped needle-stylet assembly, inside an outer flexible sheath. This is the so-called translumbar aortogram needle described by Amplatz in 1963. Once the needle penetrates the collecting system, a guide wire is passed, and then the sheath is pushed off the needle, over the guide wire, into the renal pelvis. The only advantage of the sheathed needle over the standard 18-gauge nephrostomy needle is a small saving in time, and then only for those who use preshaped or steerable guide wires for maneuvering within the kidney. For those who maneuver with shaped catheters, the sheathed needle offers no advantage, only the disadvantage of a larger assembly for puncture.

Radiolucent Needle Holder

The use of a radiolucent handle allows continuous fluoroscopic monitoring "down the barrel" of the needle during insertion, while keeping the operator's hands out of the x-ray beam. Such handles have been developed both for the standard 18-gauge nephrostomy needle and also for the 21- to 23-gauge "skinny" needles. These offer the advantage of perfect control, particularly of the rigid 18-gauge needle, with the disadvantage of some loss of direct "feel."

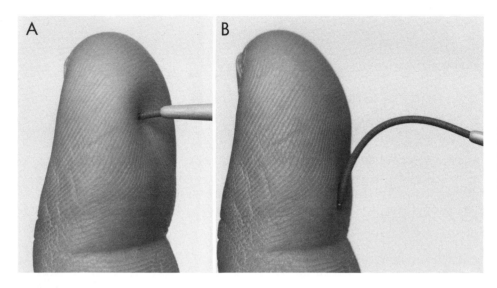

Fig 6–8. The "lance effect." **A,** for the first few millimeters, a guide wire acts like a lance. **B,** once the wire is able to bend, it exerts less pressure on the tissue, reducing chances of perforation.

Guide Wires

The choice of a guide wire is necessarily a compromise. The stiffer a wire, the better it guides a dilator, but the more likely it is to perforate the pelvicalyceal system. Most wires, therefore, have a tapered core, which makes a more flexible tip. It is important to remember that when any guide wire, no matter how soft, is passed out of a catheter or needle, it acts as a lance for the first few millimeters, until enough protrudes beyond the tip of the needle or catheter to allow the wire to bend (Fig 6–8). In tight situations, pulling the catheter back over the wire for a few millimeters instead of advancing the wire allows enough wire to protrude, and so avoids this lance effect.

Standard guide wires include the following (Fig 6–9):

The 0.035-in. floppy-tipped guide wire (Bentson wire). This has a long flexible tip, which is less likely to perforate the urothelium. Therefore, it is usually the first wire passed out of the nephrostomy needle into the kidney, and is also the best wire for use when probing and maneuvering with a catheter. This wire is also generally adequate for passing dilators and 8 F nephrostomy catheters.

The 0.038-in. "regular J" wire is somewhat stiffer, which facilitates passage of dilators and catheters, and this is our regular "working wire." The lack of a long floppy tip, however, requires caution during passage out of a needle or catheter. Furthermore, the shaft may not be stiff enough for passage of dilators.

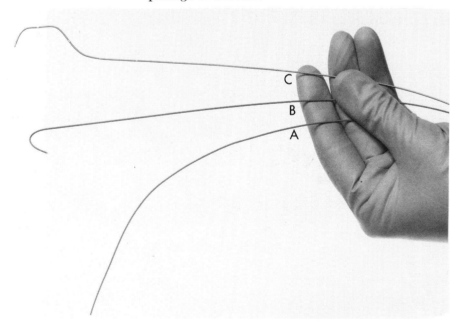

Fig 6–9. Commonly used guide wires. **A,** the 0.035-in. floppy-tipped guide wire (Bentson wire) is the least traumatic wire used during nephrostomy. **B,** the 0.038-in. "regular J" wire is somewhat stiffer, and is the standard wire for passing dilators and catheters. **C,** the Lunderquist-Ring steerable guide wire has torsional stiffness so that its tip may be preshaped and rotated within the collecting system and ureter.

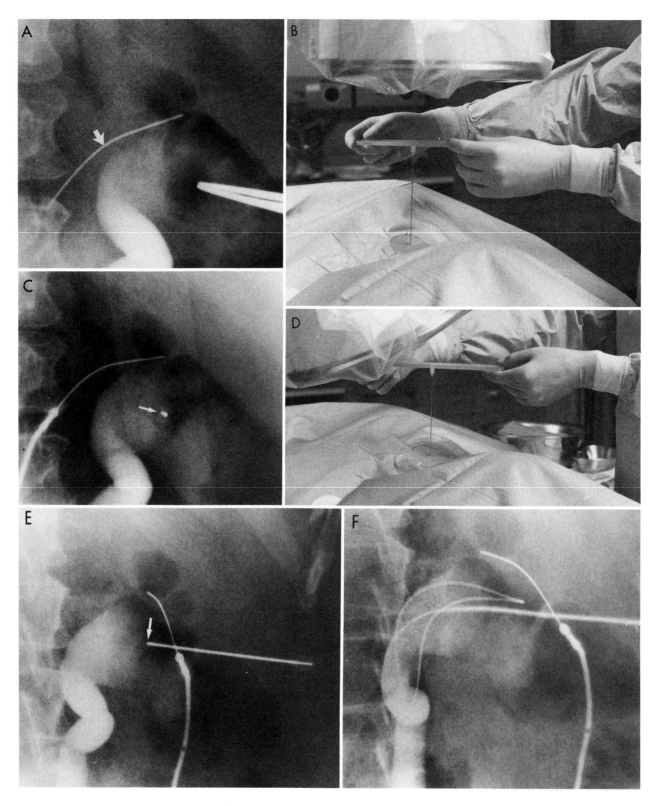

The Lunderquist-Ring steerable guide wire has torsional stiffness. The tip can, therefore, be pre-shaped and then rotated within the kidney for probing the collecting system and ureter, instead of using preshaped catheters. Coupled with the sheathed nephrostomy needle, these allow rapid passage of the initial guide wire down the ureter.

Moveable-core guide wires have been advocated. The core of these wires can be withdrawn to provide a floppy tip for manipulation, and then replaced to provide increased stiffness. This is sound in theory, but in practice it is often impossible to reinsert the core beyond any significant curve along the tip.

The stiff Lunderquist wire is a particularly rigid solid wire soldered to a flexible tip, and is used solely as a guide for passage of a catheter or dilator. It is never advanced outside the lumen of a catheter due to the likelihood of perforation. These wires are used only for difficult dilation and placement of soft stents, when conventional wires may buckle.

A special guide wire (Cook Inc., Bloomington, Ind., THSF, 0.038-in., 145-cm Amplatz Stiffening Guide [ASG]) has been developed, combining the properties of the Bentson and Lunderquist wires. This wound wire has a superstiff shaft and a floppy tip, and is very suitable for use during nephrostomy insertion. The transition from floppy to very stiff is gradual, making the Amplatz Stiffening wire very useful and safe for many interventional procedures.

More delicate wires are available for passage out of fine needles. A 0.018-in. wire fits through a 22-gauge Chiba needle, and through the 21-gauge needle of the single-stick systems. These wires, although difficult to see, are useful because they allow definitive nephrostomy to be achieved through a skinny needle tract.

Fig 6–10. Technique of nephrostomy puncture. **A,** hemostat marks the selected entry point into a posterior carbon dioxide (CO_2)-filled calyx; CO_2 and positive contrast have been injected through a Chiba needle *(arrow)*. **B,** the 18-gauge needle has been assembled in the radiolucent handle and positioned in the dermatotomy, beneath the image intensifier. The "down-the-barrel" technique is the ideal puncture method, eliminating multiple passages as in the oblique puncture technique. **C,** the needle is projected as a dot *(arrow)* over the targeted calyx. Radiolucent needle-holder is barely visible. **D,** progress of needle is checked with parallax, utilizing rotation of the C-arm. **E,** parallax imaging shows the needle to lie within the gas-filled calyx, confirming suitable location *(arrow)*. Puncture of the anterior wall of the collecting system is avoided. **F,** a 0.035-in. floppy-tipped guide wire is carefully passed beyond the needle and coiled in the collecting system.

General-Purpose Catheters

The 7 F Cobra 1 catheter, available from many manufacturers, has, in our experience, been the most versatile of all catheters for negotiating around the upper urinary tract. Coupled with the 0.035-in. floppy-tipped guide wire, access can be gained into virtually any calyx or through any ureteropelvic junction that is large enough to take a wire. Catheters of other shapes may also be used, particularly in the very dilated pelvicalyceal system, where the lordotic tertiary curve of the Cobra 1 pulls the tip away from the wall of the collecting system.

Polyethylene tubing, 5 F, is commonly used as an aid to secure the "safety" wire to the skin. Regular angiographic guide wires have a Teflon coating, and even when sutured to the skin with a tight ligature may slip out during manipulations in the nephrostomy tract. However, when a polyethylene catheter is passed over the wire, the ligature crimps the soft catheter, preventing accidental loss of the "safety" wire. These catheters are left in place down the ureter for several days following complex endourologic procedures, and this allows sure access to the upper urinary tract should unforeseen complications occur.

PUNCTURE TECHNIQUE

Described below is the conventional method of nephrostomy insertion using the 18-gauge diamond-tip nephrostomy needle. The patient has been sedated and is lying on the table with the affected side elevated approximately 20 to 30 degrees. The collecting system is visible because of the prior introduction of either positive or negative contrast. The entry point into the collecting system and the skin puncture site have been selected, as outlined previously (Fig 6–10).

Local Anesthesia

The skin around the puncture site is infiltrated using 1% lidocaine solution injected through a 25-gauge needle. A small dermatotomy is then made, and a 21- to 23-gauge skinny needle is passed along the projected nephrostomy tract. Use of the radiolucent split handle facilitates this part of the procedure. If no handle is used, the needle tract has to be observed fluoroscopically, since skinny needles may deviate considerably. The tract is then infiltrated with approximately 20 ml of 1%

lidocaine, with particular attention paid to the region of the renal capsule.

Needle Puncture

The 18-gauge nephrostomy needle is then assembled in the radiolucent handle and the tip positioned in the dermatotomy (Fig 6–10,B). The needle is aligned so that it is seen as a dot on the fluoroscopic monitor. The degree of rotation of the patient or of the C-arm unit is adjusted so that this dot is projected exactly over the predetermined entry site into the kidney (Fig 6–10,C). During quiet respiration, and with continuous fluoroscopy, the needle is advanced, and after 5 cm or so the position of the needle is frequently checked using parallax, either by rotating the patient or the C-arm (Fig 6–10,D). Often two distinct "pops" are felt as the renal capsule and then the collecting system are penetrated. In addition, it is common to recognize the distortion of the calyx by the immediate proximity of the advancing nephrostomy needle. When it is shown with parallax that the needle is within the collecting system (Fig 6–10,E), the stylet is removed and urine, or bubbles of gas when negative contrast has been used, will spontaneously erupt from the hub of the needle. If this does not occur, fluoroscopy is repeated and the needle adjusted accordingly. If there is any doubt as to position, contrast should be injected in small quantities for confirmation. Significant extravasation should be avoided, because this may obscure further attempts at entering the collecting system in the same vicinity.

Passage of the Guide Wire

The initial guide wire used is the 0.035-in. floppy-tipped guide wire. This is very carefully passed beyond the tip of the nephrostomy needle, and usually it will be seen to coil within the renal pelvis (Fig 6–10,F). It is possible, however, for guide wires to pass with surprising ease into the renal sinus and even down the periureteric tissues. Alternatively, the wire may pass into a vein or artery. If there is any doubt about the location of the guide wire, a 5 F catheter is passed over the wire, and contrast medium is judiciously injected.

It is important to pass enough wire so that the stiffer portion of the wire is within the renal collecting system. The purpose of the floppy end of a wire is to avoid piercing the collecting system. It is not a reliable guide for the passage of dilators and catheters.

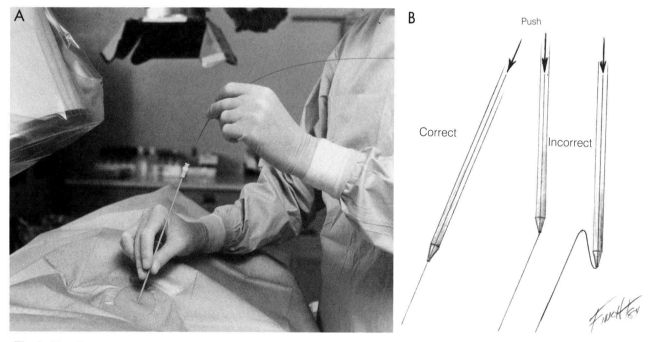

Fig 6–11. Proper dilation technique. **A,** the dilator is held close to the skin and is rotated down between the thumb and first two fingers whilst the other hand holds the guide wire taut. Intermittent fluoroscopy should be performed to ensure the dilator is being pushed in the direction of the tract. **B,** pushing off the direction of the tract, and failure to maintain tension on the guide wire leads to buckling of the guide wire and false passage of the dilator. The dilator has to be advanced in small increments using a screwing motion.

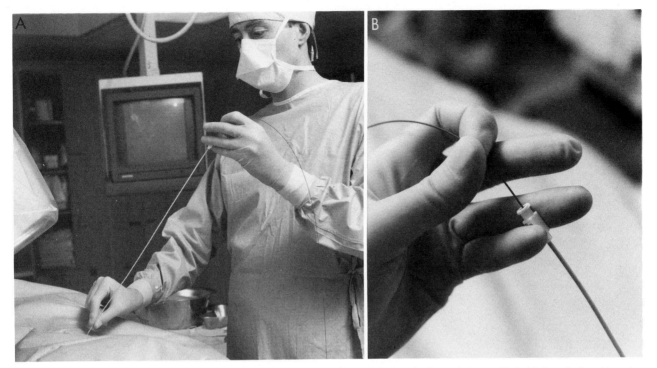

Fig 6–12. Proper technique for manipulating the catheter. **A,** the right hand controls the catheter and is held close to the skin entry point. The left hand controls movement of the guide wire. **B,** the hub of the catheter is held between the fourth and fifth fingers while the guide wire is flicked in and out of the catheter using the thumb and forefinger.

Dilatation of the Tract

In order to facilitate the insertion of a 7 or 8 F catheter into the collecting system, the tract must first be dilated. Sequential fascial dilators are used. These are commonly 6, 8, and 10 F in size. Another technique is the introduction of a dual-guide introducer, which consists of a 6 F inner catheter and a coaxial outer 11 F dilator (Cook Inc., Bloomington, Ind.). By this final step of dilatation two guide wires can be introduced through the 11 F Teflon sheath.

When a dilator is passed, it is held between the thumb and forefinger of the right hand, close to the skin, and is rotated down the tract, like a wood screw. Countertraction is applied to the guide wire with the other hand (Fig 6–11,A). It is essential that the dilator be passed in the same direction as the guide wire, and that this be checked by intermittent fluoroscopy. Otherwise, buckling of the dilator, or kinking of the guide wire, may lead to compounding difficulties at subsequent manipulations (Fig 6–11,B). The dilator is rotated down until its tip is just past the entry point into the pelvicalyceal system. It is important not to advance it too far, for fear of perforating the anterior wall.

Manipulation Down the Ureter

Following dilatation of the tract to 10 F, the 7 F Cobra 1 catheter is inserted over the wire, and this is used to manipulate the guide wire down the ureter. The right hand holds the catheter close to the skin, and is used to rotate and advance the catheter. The left hand holds the hub of the catheter between the ring and little fingers, and the wire between the thumb and forefinger. In this way the floppy-tipped guide wire can be flicked in and out of the tip of the Cobra like a snake's tongue (Fig 6–12). By advancing the guide wire, and following up with the catheter, it is almost always a simple task to pass the wire well down the ureter, or into any calyx of the kidney, if so desired. As in the passage of dilators, countertension on the guide wire is crucial, particularly when negotiating strictures. Once the guide wire is well located in the ureter or in the pelvicalyceal system it can be used for the introduction of a definitive nephrostomy drainage catheter, or in the more complex endourologic procedures, for the introduction of a second guide wire followed by dilatation up to 30 F.

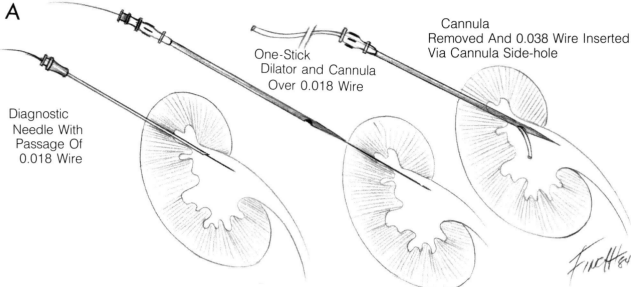

A

Diagnostic
Needle With
Passage Of
0.018 Wire

One-Stick
Dilator and Cannula
Over 0.018 Wire

Cannula
Removed And 0.038 Wire Inserted
Via Cannula Side-hole

Fig 6–13. "Cope" single-stick system. **A,** the steps are outlined for inserting a 0.038-in. guide wire using a 21-gauge needle,
and the special tapered dilator-cannula assembly. **B,** equipment
detail: *(left)* dilator-cannula assembly is passed over the stiff
0.018-in. wire. *(upper right)* the stiffening cannula has been removed, causing the dilator to bend. *(lower right)* the 0.018-in. wire
is removed and a 0.038-in. "J" wire is passed and exits the large
side hole.

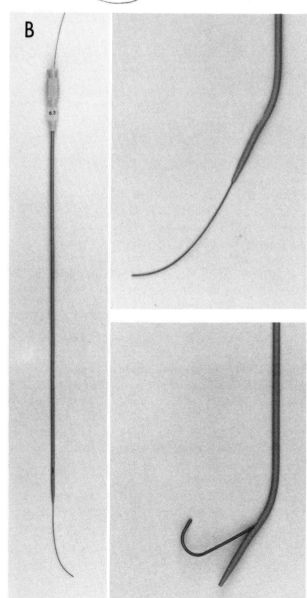

B

"SINGLE-STICK" SYSTEMS

Single-stick systems are so called because the
nephrostomy tube is inserted through the tract of
the initial fine-needle puncture, performed for
opacification, obviating the requirement for a second puncture using the larger 18-gauge needle.

The most compelling indication for this system
is when there is a good chance of missing the targeted entry point into the pelvicalyceal system,
with the potential for multiple passes. Examples
include drainage of a nonopacified obstructed kidney using ultrasound guidance, or angled puncture
into an opacified system using a nonangulating
fluoroscopic unit that does not allow visualization
"down the barrel" of the needle. Because the initial puncture is made with a 21- to 22-gauge needle, there is less likelihood of significant trauma
to the kidney from multiple unsuccessful puncture attempts. These needles, however, are more
flexible than the standard 18-gauge nephrostomy
needles, and this makes it more difficult to aim
them accurately onto a small target. If the collecting system is adequately opacified, and a C-arm is
available, then the single-stick system offers no

real advantage over the conventional 18-gauge nephrostomy needle. On the contrary, the puncture may be inappropriately placed in relation to the calculus.

Techniques

'Cope' Single-Stick System (Fig 6–13).

The puncture is made with a 21-gauge diamond-tipped needle-stylet assembly. A special, stiff 0.018-in. guide wire with a flexible tip is passed, the needle is removed, and over the wire a special tapered dilator is carefully rotated down into the collecting system. This dilator has a side hole back from the tapered tip; once the side hole is in the collecting system, the fine wire is removed and a regular 0.038-in. "J" guide wire is passed. This wire exits the side hole and enters the pelvicalyceal system, following which the special dilator is removed and sequential fascial dilatation performed in the usual way.

Problems which may be encountered with this system include: (1) difficulty seeing the fine guide wire on the fluoroscopic monitor, (2) inability to pass the 0.038-in. guide wire out of the side hole. Careful rotation of the dilator usually resolves this problem, and (3) incorrect location of the entry site.

The 'Backloaded' Single-Stick System (Fig 6–14)

With this system, a sheathed 19-gauge needle is backloaded over a longer 22-gauge needle-stylet assembly. The tip of the 22-gauge needle is advanced until it enters the collecting system. The stylet is withdrawn and the position is confirmed by aspiration of urine and the injection of contrast. Then, holding the 22-gauge needle in place, the sheathed 19-gauge needle is advanced down to the tip of the 22-gauge needle, so that the end of the sheath is also within the collecting system. Both needles are then removed and a 0.038-in. wire is passed through the sheath into the renal pelvis. The tract is dilated in the usual way.

A major disadvantage of this system without a guide wire is that the 22-gauge needle may either pull out of the calyx, or else perforate the anterior

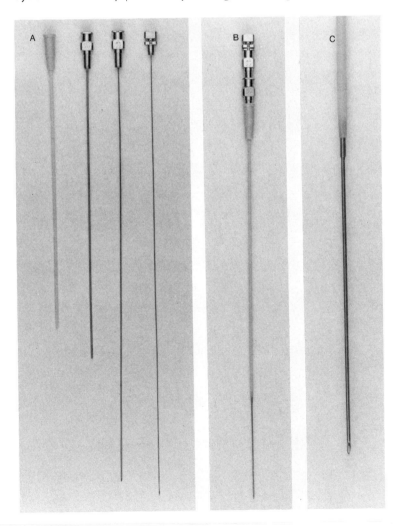

Fig 6–14. "Backloaded" single-stick system. **A,** the components of the system include the 22-gauge needle and stylet, and the 19-gauge needle and sheath. **B,** the assembled system is shown ready for puncture. **C,** close-up view of the puncturing end of the system showing the sheathed 19-gauge needle backloaded over the 22-gauge needle-stylet.

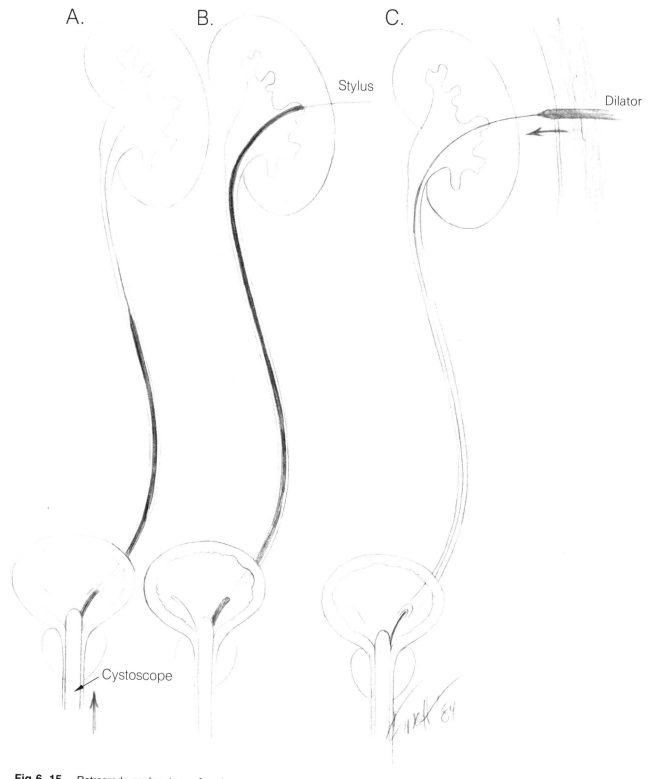

Fig 6–15. Retrograde nephrostomy. **A,** using a system of coaxial catheters, a Teflon sheath is placed in a calyx. **B,** a long stylus is passed posterolaterally through the renal parenchyma to the skin surface. **C,** antegrade dilation is then performed down onto the kidney in the conventional manner.

wall during advancement of the sheathed needle, so that the sheath ends up outside of the collecting system, resulting in lost access. This is most likely to occur in the nondilated system.

RETROGRADE NEPHROSTOMY

Retrograde nephrostomy is an experimental technique whereby a tract from the pelvicalyceal system to the flank is created using a 110-cm long 20- or 21-gauge needle, which is passed retrograde from the urethra to the targeted calyx using a coaxial system of catheters. The needle is then passed from the calyx into the soft tissues of the flank and through the skin. A 0.020-in. extra stiff "rocket wire," 250 cm in length, is then passed through the 21-gauge needle; the coaxial catheters are removed via the urethra and the needle and wire are used for the antegrade passage of dilators in the conventional manner (Fig 6–15).

Advantages

- The retrograde approach guarantees access to the collecting system because the tract originates from a calyx.
- Because the "rocket wire" extends from the

flank to the urethra, dilatation of the tract is facilitated by tension to both ends of this wire. It also guarantees a secure access at all times.

Disadvantages

The one compelling disadvantage of this technique is that the operator has only limited control over the direction of the soft tissue tract. Trauma to organs adjacent to the kidney causes a small but significant incidence of complications from nephrostomy placement. In most cases, the cause is puncturing the kidney too laterally. With this technique, rotating the retrograde catheters allows some degree of control over the soft tissue tract, but this has yet to be shown to be sufficiently reliable or as safe as the conventional antegrade puncture.

OTHER TECHNIQUES

Nephrostomy through a Cannula

Inserting a nephrostomy catheter through a metal cannula was the original technique for percutaneous nephrostomy (Fig 6–16). An 8 F silicon rubber catheter may be inserted into the renal pel-

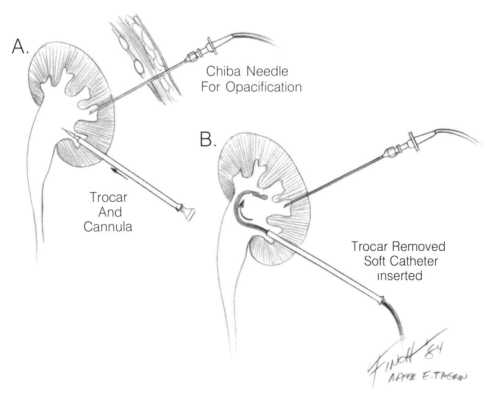

Fig 6–16. Nephrostomy through a cannula. **A,** following Chiba needle opacification, the blunt cannula and sharp trocar are inserted into the collecting system. **B,** the trocar is removed and a soft silicone catheter is inserted into the renal pelvis.

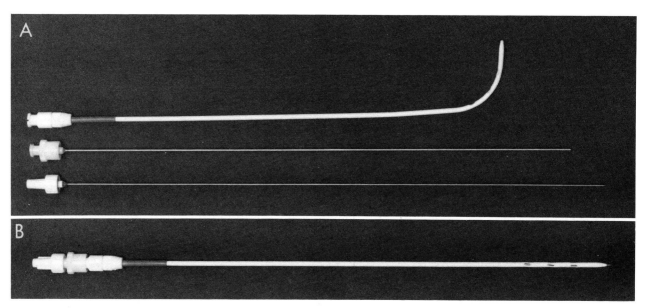

Fig 6–17. Catheter-over-needle nephrostomy: equipment detail. **A,** the components; **B,** the assembly ready for puncture.

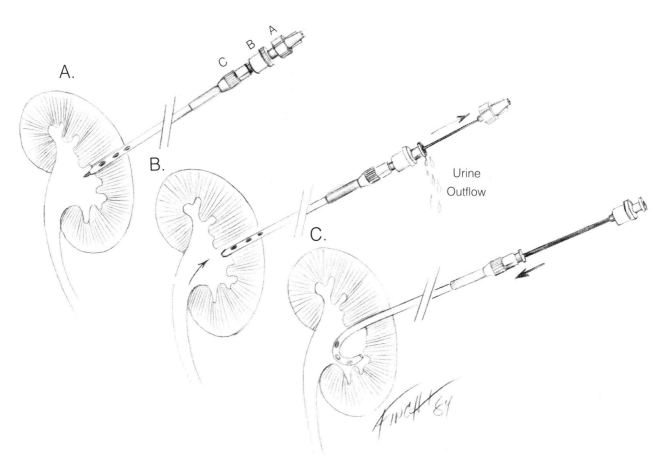

Fig 6–18. Catheter-over-needle nephrostomy. **A,** assembly consists of a taper catheter with side holes, which is stretched over a stiffening cannula. A sharp trocar protrudes beyond the tip. The assembly is positioned into the collecting system. **B,** position is confirmed by removing the stylet and aspirating urine. **C,** the catheter is then pushed off the cannula into the collecting system.

vis through a 10.5 F thin-walled cannula. The cannula is initially inserted into the collecting system with the help of a pencil-tipped trocar.

Advantages

- In experienced hands, the technique is rapid.
- Once the cannula is in place, soft silicon catheters are easily inserted into the kidney. This is in contrast to angiographic techniques in which the nature of the catheter material is very important in determining the ease with which it passes over a wire into the collecting system. Generally, stiff catheters are easier to insert than the softer, perhaps more biocompatible types.

Disadvantages

The major disadvantage is that the trocar-cannula assembly is large, and more traumatic to the kidney. The coaxial dilators and sheaths developed for stone removal, and the "peel-away" catheter introduction systems now available, allow passage of soft catheters and stents, and seem to have made this early technique obsolete.

Catheter-Over-Needle Technique (Figs 6–17 and 6–18)

Other systems are available whereby a catheter is stiffened with a needle-stylet assembly whose pointed tip protrudes beyond the tapered end of the catheter. The system is advanced into the kidney, and when the tip is in the collecting system (confirmed after removal of the stylet), the catheter is pushed over the needle and into the collecting system. Again, the disadvantage of this system is the large size of the initial puncturing instrument compared with the conventional 18- or 21-gauge angiographic systems. Such a system may be used for the percutaneous drainage of accessible abscesses, but is not recommended for the establishment of a nephrostomy.

CHAPTER 7

Percutaneous Nephrostomy: Tube Placement—Types and Techniques

David W. Hunter, M.D.

Percutaneous nephrostomy drainage catheters can be divided into three groups based on the type of drainage which they afford: (1) external drainage only, (2) internal and/or external drainage, and (3) internal drainage only.

Within each of these groups there has been a veritable explosion of new catheter designs and materials in the last several years. Several of the more commonly used catheters in each group will be discussed and the advantages and disadvantages of each will be indicated.

EXTERNAL DRAINAGE

The "standard" catheter against which other external drainage catheters must be compared is the short, 8 F angiographic polyethylene pigtail (Fig 7–1) provided in many of the percutaneous nephrostomy kits. Its stiffness and tapered tip make it relatively easy to place through a new tract with minimal (9 F) dilation. The pigtail re-forms easily even in small, nondilated systems, and the side holes and lumen are more than adequate for normal urine flow. This type of catheter, however, has some shortcomings, which in certain special circumstances make it less than optimal. In patients requiring long-term drainage, its stiffness can make it uncomfortable and encrustation and obstruction can be frequent problems. In patients who are obese or in whom reliability or catheter fixation are a problem, the pigtail provides almost no resistance to dislodgment. In patients who have debris or infection in their urine, the side holes and lumen are usually inadequate. In pediatric patients, on the other hand, the catheter is too large.

The most widely used alternative external drainage catheter is the Cope loop, or any of its modifications (Fig 7–2). The softer material makes it quite comfortable even for long-term use and the self-retention property both provides security against dislodgment and obviates the need for sutures or tapes to fix the catheter to the skin. Its softness makes it somewhat more difficult to introduce, but this problem can be overcome by overdilating the tract (approximately 2 F larger than the catheter size), allowing the tract to mature by leaving a similar size but stiffer catheter in it for two or three days, or by using an internal stiffening cannula or an external peel-away sheath (Figs 7–3,A and B). Encrustation and obstruction have still been an occasional problem with this softer material. Encrustation is of particular concern when it occurs at the point where the string holds the catheter against itself to make the loop. This can make it impossible to straighten the catheter for removal. In such circumstances, a

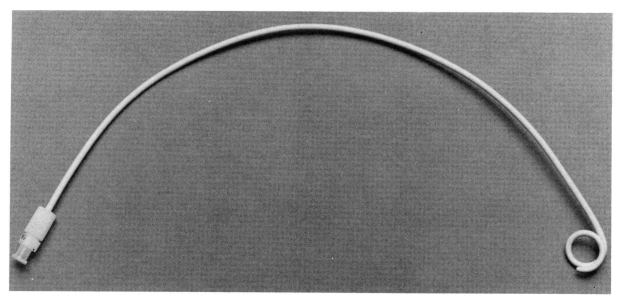

Fig 7–1. "Standard" catheter: angiographic polyethylene pigtail.

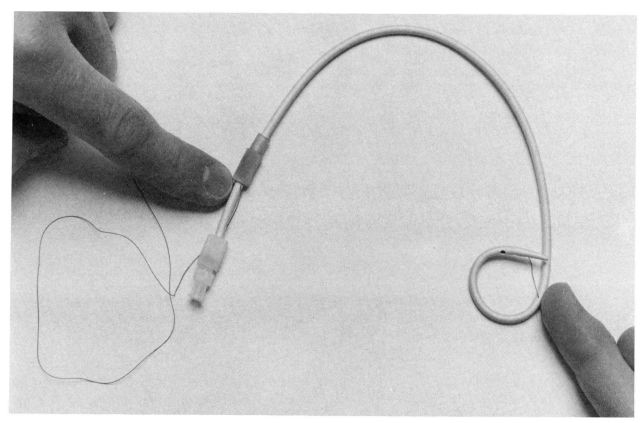

Fig 7–2. Cope loop demonstrating its flexibility and self retentive characteristics.

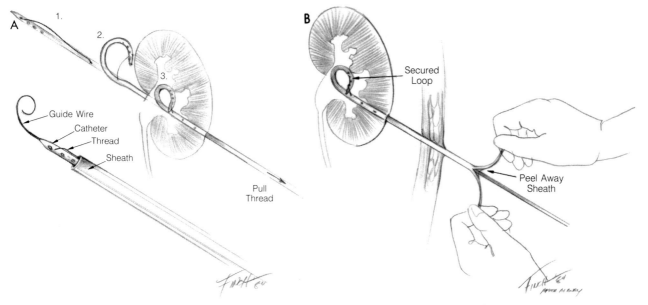

Fig 7–3. Design and placement of Cope loop via a peel away sheath.

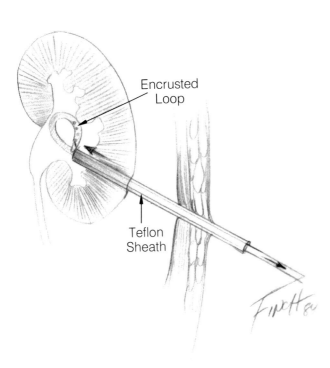

Fig 7–4. Encrusted Cope loop can be forcibly straightened and removed through a Teflon sheath.

stiff Teflon sheath (or dilator) placed over the catheter can act as a brace against which the loop can be forcibly straightened and pulled out (Fig 7–4). Catheter exchange at three- to six-month intervals will usually prevent this problem.

In patients with infected, bloody, or debris-filled urine, a catheter with a large internal diameter and large nonobstructable entry holes is required. We have frequently used a Stamey (VPI, Spencer, Indiana) 12 or 14 F catheter (Fig 7–5) in such cases. The wide Malecot tip and large internal lumen (a 14 F Stamey has approximately the same lumen size as a 20 F Foley [Bard Urological, Billerica, Massachusetts]) ensure free drainage in almost any circumstance. Stamey catheters were intended for use in suprapubic punctures and originally came with a sharp, rigid obturator (Fig 7–6), which was unacceptably dangerous for percutaneous renal work. Flexible obturators were soon developed to facilitate safe passage over a guide wire (see Fig 7–6). The main drawback of the Stamey catheter was the extreme stiffness of the shaft, which made it very uncomfortable for patients even for short-term use. A recent modification that has made this catheter our first choice for any difficult or complicated drainage is the bonding of a soft, flexible shaft to a stiff Malecot tip (Fig 7–7). The stiffer tip facilitates introduction and affords a degree of self-retention, while the soft shaft promotes patient comfort and acceptance.

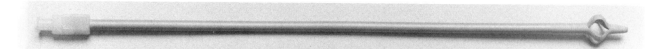

Fig 7–5.   Stamey catheter which has a large internal diameter for draining infected, bloody, or debris-filled urine.

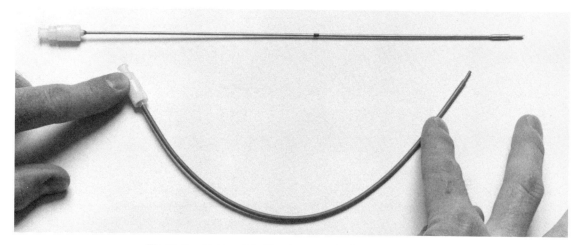

Fig 7–6.   Rigid and flexible obturators for Stamey catheters.

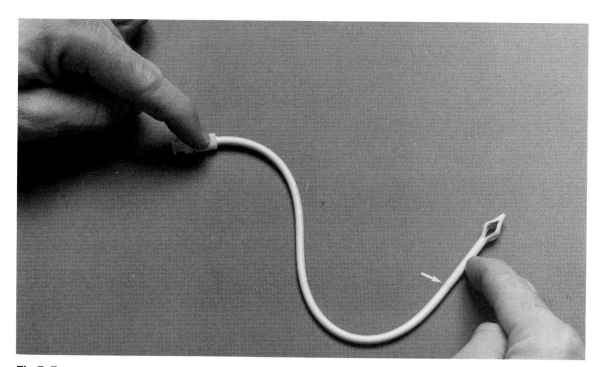

Fig 7–7.   The junction between the stiffer tip and the softer, more flexible shaft can be faintly seen as a change in texture *(arrow).*

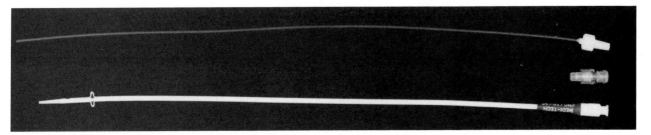

Fig 7–8. This design has the Malecot opening near the tip. This is most useful for external drainage in normal patients or external-internal drainage in transplant patients.

The wings of a Malecot catheter irritate the adjacent urothelium, which results in a slow ingrowth of granulation-like tissue around the wings and into the spaces between them. The granulation tissue may necessitate surgical removal of the catheter. To avoid this complication, any Malecot catheter should be exchanged at three-month intervals.

Modifications of the Malecot design in smaller French sizes are also available. One such, the Castaneda nephrostomy catheter (Medi-Tech, Watertown, Massachusetts) (Fig 7–8), has a tapered angiographic tip and an internal polyethylene stiffener, which make introduction very easy. The *Trillium* spring lock (Fig 7–9) does not seem to cause any increased problem with encrustation but it does limit flow of particulate or purulent matter. The shaft is comfortably soft and therefore acceptable to patients. As with all of the softer catheters, if extra side holes are desired a paper punch (Fig 7–10) must be used to create them. A scissors can be used instead, but the holes are usually much more ragged.

In a patient who may require particularly long-

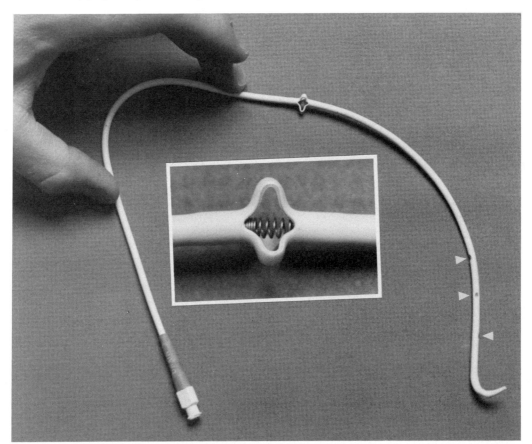

Fig 7–9. This design has the Malecot opening in the middle of the catheter. The long segment of catheter between the Malecot opening and the tip makes this an excellent catheter for internal-external drainage in normal patients. The slight "J" configuration of the tip ensures that there is minimal irritation in the bladder. Side holes *(arrowheads)* can be cut in the catheter at any level.

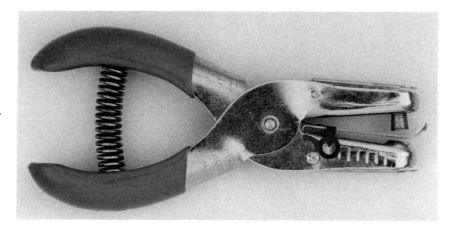

Fig 7–10. Standard paper punch creates smooth, even side holes in softer catheters.

term or lifelong external drainage, all of the above catheters may prove inadequate or difficult to manage. In such a case we have occasionally turned to a "U-loop" or "circle" nephrostomy catheter (Fig 7–11). Insertion is technically difficult requiring two tracts into widely separated calyces (Fig 7–12,A), careful dilation of both tracts, 2 F larger than the desired "U" loop, establishment of a through-and-through guide wire using a snare or basket through one tract (see Fig 7–12,A) and then passage of a tapered dilator over the wire leading the "U-loop" in one tract and out the other (Figs 7–12,B and C). Excessive force or back-and-forth motions on the catheters, or particularly on the through-and-through guide wire, can "saw" into or through the renal parenchyma. Introducer sheaths, as are used for Cope loop placement or

percutaneous stone removals, can be helpful in difficult situations. Once a "U" loop is properly positioned it is essentially impossible to remove it accidentally. Catheter repositioning and exchange are very simple.

External drainage catheters are also used following percutaneous stone removals or other percutaneous endourologic procedures. These will be discussed in Chapter 23.

In pediatric patients, 5 or 6 F pigtail catheters are usually used. Several such catheters are available commercially but are often quite stiff and occasionally, therefore, have problems with kinking. We often create our own 5 or 6 F pigtails (Fig 7–13) out of the somewhat softer, standard 5 F polyethylene catheter material.

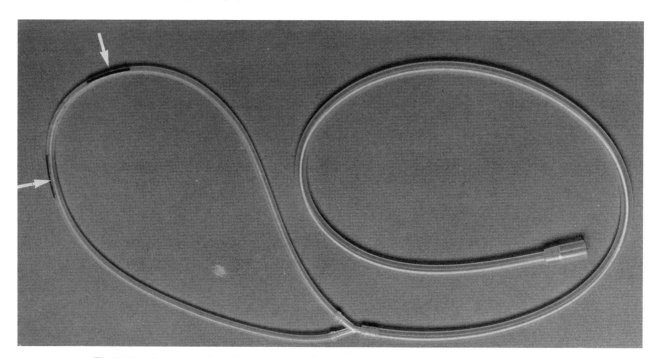

Fig 7–11. The side holes in this catheter are located between the two radiopaque markers *(arrows)*.

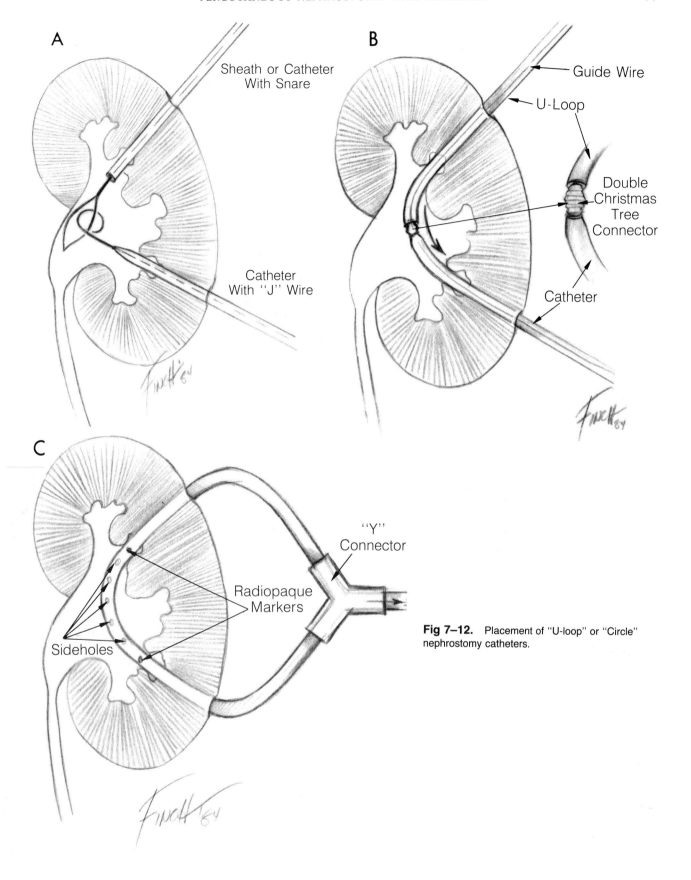

A

Sheath or Catheter
With Snare

Catheter
With "J" Wire

B

Guide Wire

U-Loop

Double
Christmas
Tree
Connector

Catheter

C

"Y"
Connector

Radiopaque
Markers

Sideholes

Fig 7–12. Placement of "U-loop" or "Circle" nephrostomy catheters.

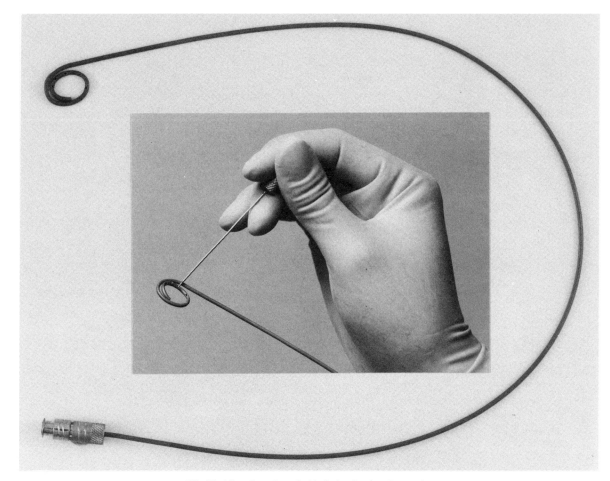

Fig 7–13.   Creation of side holes in pigtail catheter.

INTERNAL-EXTERNAL DRAINAGE

The most common "first" catheter placed for combined internal-external drainage is a standard polyethylene, 8 F, long angiographic pigtail catheter in which extra side holes are placed at the level of the bladder and collecting system (Fig 7–14). The stiffness and tapered angiographic tip facilitate introduction through what are often very resistant stenoses. Side holes are created with a standard hole punch (Fig 7–15) and are therefore quite small and unmarked, which can make accurate placement in the collecting system a problem. Lumen size can be restrictive and the catheter is uncomfortably stiff for long-term use. The pigtail provides minimal retention capability and therefore a securing system at the skin is often necessary. Long Cope loop–type catheters are available with a single loop in the bladder. They prevent dislodgment and are very comfortable to patients. However, they can be extremely difficult to introduce even with added internal stiffeners,

and if extra side holes are necessary, the string may be inadvertently cut while the side holes are being created.

A "double loop" or "Cope loop plus pigtail" catheter (Fig 7–16) simplifies accurate placement of side holes in the collecting system and offers some retention security. Since the position of the proximal side holes cannot be varied, the catheter must be carefully sized to the patient. Some catheters of this design are soft, which is good for patient comfort but makes them quite difficult to introduce. Most of these catheters come in sizes up to 8 F, which can limit flow and result in problems with recurrent obstruction. A modification of this type of catheter has recently been introduced, a one-size-fits-all, multiple-loop catheter (Fig 7–17). This obviates problems of side hole placement and catheter length, but is limited to a soft Silastic material and only up to 8 F size.

An extended Malecot variation of the Castaneda nephrostomy catheter (see Fig 7–9) comes in a 10 F size, which significantly decreases problems

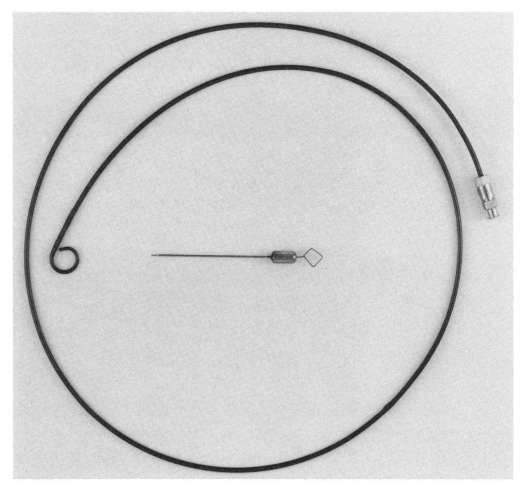

Fig 7–14. Long angiographic pigtail catheter with hole punch. Side holes can easily be created for placement in the renal pelvis with distal tip of catheter in bladder, creating an internal-external drainage catheter design.

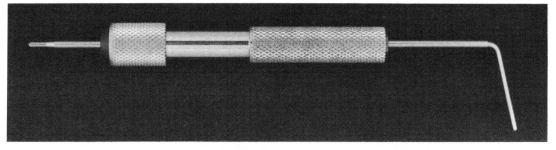

Fig 7–15. Standard hole punch.

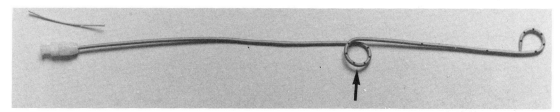

Fig 7–16. The proximal loop, which is positioned in the renal pelvis *(arrow)*, is created by pulling on the string at the hub, which pulls the catheter into a "Cope loop" configuration. The tip of the catheter is a simple pigtail.

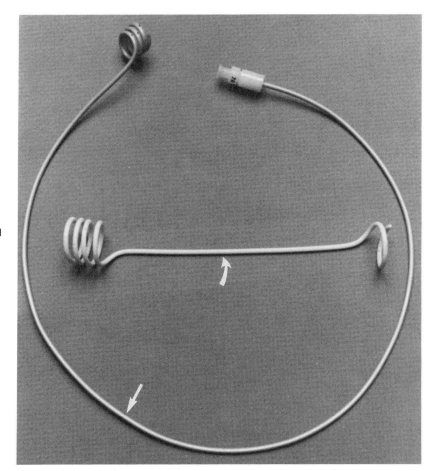

Fig 7–17. For internal-external drainage with the catheter, side holes can be punctured at the level of the renal pelvis *(arrow)*. The side holes in the distal coil will be in the bladder. The coil can contract or expand to fit the length of the ureter. The same principles apply for the internal stent *(curved arrow)*.

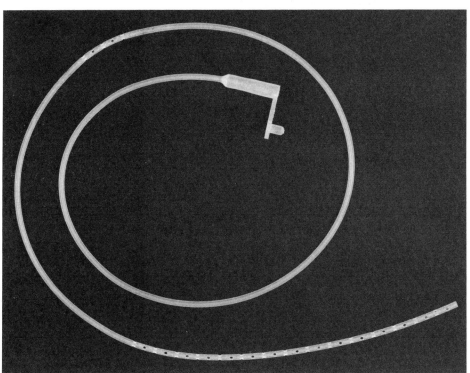

Fig 7–18. An extremely comfortable catheter for extended use is the Silastic universal stent shown above. However, due to its inherent softness, placement and replacement can be difficult.

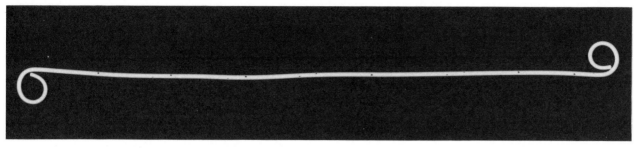

Fig 7–19. Most commonly used internal stent is the polyethylene "double-J."

with obstruction. Its tapered tip and internal polyethylene stiffener make introduction easy. The Malecot opening simplifies side hole placement in the collecting system and provides a small amount of self-retention. Extra side holes can be created with a paper punch. The larger size is particularly useful when stenting either dilated ureteral stenoses or across an area of ureteral leak. The catheter is soft enough to be comfortable but strong enough to resist encroachment by periureteral masses.

For very extended use, the soft Silastic universal stent (Fig 7–18) is extremely comfortable and does a fairly good job of resisting encrustation. It is so soft, however, that it must be pulled into position,

which means that once an angiographic catheter has been placed to the bladder, the patient must undergo cystoscopy to create a through-and-through guide wire. Proximal side holes for the collecting system are indicated by radiopaque markers, which makes the catheter easy to position. If the catheter becomes obstructed, it can be very difficult to replace since a guide wire will not force its way through the obstructing debris as it would in an angiographic catheter. Instead, it will stretch and possibly rupture the Silastic. A smaller guide wire may exit through a side hole. A guide wire and a 5 F catheter can occasionally be maneuvered down the tract adjacent to the Silastic catheter. Or, if all else fails, a sheath can be

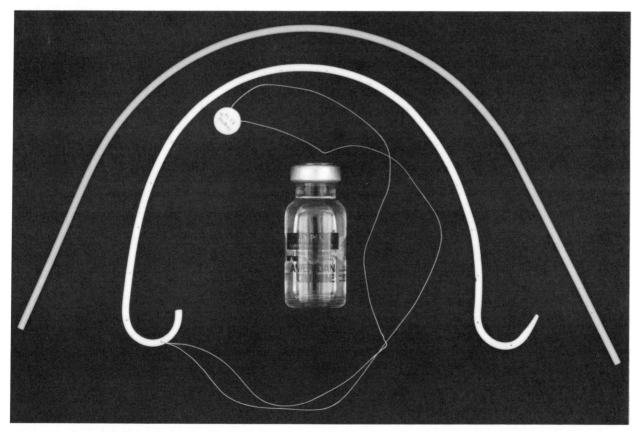

Fig 7–20. Softer, Silastic "double-J" stents are comfortable for the patient, but can be very difficult to place in an antegrade fashion.

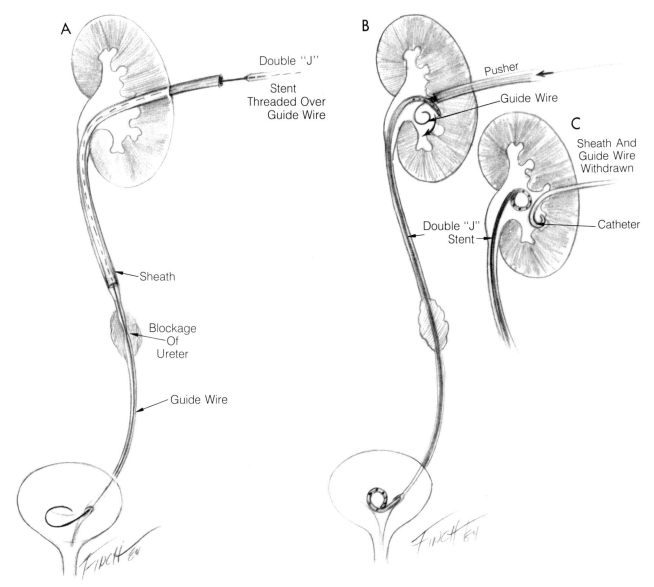

Fig 7–21. **A, B, C,** placement of the Silastic "double-J" stents may require introducer sheaths.

passed over the outside of the Silastic catheter into the collecting system, the Silastic catheter can be removed, and a guide wire inserted. In any case, a new angiographic catheter and another visit to the cystoscopy suite are invariably necessary.

INTERNAL STENTS

Internal stents are used in those patients who do not wish to have an external catheter or who are immunosuppressed and would therefore have greater difficulties with infection. The most widely used internal stent is the polyethylene "double-J" (Fig 7–19). The stiffer polyethylene stents are easier to advance through stenoses, but can be irritating to the bladder. When placing a polyethylene stent antegrade, it is often very difficult to get the upper pigtail to form so that the tip is not impaling or eroding through the urothelium. Once properly positioned, however, the stiffness of the curled ends usually prevents migration. The softer Silastic "double-J" stents (Fig 7–20) have recently been modified so that one end has a tapered angiographic tip for antegrade placement. Nonetheless, they can be difficult to advance through stenotic areas and may require a sheath for introduction (Fig 7–21,A-C) or a mature tract. The softer ends are not irritating or dangerous to the urothelium, but also do not seem to afford as much security against migration. All

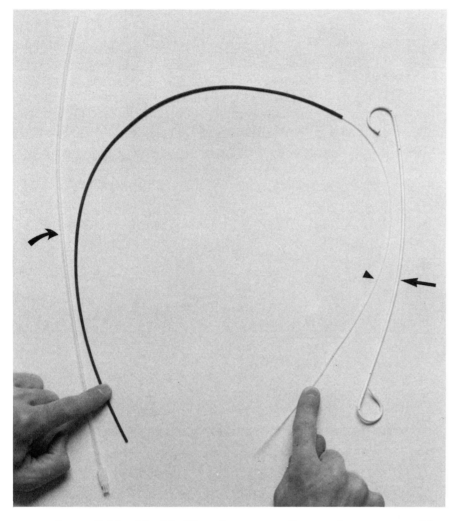

Fig 7–22. The 10 F double-J stent *(arrow)* is mounted on the clear Teflon introducer *(arrowhead)* with the tapered tip of the double-J stent leading over the guide wire and the nontapered tip firmly mounted on the larger black Teflon introducer and "bead." The clear Teflon pusher *(curved arrow)* is mounted on the large black Teflon introducer and butted firmly against the blunt end of the double-J stent. The entire three-piece unit is then advanced over the guide wire.

currently available "double-J" catheters are limited to 8 F in size. This has resulted in significant problems with obstruction and is also an inadequate size to stent freshly dilated stenoses.

Recently we have developed 10 and 12 F "double-J" catheters out of a more slippery, hopefully less encrustable, material—C-Flex (Cook Inc., Bloomington, Ind.) (Fig 7–22). The larger side holes and lumen have excellent flow and the unique introducing system, including a Teflon stiffener with a bead to hold the proximal end of the "double-J" (Fig 7–23), can be accurately posi-

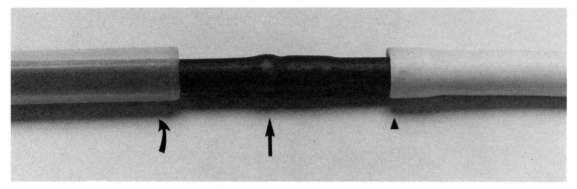

Fig 7–23. A close-up view of the region of the bead *(arrow)* shows the blunt end of the 10 F double-J stent *(arrowhead)* being mounted backward onto the bead and the clear plastic pusher *(curved arrow)* being brought down forward toward the bead, so that eventually it will be firmly pressed against the blunt end of the double-J stent.

tioned without the need of an attached monofilament thread. The catheter can be pushed off but
not pulled off the bead. "Double-J" stents can be
removed percutaneously using a snare, basket, or
graspers (with or without a scope), but are usually
removed and replaced cystoscopically.

THE FUTURE

New designs are constantly emerging and old
designs are being improved. The most interesting
changes, however, will probably be in catheter
materials. Superslippery or biocompatible plastics
or coatings may permit the development of a catheter that may never encrust or obstruct.

CHAPTER 8

Percutaneous Nephrostomy: Reestablishment of the Tract

Wilfrido Castaneda-Zuniga, M.D.

Replacement of an accidentally dislodged nephrostomy drainage catheter may be an emergency, particularly in patients with only one functioning kidney. Symptoms and a rise in creatinine level start almost immediately, since the ureter is obstructed and the nephrostomy tract usually closes within hours after dislodgment.

There are three important rules to remember in the management of patients with a dislodged nephrostomy drainage catheter: (1) Do not attempt blind manipulations through the tract, regardless of its age. The tracts are invariably tortuous. Although they were originally straight, the soft tissue has shifted. (2) Once a false passage is created by blind manipulations, it becomes almost impossible to successfully find the true tract. (3) Do not infiltrate the tract with local anesthesia prior to catheterization; this can narrow or even obstruct the tract. It is preferable to administer only heavy sedation and use local anesthesia after the tract has been catheterized with a small catheter.

The patient is placed in the prone position and, after preparation and draping, a "Christmas tree" adapter (or the tip of an angiographic catheter) is inserted into the nephrostomy tract opening; 25% contrast medium is then injected to opacify the tract (Fig 8–1). Still-framing by videotape or digital recording allows the image to freeze; this is used as a "road map." A film of the abdomen or the

memory of the operator is also sufficient if modern radiographic equipment is not available.

Once the tract is opacified, a floppy-tipped 0.035-in. guide wire (Cook Inc., Bloomington, Ind.) is gently manipulated through the bends in the

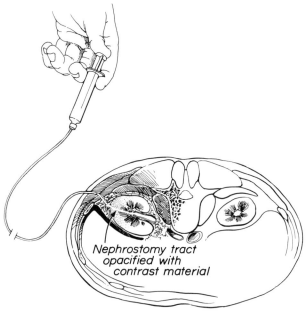

Nephrostomy tract opacified with contrast material

Fig 8–1. Catheter tip in nephrostomy tract outside opening for injection of contrast medium to opacify the tract.

tract. With the help of a gently curved steerable angiographic catheter, the wire usually reaches the collecting system quickly (Fig 8–2). From there it is manipulated in the usual fashion into a position for drainage-catheter placement.

If the patient is referred more than 72 hours after accidental dislodgment, the tract is frequently closed. Attempts to reopen it are only rarely successful. In these cases, and in those referred after blind manipulations that have resulted in one or more false passages, placing a new nephrostomy tract will be faster and safer than manipulating through a traumatized and possibly infected tract.

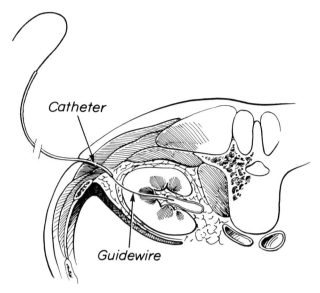

Fig 8–2. Guide wire has been passed through the opacified tract into the renal pelvis.

CHAPTER 9

Percutaneous Nephrostomy in Transplanted Kidneys—Techniques

David W. Hunter, M.D.

Percutaneous techniques have become increasingly important in the diagnosis and treatment of urologic complications in renal transplant patients. When performing a percutaneous procedure on a transplant patient, meticulous attention must be paid to technical details since the two major complications, bleeding and infection, are a significant threat to an immunocompromised patient with a solitary kidney.

ANATOMY

The most common surgical anatomy is for the donor left kidney to be placed extraperitoneally into the recipient's right iliac fossa. The renal pelvis must still be medially located and pointing down toward the bladder, which requires that the kidney be rotated 180 degrees on its axis (flipped over) reversing the anterior-posterior relationships (Figs 9–1,A and B). In particular, the larger and more numerous anterior segmental arteries are now posterior, and the renal pelvis is directed posteromedially.

VISUALIZATION AND PUNCTURE

The first step is visualization of the collecting system. The most common technique that we use is a blind puncture with a "skinny" needle. The most recent ultrasound examination is studied to determine the precise collecting system anatomy. If the collecting system is dilated and the transplanted kidney easily palpable, a thin (22-gauge) needle is passed obliquely through the middle of the transplant toward the pelvis (Fig 9–2). When gentle aspiration during withdrawal yields urine, a small sample is taken for routine cultures. Contrast and carbon dioxide (Fig 9–3) are then injected to outline suitable, anteriorly directed (posterior) calyces for the definitive puncture.

Alternatively, in dilated systems, a suitable calyx for definitive puncture can be chosen by ultrasound, and direct ultrasound guidance used to perform a "single-stick" puncture. Although theoretically appealing, this method has some practical limitations. It has often proved difficult to precisely identify the calyces. This is particularly true in cases in which rejection has resulted in compressed calyces and the only part of the ob-

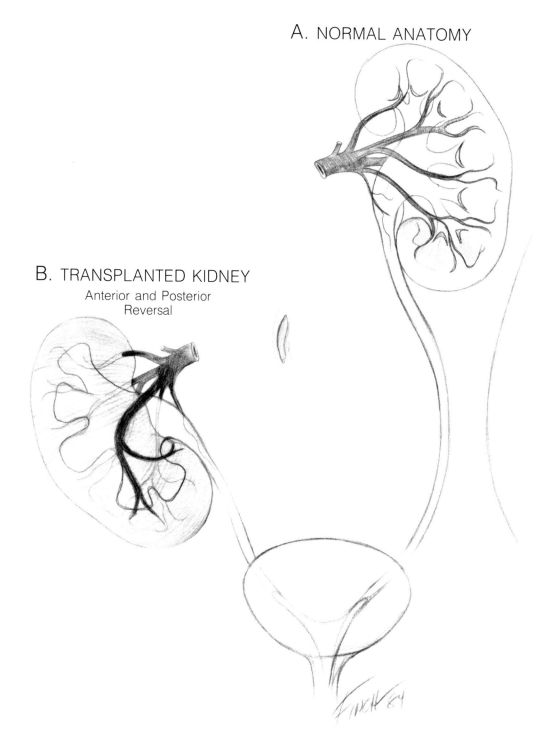

Fig 9–1. Illustration of transplant and native renal vessel and pelvic relationships.

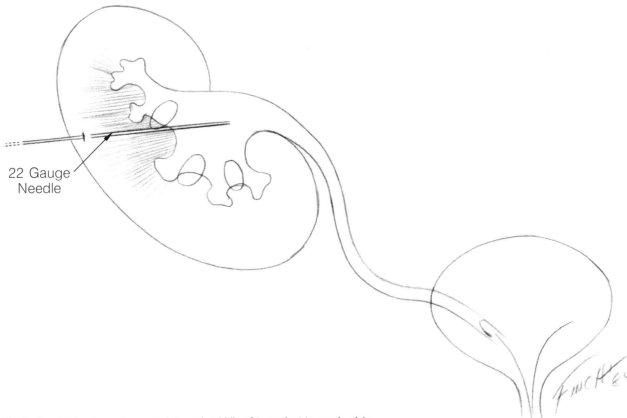

Fig 9–2. "Skinny" needle passed through middle of transplant to renal pelvis.

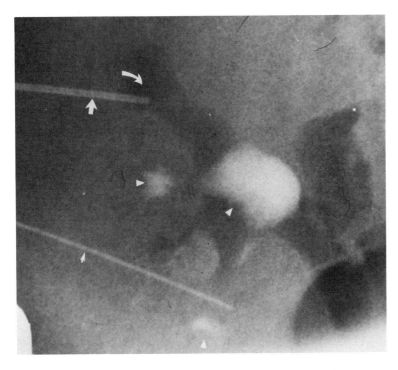

Fig 9–3. The smaller 22-gauge needle *(small arrow)* has entered the lower-pole calyx. Contrast was injected and has opacified the more dependent portions of the collecting system including two calyces *(arrowheads)* and renal pelvis *(arrowhead)*. Carbon dioxide was injected, opacifying the more anteriorly located calyces, especially in the upper pole *(curved arrow)*. The definitive puncture was then made with an 18-gauge needle *(large arrow)* directly into the upper-pole calyx.

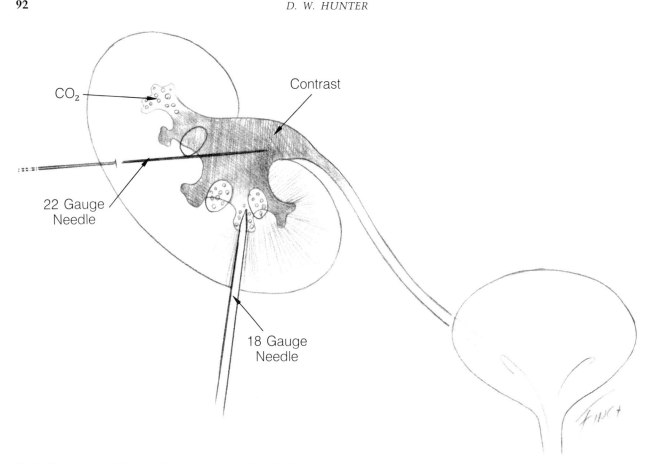

CO₂

Contrast

22 Gauge
Needle

18 Gauge
Needle

Fig 9–4. After opacification with contrast and carbon dioxide by the "skinny," 22g needle, the definitive puncture is made with a large, 18g needle.

structed system that is dilated is the ureter and the portion of the renal pelvis that is extrarenal. Additionally, the technical problems associated with the use of the ultrasound probe on a sterile field, and difficulty visualizing the skinny needle, have usually increased both the number of needle sticks and the time required to complete the procedure compared to the palpation technique.

In patients whose kidneys are difficult to palpate or who have nondilated collecting systems, ultrasound guidance or intravenous contrast becomes necessary. Even in these cases a two-stick technique is usually used with the first puncture made with a skinny needle into the renal pelvis. The calyces can then be more completely opacified and the definitive calyceal puncture made with the larger needle (Fig 9–4).

When making the definitive puncture, a C-arm or biplane fluoroscopy is extremely helpful because it allows accurate placement of the needle into the calyx on the first pass. Repositioning or multipass "triangulation" techniques are unacceptable in transplanted kidneys.

Since the transplanted kidney and surrounding capsule are denervated, there is very little pain associated with punctures or catheter placement. Most percutaneous procedures can therefore be performed with local anesthetics and little or no intravenous sedation.

ANTEGRADE PYELOGRAPHY

In some patients, external drainage will be unnecessary. The diagnostic evaluation in such cases can usually be completed with the skinny needle. The needle can be placed using any of the above techniques into any part of the collecting system. Antegrade pyelography is performed by gently injecting contrast until the collecting system, ureter, and bladder are adequately visualized.

If severe problems are found, such as a major leak (Fig 9–5), surgery usually follows rapidly and external drainage is not required. However, external drainage may be helpful in such patients for preoperative diversion while the patient is medi-

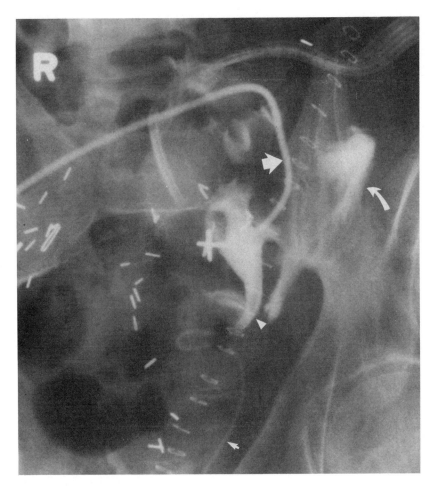

Fig 9–5. In this patient, following reoperation for ureteral obstruction, an anastomosis has been created between the native ureter and the transplanted renal pelvis. An 8 F pigtail catheter *(large arrow)* is in the renal pelvis for external drainage. A 5 F ureteral stent *(small arrow)* has been placed across the anastomosis to the bladder. Injection of contrast demonstrates a leak from the anastomotic site *(arrowhead)* with extravasation into the extraperitoneal soft tissues *(curved arrow)*.

cally stabilized, or for postoperative decompression while the new anastomoses heal.

If abnormalities are found that are of questionable significance, such as a minor stenosis or kink (Fig 9–6), a more precise quantitative assessment of ureteral patency can be obtained with a Whitaker test. Dilute (20%) contrast is injected at the same rate of 10 ml/minute as in nontransplant patients. Pressures are measured every minute in the collecting system and bladder and a pressure differential of greater than 20 cm H_2O is considered diagnostic of a significant obstruction. The collecting system pressure measurements are more accurate if a 21-gauge or larger needle is used. If necessary, a small 4 or 5 F catheter can be placed in the collecting system for this test. However, if either catheter placement or needle puncture causes hematuria, the results of the Whitaker test must be cautiously interpreted, since small clots may cause obstruction and give a false-positive result.

If antegrade pyelography reveals no abnormalities and there is free flow of contrast to the blad-

der with small, low-pressure injections, no further testing is required and the needle may be removed.

One recurrent finding on transplant antegrade pyelography that deserves special comment is the midureteral kink (Fig 9–7). In the opinion of the transplant surgeons at the University of Minnesota this kink occurs at the point where the ureteral attachment to the lower pole ends and the ureter swings toward the bladder (Fig 9–8). For reasons that are unclear, stenoses seem to develop at this kink very commonly (Fig 9–9), but should be evaluated by a Whitaker test before being treated, since they are often not urodynamically significant.

Drainage Catheter Placement

The type and size of the drainage catheter, the point at which it enters the collecting system, and the position in which it is placed will depend on the pathology and therapeutic plans.

In patients with clear urine and only question-

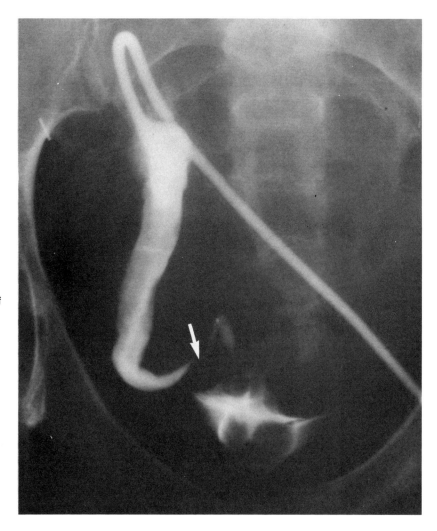

Fig 9–6. There is antegrade flow of contrast through the ureter to the bladder. The distal third of the ureter has a short segment that is quite stenotic *(arrow).* Although the ureter above the stenosis is dilated, antegrade flow was not severely impeded and, therefore, the significance of the stenosis was in doubt.

ably significant pyelographic abnormalities, a catheter is occasionally placed for future Whitaker testing and as a trial to see if external drainage will improve renal function tests. In such cases, a small (5 or 6 F) pigtail is used and is placed in the renal pelvis or in a calyx remote from the entry site. Care should be taken to avoid entering the ureter with either the guide wire or the catheter, since transplanted ureters are very irritable and can remain obstructed by spasm and edema 24 to 48 hours after minimal manipulation.

In patients with obstruction or a leak who require a catheter for drainage or diversion, larger catheters (8 to 12 F) are used. The increased size of the side holes and lumen offers less resistance to drainage and has less of a tendency to clog. The most commonly used catheter is the standard 8 F short pigtail. A commonly used alternative is the Cope loop, which more adequately resists dislodgment and is softer and more comfortable. In extreme cases with large amounts of debris, clots, or pus, our favorite catheter has been the dual stiffness Stamey (Cook Inc., Bloomington, Ind.) (Fig 9–10), which has a large mushroom-type entry site and a large lumen. Larger catheters are usually placed in the pelvis and not in a remote calyx since the catheter shaft can partially obstruct the infundibulum, preventing adequate drainage (Fig 9–11).

Patients with a short-segment stenosis who are candidates for dilation and stenting will need an internal-external drainage catheter placed to the bladder. Several technical considerations should be kept in mind when planning such a procedure.

The renal pelvis and ureter point inferiorly as well as posteromedially. In order to provide the straightest and easiest tract, the definitive calyceal puncture should be into an upper-pole anterolaterally directed calyx (Fig 9–12). When first traversing the ureter we always lead with a soft, floppy-tipped or tight "J" guide wire, especially in cases with recently created anastomoses. Prior to

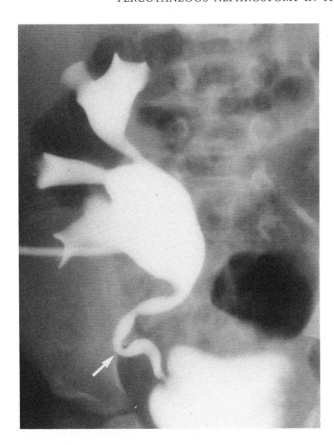

Fig 9–7. The antegrade nephrostogram is normal following dissolution of an obstructing thrombus that occurred following biopsy. The midureteral kink *(arrow)* is very nicely seen.

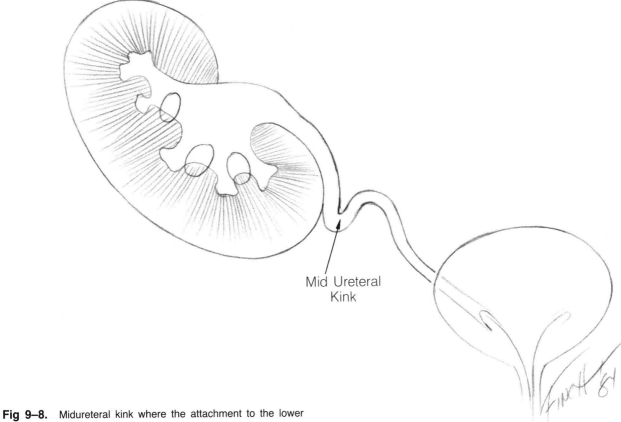

Mid Ureteral
Kink

Fig 9–8. Midureteral kink where the attachment to the lower renal pole ends and the ureter swings toward the bladder.

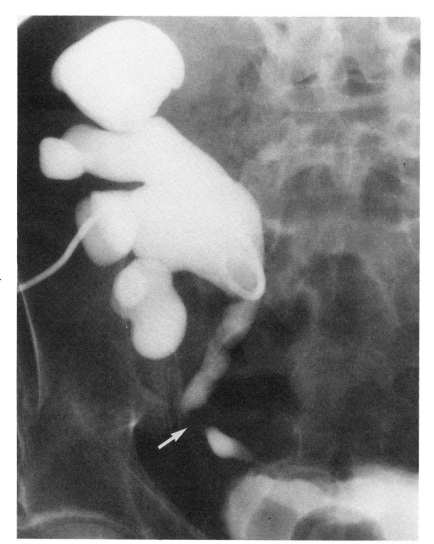

Fig 9–9. Midureteral kink *(arrow)*.

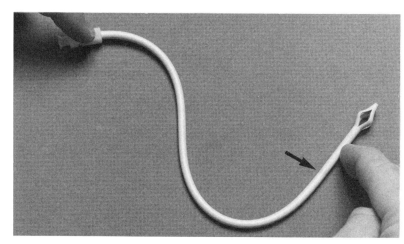

Fig 9–10. Stamey catheter. *Arrow* marks the junction between the stiffer tip and the softer, more flexible shaft.

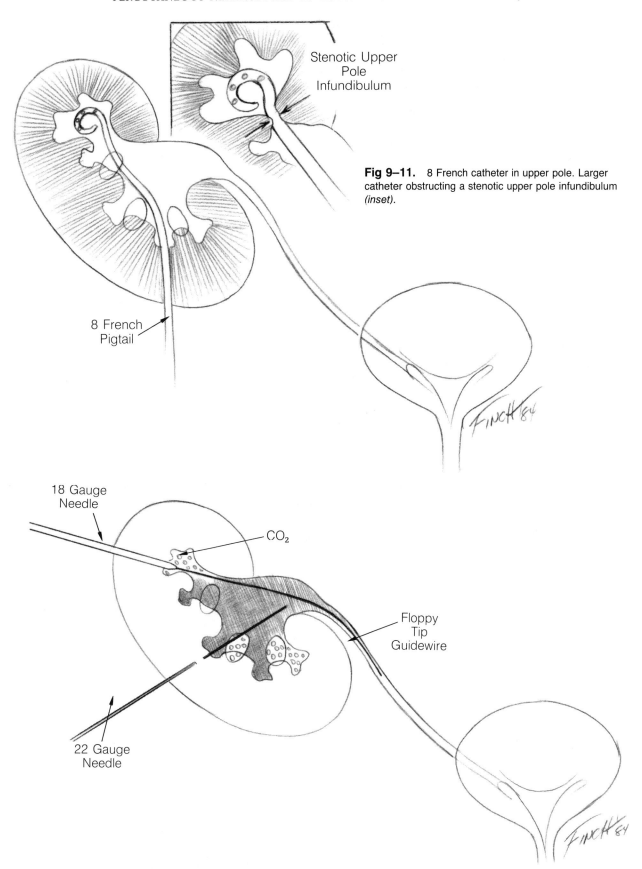

Fig 9–11. 8 French catheter in upper pole. Larger catheter obstructing a stenotic upper pole infundibulum *(inset).*

Stenotic Upper Pole Infundibulum

8 French Pigtail

18 Gauge Needle

CO_2

Floppy Tip Guidewire

22 Gauge Needle

Fig 9–12. Carbon dioxide injected through the smaller needle in the renal pelvis has opacified several calyces, in particular the anterolaterally directed upper-pole calyx *(arrow)* through which the definitive puncture has been made.

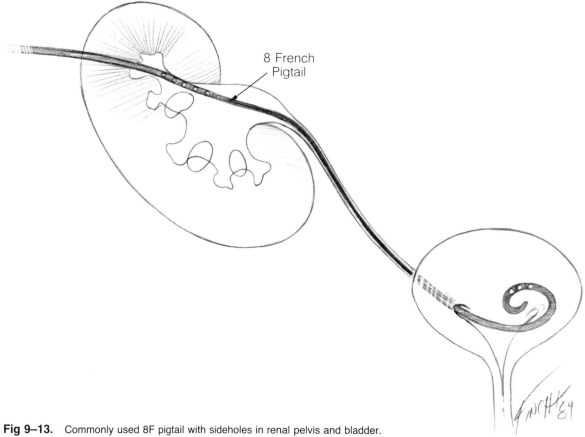

Fig 9–13.   Commonly used 8F pigtail with sideholes in renal pelvis and bladder.

Fig 9–14.   Side holes have been cut in the catheter at the level of the renal pelvis *(small arrow).* The Malecot opening in the catheter *(large arrow)* is positioned in the bladder just beyond the ureteroneocystostomy.

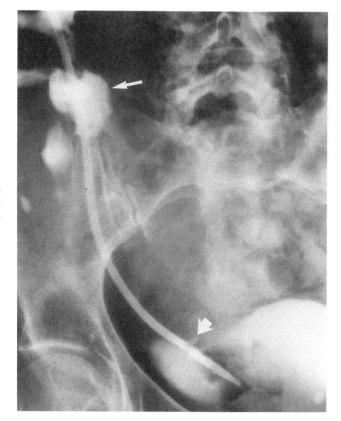

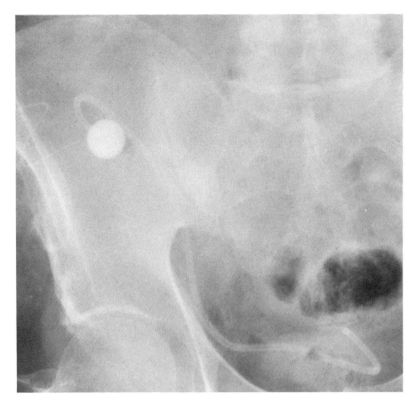

Fig 9–15. Amplatz "Double-J" stent.

dilation the commonest internal-external drainage catheter that we use is an angiographic 8 F pigtail with side holes in the pelvis and bladder (Fig 9–13). Following dilation we have used the Castaneda nephrostomy catheter (Medi-Tech, Watertown, Massachusetts) (Fig 9–14), which is 10.3 F in diameter and therefore distends the ureter to a size that should be more than adequate. The tapered tip and internal stiffener make it very easy to introduce. Large side holes are cut at the level of the renal pelvis with a sterile paper punch. After two or three days, when all hematuria has cleared, urinalysis and cultures are negative, and the patient is pain free and clinically stable, the Castaneda catheter is replaced with an Amplatz 10 F double-J stent (Fig 9–15). A stent length of 16 cm has been adequate in every case except one, in which a long redundant ureter required a 20-cm stent. The stent is removed cystoscopically after six weeks (a time that was chosen somewhat at random). This is a short enough period to keep secondary problems of mechanical bladder irritation and infection to a minimum, but long enough to allow some permanent healing at the dilated site.

On the basis of surgical reports, stenosis of the transplanted ureter or ureteroneocystostomy has been assumed to be fibrotic and dilation has therefore been done with slightly oversized (6- to 8-mm diameter), high-pressure (maximum, 12 to 17 atm) balloons (Fig 9–16). The balloons are inflated slowly so that the minimal possible effective pressure is used.

COMPLICATIONS AND THEIR MANAGEMENT

In percutaneous procedures on transplant patients, infection has been our greatest concern. All transplant patients at the University of Minnesota have been routinely given maintenance therapy with trimethoprim-sulfamethoxazole (Bactrim), which is continued. In addition, we have routinely added two extra antibiotics, usually an aminoglycoside plus a penicillin or chloramphenicol for the period from 12 hours before to 48 to 72 hours after each procedure. All procedures, even simple nephrostograms, are done using sterile technique. We also try to keep each drainage system as "closed" as possible. Therefore, in every case of internal-external drainage we try to cap the external end of the catheter as rapidly as possible and rely on internal drainage alone. Overall, infection has not been as serious a problem as we feared, since patients with obstruction usually do not have as-

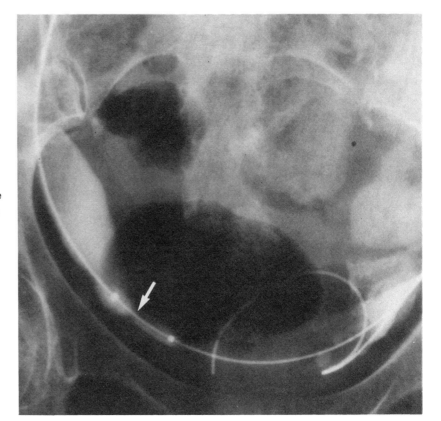

Fig 9–16. The defect in the balloon at the site of the stenosis *(arrow)* can still be seen, even with inflation pressures of 15 to 17 atm.

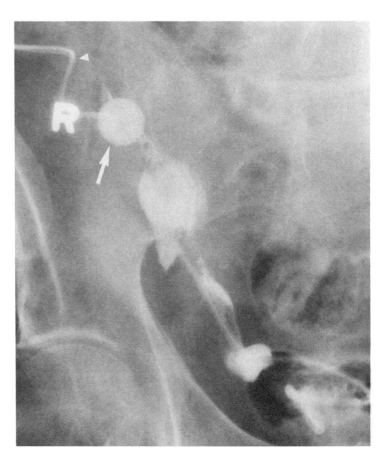

Fig 9–17. The inflated Foley balloon *(arrow)* has been placed in the upper-pole calyx. The patient's very large and very mobile panniculus has kinked the catheter *(arrowhead),* but unlike all of the other catheter types that were tried, the tip of the catheter remains in the collecting system because of the balloon.

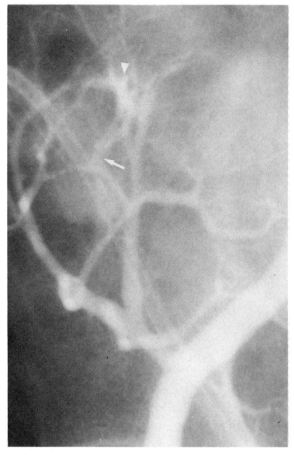

Fig 9–18. One arterial branch *(arrow)* led to an arteriovenous fistula *(arrowhead),* which intermittently bled into the collecting system.

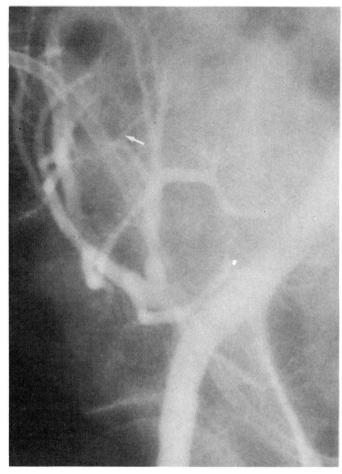

Fig 9–19. Following Gelfoam embolization, the arterial branch that fed the fistula *(arrow)* has been completely occluded.

sociated rejection or medical problems and patients who develop a positive urine culture can usually be easily treated with an appropriate parenteral antibiotic.

Catheter dislodgment or kinking may be a severe problem in obese patients with a large panniculus or patients with an altered mental status. In one such case a Silastic Foley catheter (Fig 9–17) proved to be the only satisfactory solution.

Minimal to moderate hematuria occurs in every case, but clears within 24 to 48 hours. Persistent or recurring hematuria after 48 hours usually in-

dicates that the procedure has caused either a pseudoaneurysm (Fig 9–18) or an arteriovenous fistula. These can be managed in the usual fashion with selective percutaneous embolization (Fig 9–19). Severe hematuria immediately following catheter placement is rare if the definitive puncture is properly made into a calyx. It most often occurs in patients who are uremic and have abnormal coagulation parameters. In such patients bleeding has been easily controlled by temporarily correcting the coagulation abnormality.

CHAPTER 10

Percutaneous Nephrostomy in Infants and Children

Ricardo Gonzalez, M.D.

Percutaneous drainage of the upper urinary tract plays an essential role in pediatric urology. In the last five years, percutaneous nephrostomy has completely replaced open nephrostomy tube placement as an isolated procedure at our institution. Furthermore, we have adapted the technical principles and instrumentation of percutaneous procedures for the placement of open nephrostomies when renal drainage is required as part of reconstructive operations.[1]

Despite the relative simplicity of percutaneous nephrostomy tube placement, the indications for the procedure should not be the mere diagnosis of hydronephrosis. It should also be remembered that to perform simple antegrade urography or pressure flow studies or to obtain cultures from renal pelvis urine, a puncture with a 22-gauge needle is sufficient. This procedure, considerably simpler than a formal percutaneous nephrostomy is virtually free of complications. Prolonged nephrostomy tube drainage in children is often poorly tolerated and tubes have a tendency to be dislodged in the active infant and child. Therefore, nephrostomy drainage is used only for relatively short periods of time, preferably less than one month.

INDICATIONS FOR PERCUTANEOUS NEPHROSTOMY DRAINAGE

The following are the indications for percutaneous nephrostomy drainage in infants and children.

Temporary Drainage in the Child With Sepsis and Obstruction, With or Without Uremia

These are usually infants with posterior urethral valves, ectopic ureteroceles, or infected ureteropelvic junction obstructions. Drainage of the urinary tract is often life-saving, but its timing should be carefully coordinated with other therapeutic measures, including correction of fluid and electrolyte imbalance, antibiotic administration, and, in some cases, hemodialysis.[2] In these sick infants intravenous injection of contrast medium can be hazardous and the use of ultrasound to perform the initial puncture is essential. As soon as the child's condition is stable the correct anatomical diagnosis should be established with contrast studies and measures should be taken to eliminate the nephrostomy tubes, either by correcting the obstruction or by resorting to a more suitable form of long-term diversion (such as cutaneous pyelostomy or ureterostomy).

Temporary Drainage for Transient Obstruction

In cases of postoperative edema early after pyeloplasty or distal ureteral reconstruction, percutaneous nephrostomy drainage for two or three weeks is useful to preserve renal function and alleviate symptoms. If the obstruction persists, endourologic dilation of the obstruction or reoperation can be undertaken with minimal loss of renal function. Prolonged intubated drainage in infants, however, can be detrimental to renal function. Other causes of temporary obstruction in which percutaneous drainage has been useful include distal ureteral obstruction in children due to cyclophosphamide (Cytoxan) cystitis after bone marrow transplantation, ureteral obstruction by retroperitoneal tumors expected to respond to chemotherapy, fungus balls, and others.

Temporary Drainage for the Treatment of Other Postoperative Complications

Percutaneous nephrostomy drainage can be a useful procedure for proximal drainage of urinary fistulas or urinary extravasation complicating reconstructive surgical procedures.

Evaluation of Individual Function of a Kidney

When such information is useful to make therapeutic decisions and cannot be obtained by less invasive means, a temporary percutaneous nephrostomy drainage can be useful. In most infants and young children with ureteropelvic junction obstructions and evidence of function on a radioisotopic renogram, early reconstruction is attended by a high rate of functional improvement.[3] Therefore, primary repair is performed without preliminary nephrostomy drainage. However, in older children and adolescents with unilateral high-grade obstruction and very poor function on renography, a preliminary percutaneous nephrostomy and assessment of renal function after one or two weeks of decompression will help decide between pyeloplasty and nephrectomy.

Drainage of Urinomas

Although not strictly a nephrostomy, percutaneous drainage of urinomas usually secondary to congenital obstruction or occurring postoperatively can be useful and requires techniques similar to those used for percutaneous nephrostomies.

PERCUTANEOUS MANIPULATION IN THE COLLECTING SYSTEM

Percutaneous nephrostomy tract dilations for the purpose of manipulation are just beginning in children. Percutaneous nephrolithotomy has been performed in children older than 8 years[4] and, as in adults, is the method of choice. This approach in children younger than 8 years is rare. Percutaneous nephrostomy for dilation or incision of anatomical defects causing ureteral obstruction has been performed with success in children. It is most successful for postoperative strictures of the ureter of recent onset.

TECHNICAL CONSIDERATIONS

The techniques for percutaneous nephrostomy and dilation are the same for children as they are in adults except for differences in anesthetic needs and in the sizes of the tubes and tracts. These techniques are discussed in other chapters in this book. For percutaneous nephrostomy, tube size is usually no greater than 8 F. We have performed large tract dilations for percutaneous nephrolithotomy or intrarenal surgery only on children more than 8 years old. In these cases, we have dilated the tract to 24 F without ill effects. In smaller children, smaller-sized tracts would be appropriate where the size of available instruments is a limiting factor, especially for lithotripsy. One alternative is to use available cystoscopes and electrohydraulic lithotripsy or the ureterorenoscope and its ultrasonic probe. Fortunately, smaller nephroscopes and probes are now being developed.

REFERENCES

1. Chiou R.K., Gonzalez R.: Operative thin trocar nephrostomy. *Urology* 22:545, 1983.
2. Gonzalez R., Sheldon C.A.: Septic obstruction and uremia in the newborn. *Urol. Clin. North Am.* 9:297, 1982.
3. King L.R., Coughlin P.W.F., Bloch E.C., et al.: The case for immediate pyeloplasty in the neonate with ureteropelvic junction obstruction. *J. Urol.* 132:725, 1984.
4. Hulbert J.C., Reddy P.K., Gonzalez R., et al.: Percutaneous nephrolithotomy: An alternative approach to the management of pediatric calculus disease. *Pediatrics* 76:610, 1985.
5. King L.R., Coughlin P.W.F., Ford C., et al.: Initial experience with percutaneous and transureteral ablation of postoperative ureteral stricture in children. *J. Urol.* 131:1167, 1984.

CHAPTER 11

The Whitaker Test

Ricardo Gonzalez, M.D.

Pressure flow studies of the upper urinary tract are often essential to differentiate between the dilated obstructed and the dilated unobstructed urinary tract. The clinician is often confronted with an asymptomatic patient with dilatation on intravenous pyelogram in whom the diuresis renogram yields equivocal results.[1] Frequent examples of such cases include persistent dilatation after surgical correction of obstructed ureteral lesion, cases of apparent megacalycosis or the nonobstructing, nonrefluxing megaureter. Pressure flow studies of the urinary tract (the Whitaker test) provide a simple objective way to correlate pressure with flow, thus fulfilling the urodynamic criteria to determine the presence or absence of obstruction. We have performed more than 150 Whitaker tests as originally described, with several modifications.[2,3] We have been generally satisfied with the interpretation of the results obtained and there have been no complications.

TECHNIQUE

In infants and adults the test can often be done with local anesthesia, with or without sedation, whereas in toddlers it often requires general anesthesia for immobilization. The apparatus needed to perform this test is shown in Figure 11–1. A bladder catheter is inserted, the patient is placed in the prone position, and the collecting system is punctured through a posterior approach with a 22-gauge needle. The needle can be directed fluoroscopically after injecting intravenous contrast medium or by ultrasonographic control. After access to the collecting system is obtained, an antegrade pyelogram is obtained, which helps delineate the anatomy. Following this, perfusion is begun with a dilute contrast medium injected with an intravenous injection pump capable of delivering flows of up to 15 ml/minute. With a three-way stopcock, pressures are measured with water manometers at one-minute intervals by briefly interrupting the perfusion. The test is continued until a steady state between inflow and outflow is reached, obstruction is demonstrated, or a plateau in the kidney pressure is reached. The perfusion is monitored with intermittent fluoroscopy in order to rule out extravasation and to make sure that useful measurements are made when the collecting system is distended to capacity.

INTERPRETATION OF RESULTS

The bladder is drained as needed. The pressures recorded at one-minute intervals are plotted. Results obtained are interpreted as follows: when the pressure differential is less than 15 cm H_2O no obstruction is present, and when the differential exceeds 22 cm H_2O obstruction is present. Differential pressures between 15 and 22 cm H_2O are seen

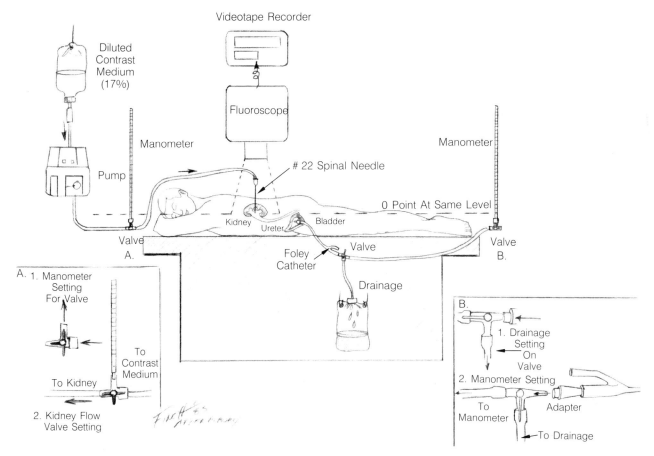

Fig 11–1. Schematic illustration of Whitaker test showing apparatus required.

in less than 10% of patients, and these are the only cases in which the Whitaker test may yield equivocal results. The test is performed with the bladder full and empty. It is useful to detect intermittent obstruction caused by angulation of the distal ureter such as is seen after some ureteroneocystostomies, and it also helps in the diagnosis of hydronephrosis secondary to bladder hypertonicity in which upper tract dilatation is caused by elevated intravesical pressures with normal differential pressures between the renal pelvis and the bladder. These values of differential pressure are given for the standard perfusion rate of 10 ml/minute. In newborns with a minimally dilated collecting system, I begin the test at 5 ml/minute, and if obstruction is demonstrated no further evaluation is needed.

Although far from perfect, the Whitaker test as described provides useful functional and anatomical information that cannot be obtained by the in-

travenous pyelogram, the retrograde pyelogram, or the diuresis renogram, even when used in combination. The test is usually performed on an outpatient basis and we have observed no complications from the puncture of the kidney and immediate removal of the needle after termination of the test, even in cases of obstruction.

REFERENCES

1. Gonzalez R., Chiou R.K.: The diagnosis of upper urinary obstruction in children: Comparison of diuresis renography and pressure flow studies. *J. Urol.* 133:646, 1985.
2. Whitaker R.H.: Pressure flow studies, in O'Reilly P.H., Goslong J.A. (eds.): *Idiopathic Hydronephrosis.* Berlin, Springer Verlag, 1982, chap. 5.
3. Pfister R.C., Newhouse J.H., Hendren W.H.: Percutaneous pyeloureteral urodynamics. *Urol. Clin. North Am.* 9:41, 1982.

CHAPTER 12

Percutaneous Nephrolithotomy: Patient Selection and Preoperative Management

Paul H. Lange, M.D.

In general, the indications for percutaneous nephrolithotomy are the same as those for standard operations; that is, the stone should be causing symptoms and/or obstruction or be in imminent danger of doing so, or it should be a source of infection. Whenever possible, other stones in the collecting system should be removed at the time of endourologic removal of a surgical stone, though this depends on the situation and, to some extent, on the physician's philosophy. The patient with purely asymptomatic stones presents a dilemma. In most cases the stones should not be removed unless they are definitely growing or unless an asymptomatic pelvic stone appears to be too large to pass spontaneously. In other special circumstances, purely asymptomatic stones can be removed. These include patients with chronic urinary tract infections or documented renal damage from the presence of the stone. Removal of asymptomatic stones is also justified among airline pilots or other professionals who cannot pursue their occupation because of the stone(s).

The contraindications to percutaneous nephrolithotomy are generally the same as those for primary percutaneous nephrostomy. Extreme obesity becomes more important in this situation because many of the instruments needed for stone removal do not exceed 20 cm. In anatomical situations in which there is increased difficulty and/or risk, the indications should be carefully reviewed, especially by those teams without extensive experience; these situations include solitary kidney, a high-lying kidney for which percutaneous access above the 12th rib will be necessary, small or bifid intrarenal collecting systems, severe kyphoscoliosis, certain congenital abnormalities (such as horseshoe or pelvic kidney), a very mobile kidney, an impacted ureteral stone, and branched and staghorn calculi (especially when the collecting system is minimally dilated or the stone extends into multiple calyces with narrow infundibuli).

Patient preparation should, of course, begin with an extensive explanation of the procedure and informed consent. The following issues should be stressed:

1. The procedure is not without complications. Emergency surgery for bleeding may be necessary and a nephrectomy may result. This bleeding may be immediate or delayed (e.g., arteriovenous fistula).

2. There is a 5% to 10% chance that the procedure will fail and an open surgical procedure may be required.

3. The procedure may take more than one session and prolonged hospitalization is a possibility. This is a relatively new procedure and the long-

term effects (while currently unalarming) are unknown, particularly with regard to its effect on kidney function and subsequent stone recurrence.

4. This is not a pain-free procedure, nor is it nonoperative.

5. There is a likelihood that the patient may leave the hospital with a nephrostomy tube and that on removal, there may be leakage of urine for some time.

The preoperative laboratory work is generally the same as for a primary percutaneous nephrostomy. More attention, however, should be paid to the location of the stone, though oblique films are not necessary since the information can usually be obtained through C-arm or biplane fluoroscopy at the time of the procedure. For a percutaneous nephrolithotomy, it is probably appropriate that serum calcium, phosphorus, and uric acid determinations be obtained prior to the procedure, though a complete metabolic evaluation can be delayed until after recovery. Blood type is deter-mined in most centers, although a formal cross-match is often not obtained. Nonetheless, the possibility of blood transfusion must be anticipated.

The patient is kept without food or drink the evening before the procedure. Again, a urine culture should be sterile, if possible, or the appropriate antibiotic or broad-spectrum antibiotics should be given. Procedures to induce diuresis are often desirable to distend the renal pelvis. Preanesthetic medications should be administered even in those patients in whom local anesthesia is used. A urethral catheter is an absolute necessity, as large amounts of irrigating fluid often distend the bladder. A retrograde ureteral catheter is used in many centers, but not all. The indications for percutaneous stone removal will certainly change with the general availability of extracorporeal shock-wave lithotripsy. The relative place of each modality, either singly or in combination, awaits more extensive experience.

CHAPTER 13

Percutaneous Nephrolithotomy: Retrograde Access

Pratap K. Reddy, M.D.

Retrograde access to the renal collecting system immediately prior to percutaneous nephrolithotomy plays an important role in the successful management of renal or ureteral calculi. It helps in the precise three-dimensional anatomical delineation of the collecting system and localization of the calculi; facilitates accurate percutaneous puncture of the collecting system, especially in nondilated collecting systems (Fig 13–1); achieves accessory drainage of the collecting system in complicated cases; and prevents fragment migration down the ureter in cases of calculus disintegration (Fig 13–2). In our experience it is unnecessary to occlude the ureter or the ureteropelvic junction with balloon catheters for this purpose.

EQUIPMENT

The following is a list of instruments that may be used to achieve retrograde access to the collecting system. Manufacturers' names are given in parentheses.

1. Rigid cystoscopes (ACMI, Storz, Olympus, Wolf).
2. Flexible scopes (Olympus, ACMI, Pentax).
3. Open-ended ureteral catheters (Van-Tec, Cook, Kifa).
4. Guide wires 0.035- and 0.038-in., floppy wires.

TECHNIQUE

Access to the collecting system is achieved by the retrograde passage of an open-ended ureteral catheter using either rigid or flexible endoscopes.

Passage of the ureteral catheter using the rigid cystoscope is routine and will not be described here. However, newer ureteral catheterization techniques using the flexible cystoscope (choledochonephroscope) will be described briefly because of its potential advantages.

The patient is prepared and draped in the supine position. Lidocaine (Xylocaine) jelly is instilled through the urethra. The flexible cystoscope is then guided under vision through the urethra into the bladder. The ureteral orifice is readily identified. A 0.035-in. floppy guide wire is threaded up the ureter into the renal pelvis. The flexible cystoscope is then removed and an open-ended ureteral catheter is passed over the guide wire into the renal pelvis. The whole procedure is aided by the use of fluoroscopy.

Two technical problems could be encountered during this procedure.

Insertion of Guide Wire Into the Ureteric Orifice

Following identification of the ureteric orifice, attempts at passing the guide wire into the orifice may be difficult due to the floppy nature of the

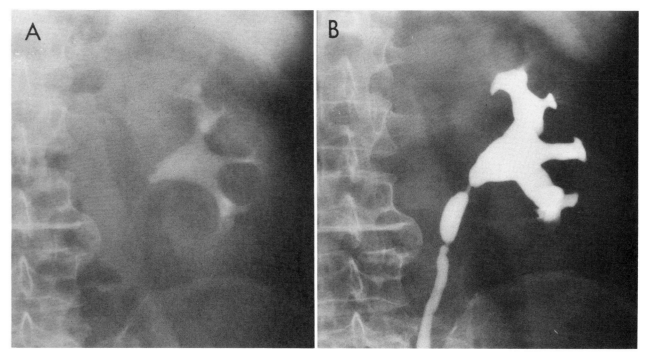

Fig 13–1.   Intravenous pyelogram **(A)** and retrograde pyelogram **(B)** showing precise anatomy and dilatation of the calyces, produced by retrograde injection.

guide wire and lack of stabilization of the tip of the guide wire. This can be overcome by keeping the tip of the flexible cystoscope very close to the ureteric orifice (to steady the guide wire) or a 5 F Kifa catheter could be passed over the guide wire through the flexible cystoscope through the ureteric orifice and the guide wire can then be easily threaded up the ureter (Fig 13–3).

Guide Wire May Be Dislodged Into the Bladder
Care must be taken while passing the open-ended ureteral catheter over the guide wire. If the ureteral catheter abuts the ureteric orifice it tends to coil in the bladder, and as it does the guide wire is lost from the ureter. Thus, this part of the procedure should be monitored by fluoroscopy (Fig 13–4).

ADVANTAGES OF FLEXIBLE OVER THE RIGID ENDOSCOPE

- The procedure is performed under topical anesthesia.
- As the patient is in the supine position the procedure can be performed on an angiographic table just prior to the percutaneous nephrostomy (we have, on occasion, performed this with the patient in the semiprone position).
- It lessens the extensive draping used in rigid endoscopy.
- It is well tolerated by the patient.

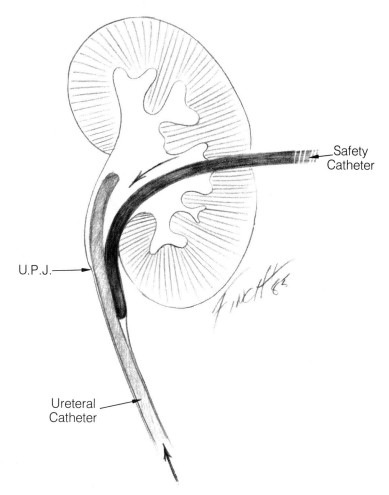

Fig 13–2. In percutaneous nephrolithotomy a retrograde catheter enhances access and drainage, and can prevent ureteral obstruction from stone fragments.

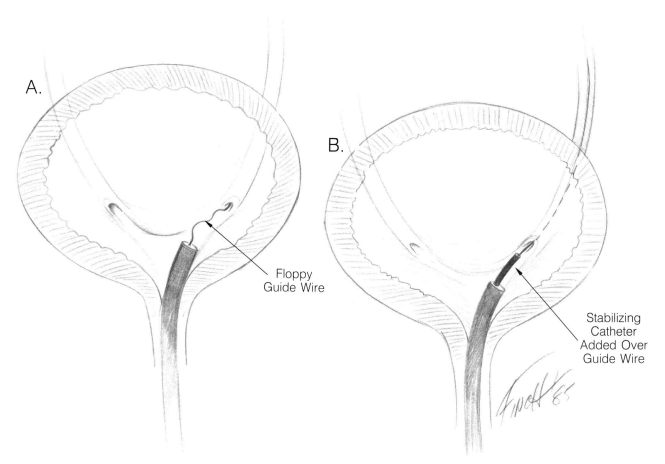

Fig 13–3.   Guide wire insertion into ureteric orifice: the problem **(A)** and solution **(B).**

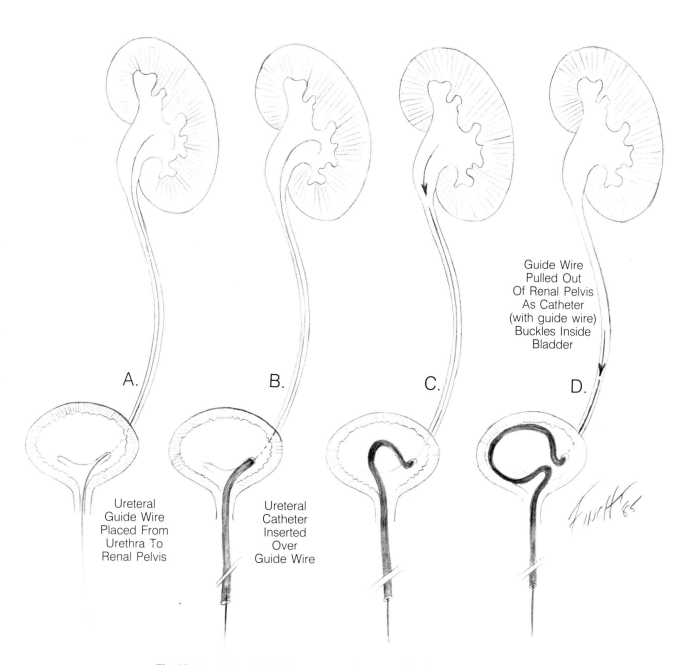

Guide Wire
Pulled Out
Of Renal Pelvis
As Catheter
(with guide wire)
Buckles Inside
Bladder

A.

B.

C.

D.

Ureteral
Guide Wire
Placed From
Urethra To
Renal Pelvis

Ureteral
Catheter
Inserted
Over
Guide Wire

Fig 13–4.   Guide wire lost from ureter when ureteral catheter is passed over it.

CHAPTER 14

Percutaneous Nephrolithotomy: Approaches

Carol C. Coleman, M.D.

The percutaneous approach to the kidney for renal stone extraction was developed as a result of percutaneous nephrostomies for relieving upper urinary tract obstruction. Percutaneous renal stone removal has been used in the past but was not well accepted until recent years. Advances in angiographic techniques and urologic instrumentation provided means to remove virtually all urinary calculi without major surgery. The availability of dilating systems allowed safe dilatation and the introduction of large instruments and scopes. From our experience gained with more than 650 stone removals we have developed an approach that has resulted in a high success rate with a low incidence of complications.

The initial puncture site in percutaneous stone removal is of paramount importance. The puncture itself can be facilitated by placing a ureteral catheter cystoscopically, allowing for good opacification and distension of the collecting system. The entrance point into the collecting system must be placed so that the guide wire can be passed into the renal pelvis and ureter for subsequent dilation. The entrance site affects dilation and also determines the accessibility of the stone for instrumentation and extraction.

It is important to anticipate the method of stone removal. The ultrasonic lithotriptor and nephroscopes are rigid and cannot make sharp turns.

Therefore, with this equipment a relatively straight path to the stone must be established. If the course to reach the stone is curved, a flexible nephroscope may be required. Another determining factor in the approach is the familiarity of the endoscopist with the flexible scope. The use and techniques of the scope can be difficult to learn at first. Therefore, early on the rigid scope may be the instrument of choice.

The entrance site also influences the incidence of complications (see Chapter 3). The renal puncture should be made as peripheral as possible and through the calyx. With calyceal stones a puncture in the infundibulum is sometimes necessary; however, there are larger vessels crossing the infundibulum and there is an increased chance of bleeding.

Once the number, type, and location of the patient's stones are identified, and the type of instrumentation is determined, the approach to the kidney can be considered. All of this information plus a thorough knowledge of the anatomy influences the puncture site selection. An error in entrance site may cause a failure of stone extraction or cause a time- and money-consuming experience. Occasionally, particularly with multiple stones, a second puncture may be needed.

We developed the following approaches after performing numerous percutaneous renal stone

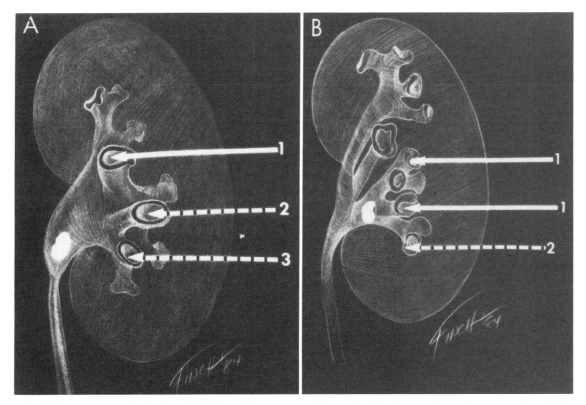

Fig 14–1. **A,** schematic drawing of a kidney with a small floating renal pelvic stone. The easiest approach would be through the posterior calyx no. 1 providing a straighter path for working the wire into the ureter and subsequent dilation. The next choices would be through the posterior calyces labeled no. 2 and 3. If the kidney is positioned high under the ribs and an infracostal approach is desired, approaches no. 2 and 3 should be successful, although no. 3 would be a little more difficult because of the more angled course of the working wire from the calyx into the ureter. **B,** free-floating pelvic stone, difficult anatomy. In this case, secondary to the bifid pelvis the anatomy is unfavorable for a high puncture. A lower posterior calyx should be punctured, those labeled no. 1 or 2.

extractions. There is a great variation in the configuration of the collecting systems and the stone size and shape, as well as in the number of stones. Therefore, each patient must be considered on an individual basis using the suggested approaches only as guidelines.

SMALL PELVIC STONES

The free-floating small (less than 1.5 cm in diameter) renal pelvic stone is the easiest to remove, and it is therefore the initial choice for an operator with early experience. With increased experience, removal of more difficult larger stones can be tried.

The posterior calyx in the midpole or a lower-pole posterior calyx is punctured (Figs 14–1,A and B). The guide wire is passed down the ureter and the tract is dilated. If the calculus is 1.5 cm or smaller it can be extracted with a forceps, grasper, or basket or by simultaneous aspiration through a

Teflon sheath and flushing through the retrograde ureteral catheter. For larger stones, fragmentation techniques are required.

LARGER PELVIC STONES AND STAGHORN CALCULI

Depending on the calyceal and infundibular anatomy, a posterior calyx is punctured (Figs 14–2,A-C). For staghorn calculi puncturing a middle- or lower-pole posterior calyx facilitates the passage of the guide wire into the ureter, since there is limited space for manipulation between the staghorn calculus and the renal pelvis. Dilation may be difficult in the reduced space. Injection of contrast medium through a retrograde ureteral catheter is most helpful for distension of the pelvis. In puncturing a collecting system containing a large staghorn calculus, the tip of the needle must be advanced several millimeters inside of the collecting system either by displacing the

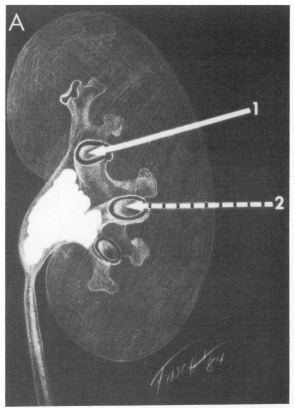

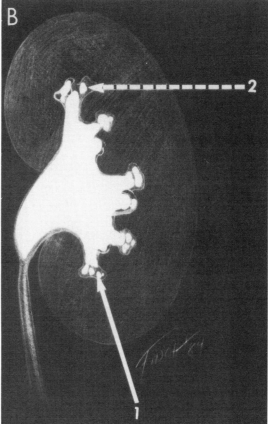

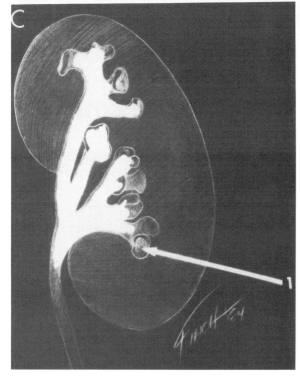

Fig 14–2. **A,** large renal pelvic stone. For non-staghorn calculi when there is room in the collecting system, a higher puncture is preferable for easy passage of the guide wire down the ureter and subsequent dilation and instrument passage. **B,** large staghorn calculus. For large staghorn calculi there is limited space for manipulation. Approach no. 1 provides the shortest route to the ureter, although it is a curved path. Either no. 1 or 2 provides the best access for the ultrasonic lithotriptor to all parts of the intrarenal collecting system. **C,** large staghorn calculus, difficult anatomy. Here, two or three punctures may be necessary to remove all parts of the calculus. Access no. 1 should allow removal of all the lower renal stone, and with skill and luck, the midrenal stone to be removed. Most likely a second puncture will be needed for the upper-pole stone segment.

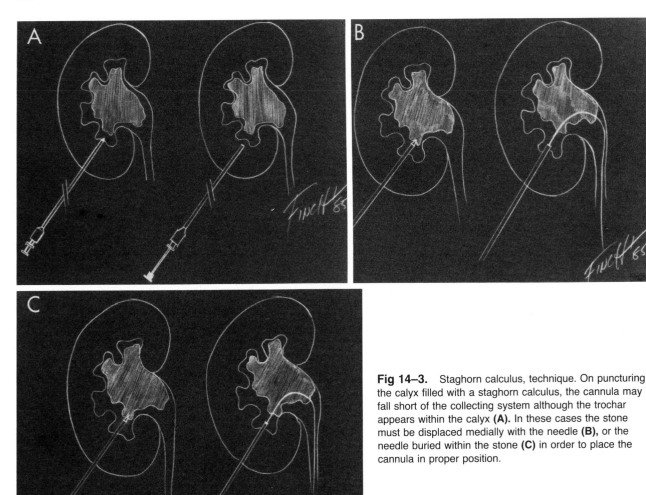

Fig 14–3. Staghorn calculus, technique. On puncturing the calyx filled with a staghorn calculus, the cannula may fall short of the collecting system although the trochar appears within the calyx **(A)**. In these cases the stone must be displaced medially with the needle **(B)**, or the needle buried within the stone **(C)** in order to place the cannula in proper position.

stone or by forcing the needle tip into the stone itself (Figs 14–3,A-C). Otherwise, if the stylus is removed the cannula may be outside of the collecting system. For these larger stones, fragmentation techniques will be needed. The ultrasonic lithotriptor is most frequently used. All of our patients have a retrograde ureteral catheter in place, which also prevents the migration of fragments into the ureter.

CALYCEAL STONES

Calyceal stones are the most difficult stones to remove. Therefore this should not be attempted until expertise has been obtained with easier cases. There are two ways to approach calyceal stones, either directly or indirectly. For the isolated lower-pole posterior calyceal stone a direct puncture is made slightly medial to the retained calculus, usually at the calyceal infundibular border (Figs 14–4 and 14–5). By puncturing slightly more medial to the stone, the stone is trapped within the calyx thus avoiding its displacement into the renal pelvis and possible migration into another calyx or ureter. Puncturing medially also facilitates the guidewire passage into the ureter and subsequent tract dilatation (Fig 14–6).

For middle- and upper-pole isolated posterior calyceal stones a direct or distant puncture can be made (Figs 14–7 and 14–8). In cases where the stone is high and a direct approach using a supracostal puncture is not desired, a distant approach can be used through a lower-pole posterior calyx.

For an isolated anterior calyceal stone in the lower pole either a direct or distant approach can be used (Fig 14–9). For a direct puncture, which is quite difficult, the patient's position must be

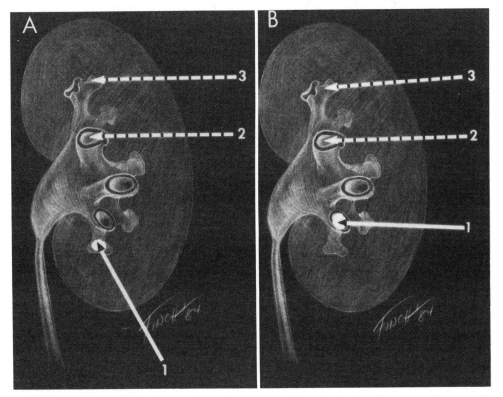

Fig 14–4. Lower pole calyceal stone. For an isolated lower-pole compound calyceal **(A)**, or lower-pole posterior calyceal stone **(B)**, a direct approach (no. 1) is best. If this is technically difficult to do then a posterior calyx somewhat removed from that of the stone can be used (no. 2 and 3) so that the angle between the two calyces is as straight as possible. The upper-pole compound calyces (no. 3) are less desirable because usually they require a supracostal puncture.

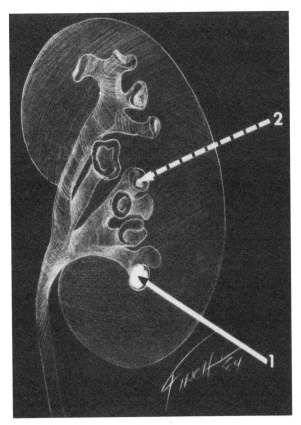

Fig 14–5. Lower-pole compound calyceal stone, difficult anatomy. An upper-pole puncture in this case would probably fail in the stone extraction. A direct puncture (no. 1) is the best. Punctures into the adjacent posterior calyces may prove to provide a difficult stone removal secondary to the acute angulation needed for manipulation into the lower-pole calyx. Approach no. 2 will give the least angulation.

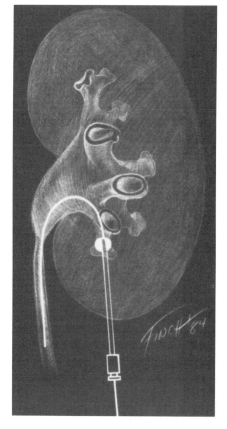

Fig 14–6. Puncturing medial to the calyceal stone traps the stone in the calyx and also facilitates the passage of the guide wire into the ureter.

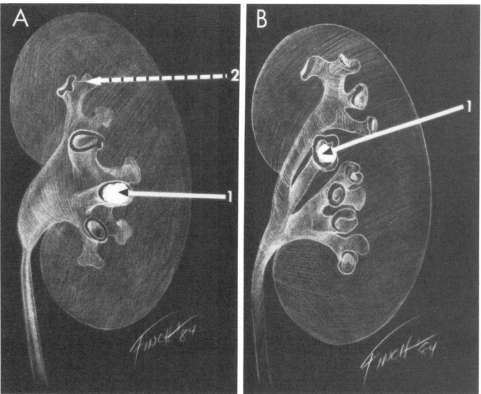

Fig 14–7. A, midposterior calyceal stone. The middle- and upper-pole posterior calyceal stones can be removed from a direct puncture (no. 1). If a distant puncture is made it should be far enough away from the stone to minimize the angle necessary for the retrieving instrument (no. 2). **B,** middle-pole posterior calyceal stone, difficult anatomy. In this case there is only one choice for puncturing, no. 1. All other entrance sites would require acute angulation of the retrieving instrument for stone removal.

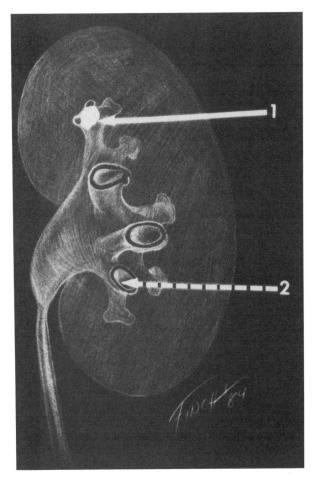

Fig 14–8. Upper-pole compound calyceal stone. *No.1*, a direct puncture onto the stone can be used. Or, if a supracostal puncture is not desired, the stone can be approached from a lower pole posterior calyx (*no.2*).

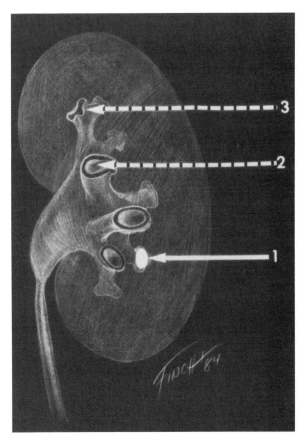

Fig 14–9. Lower-pole anterior calyceal stone. Anterior calyceal stones can be approached directly or indirectly. In this case no. 1 indicates the direct puncture, which can be quite difficult. No. 2 is an indirect approach through a posterior calyx slightly remote from the stone in order to straighten the path for the retrieving instrument. No. 3 probably would require a supracostal puncture.

steeply oblique to gain access to the infundibulum (Fig 14–10). With anterior calyceal stones a very precise puncture is required. If the puncturing needle is introduced facing the anterior calyx or its infundibulum the guide wire will consistently enter the calyx making the dilation almost impossible. Either a more medial puncture is necessary at the junction of the infundibulum with the renal pelvis (which is further away from the stone, increasing its difficulty of removal) or a medially angled puncture of the involved anterior infundibulum must be made. This will allow passage of the guide wire into the ureter. After dilation the endoscopist can then manipulate the flexible nephroscope into the anterior calyx. Once the puncture is made and it is found that it is difficult to advance the guide wire out of the infundibulum, there are two techniques we have used to resolve the situation. For perpendicular punctures the needle can be tilted slightly laterally, angling the

needle tip more medially for easier passage of the guide wire (Fig 14–11). Or, the guide wire (floppy-tipped) can be bounced off the stone, forming a loop that can be passed into the pelvis and then straightened (Fig 14–12). A sometimes easier approach is to puncture a posterior calyx that has favorable anatomy (Fig 14–13), and then to use either a rigid or flexible scope for extraction, depending on the angles that need to be traversed.

In the case of an anterior calyceal stone in the upper pole or above the 12th rib, the size of the stone and the anatomy of the collecting system will dictate the entrance point. For larger stones requiring fragmentation the direct approach is better than a distant puncture using a flexible scope from below (Fig 14–14). It is difficult to fragment a stone using the flexible scope. Either mechanical means, such as a grasper, or the electrohydraulic lithotriptor must be implemented. The mechanical devices are generally inefficient. The electro-

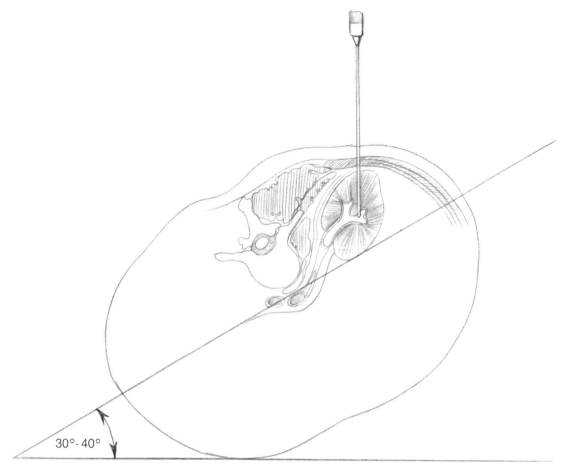

30°- 40°

Fig 14–10. Cross section of the body at the level of the kidneys. For an anterior calyceal puncture, sometimes the body must be steeply angled to approach the calyx. Also note that more parenchyma is traversed than with a posterior calyceal puncture, theoretically increasing the bleeding potential.

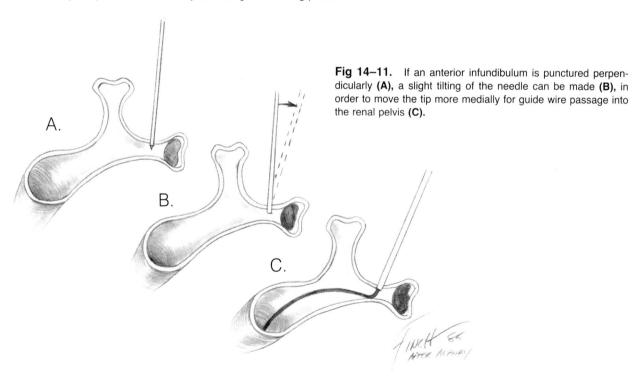

A.

B.

C.

Fig 14–11. If an anterior infundibulum is punctured perpendicularly **(A)**, a slight tilting of the needle can be made **(B)**, in order to move the tip more medially for guide wire passage into the renal pelvis **(C)**.

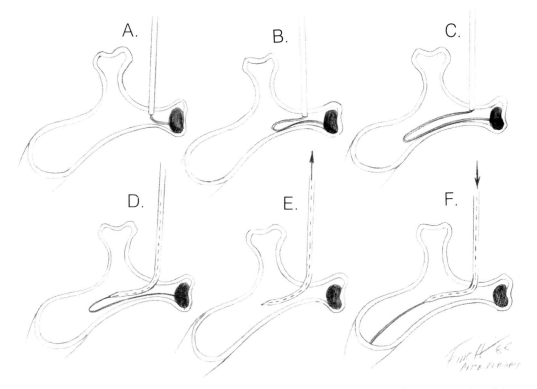

Fig 14–12. An additional technique for passing the guide wire into the ureter is by bouncing a floppy-tipped wire off the stone **(A** and **B)**, looping the wire into the renal pelvis **(C)**, then straightening the loop with a small, curved catheter **(D, E,** and **F).**

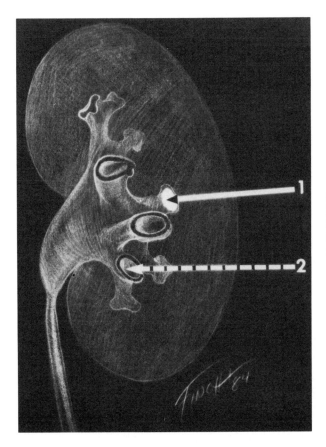

Fig 14–13. Middle-pole anterior calyceal stone. The direct approach (no. 1), or distant approach (no. 2) are again the options available for removal of middle- and upper-pole stones. If the direct approach appears to be difficult, a posterior calyx distant from the stone (to minimize the angulation) should be punctured (no. 2).

hydraulic lithotriptor has a 5 F electrode, which can be passed through the flexible scope but is generally not powerful enough for effective fragmentation. The larger electrodes must somehow be attached to the outside of the scope, which decreases its maneuverability. For smaller stones, upper-pole anterior calyceal stones that can be grasped, either a direct or a distant approach can be used (Fig 14–15). The anatomy and scopes available again dictate the choice. For punctures above the 12th rib, caution must be used not to puncture the lung or adjacent organs, as previously discussed (see Chapter 3). Also, the higher the puncture the more medial it must be, therefore making an anterior infundibular puncture more difficult.

Multiple calyceal stones pose a difficult problem. Depending on their location, the calyceal anatomy and the scopes used, each case may have a different approach (Fig 14–16). Commonly, more than one puncture may be required (Figs 14–17,A and B).

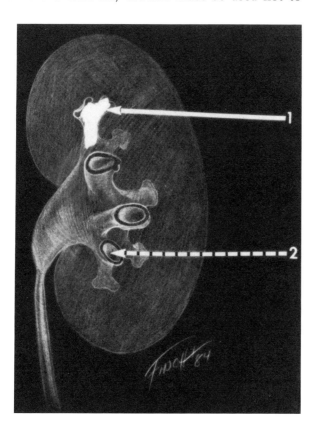

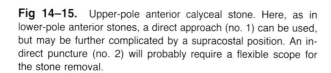

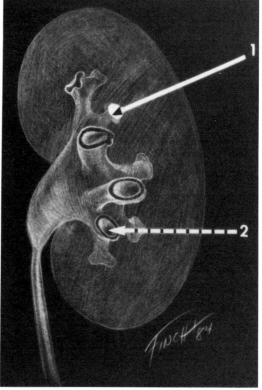

Fig 14–14. Larger upper-pole calyceal stone. The best approach is directly onto the stone for mechanical fragmentation. Fragmentation is difficult to perform with a flexible scope or flexible instrumentation from a remote entrance site such as no. 2.

Fig 14–15. Upper-pole anterior calyceal stone. Here, as in lower-pole anterior stones, a direct approach (no. 1) can be used, but may be further complicated by a supracostal position. An indirect puncture (no. 2) will probably require a flexible scope for the stone removal.

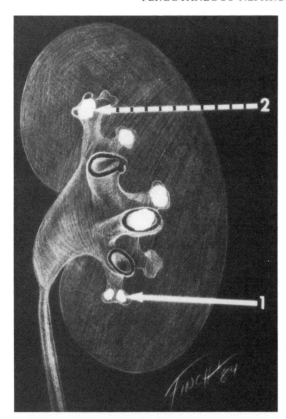

CALYCEAL STONES WITH STENOTIC INFUNDIBULA OR DIVERTICULAR STONES

Generally, the approach is directly onto the stone, since there is little risk of displacing fragments into the renal pelvis because of the small outlet (Fig 14–18). A guide wire is manipulated through the stenotic segment and the infundibulum or infundibular neck is dilated either with a semirigid dilator or balloon catheter. After the stone removal a stent is left in place for an extended period of time. For difficult anteriorly located stones or stones above the 12th rib one can enter the lower-pole calyceal region to dilate or cut the stenotic infundibulum with cautery, and thus gain access to the stone. These stones are difficult to remove and are commonly asymptomatic, in which case we do not remove them.

Fig 14–16. Multiple calyceal stones. For multiple calyceal stones either a lower (no. 1) or upper-pole (no. 2) puncture will provide the best access to all the stones. No. 1 is preferable, avoiding a supracostal puncture.

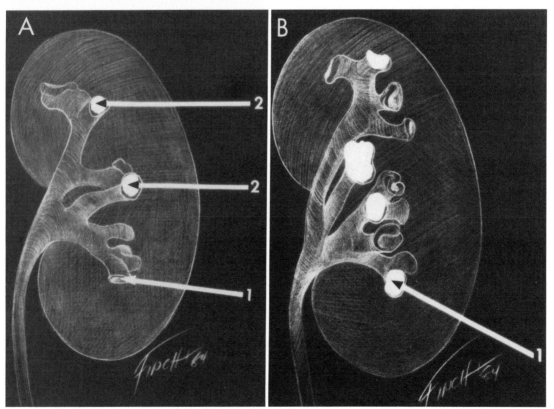

Fig 14–17. **A,** multiple calyceal stones, difficult anatomy. A distant approach (no. 1) will be the most successful in removing both the calyceal stones from a single entrance site. Direct punctures (no. 2) can be utilized but may require punctures through both calyces to remove both stones. **B,** multiple calyceal stones, difficult anatomy. The lower-pole provides the best access to all parts of the kidney. However, one or two more punctures may be needed to remove all of the stones.

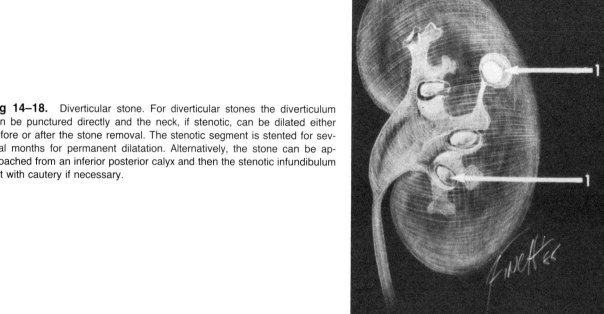

Fig 14–18. Diverticular stone. For diverticular stones the diverticulum can be punctured directly and the neck, if stenotic, can be dilated either before or after the stone removal. The stenotic segment is stented for several months for permanent dilatation. Alternatively, the stone can be approached from an inferior posterior calyx and then the stenotic infundibulum cut with cautery if necessary.

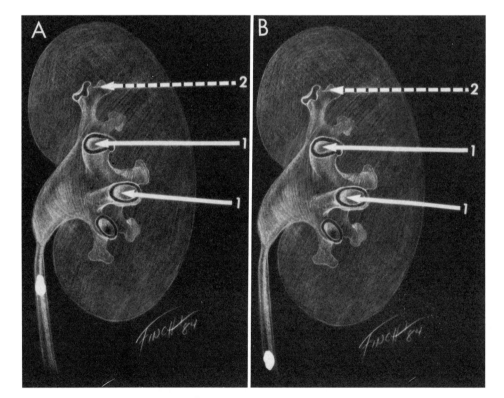

Fig 14–19. Ureteral stones. If using graspers under fluoroscopy or direct vision for a stone extraction in upper **(A)** and middle **(B)** ureteral stones, a high puncture should be made for easiest access to the stone no. 1. No. 2 usually requires a supracostal puncture and may create a problem with limitation of instrument length.

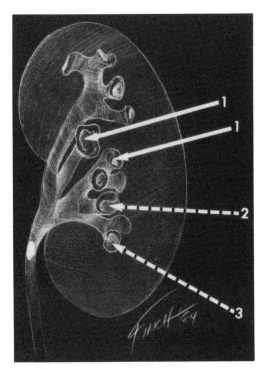

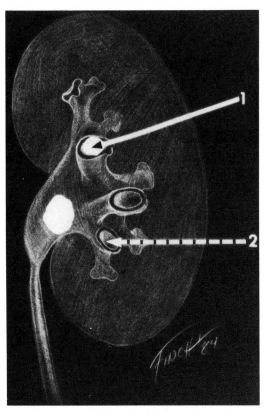

Fig 14–20. Ureteral stone, difficult anatomy. Because of the bifid pelvis and long infundibula either middle-pole posterior calyces (no. 1) provide the best access to the stone. The lower-pole calyces (no. 2 and 3) can be used but the manipulation may be slightly more difficult for the retrieving instrument.

Fig 14–21. Combination stones—upper posterior calyceal and free-floating pelvic stones. The preferred puncture in this case is directly onto the posterior calyceal stone, trapping it, removing the pelvic stone first, then removing the calyceal stone. A distant approach (no. 2) could be used, however the dilation and calyceal stone extraction may be more difficult than with approach no. 1.

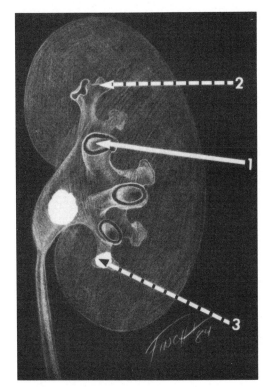

Fig 14–22. Combination stones—lower-pole compound calyceal stone and pelvic stone. Because of the angle between the lower calyx and the ureter, an upper-pole puncture (no. 1 or 2) is preferable, giving easy access to both the stones.

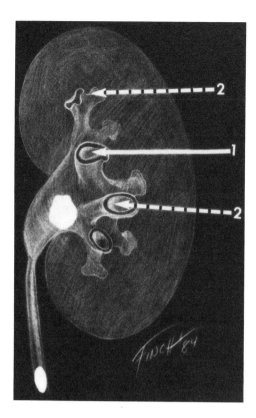

Fig 14–23. Combination stones—free-floating pelvic stone and ureteral stone. A higher puncture (no. 1) is made, giving access to both the ureter and pelvis. No. 2 in the upper pole gives good access; however, it probably will be above the 12th rib and will require long instruments if using graspers and baskets or a flexible scope in the ureter. With no. 2 in the lower pole there is a slight increase in angulation between the calyx and ureter when compared to no. 1.

Fig 14–24. Combination stones—lower-pole anterior calyceal stone and ureteral stone. The mid-upper pole provides the best access to the ureteral stone and the anterior calyceal stone (no. 1). A puncture onto the calyceal stone is difficult as well as subsequent manipulation into the ureter (no. 3).

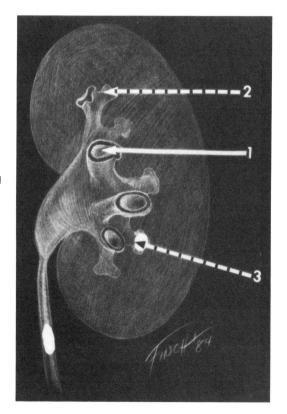

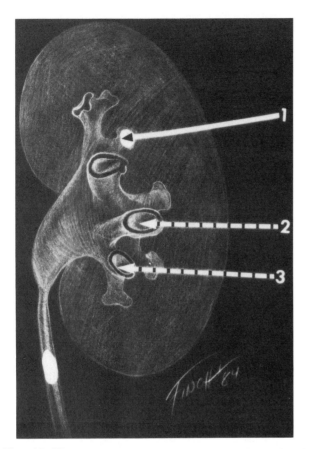

Fig 14–25. Combination stones—upper anterior calyceal stone and ureteral stone. This is a difficult situation. A direct puncture onto the calyceal stone (no. 1) gives the straightest access to the ureter, but is a difficult puncture. Alternatively, a lower posterior calyx can be chosen (no. 2 and 3) using a flexible scope to manipulate into the anterior calyx and ureter, if not using the flushing technique.

URETERAL STONES

For high-lying ureteral stones the classic teaching has been not to approach them from below cystoscopically because of the possibility of avulsion of the ureter. In our opinion, proximal ureteral stones are very difficult to remove and preferably approached from above percutaneously. Originally we used a calyceal puncture as high as possible, either above or below the 12th rib, to obtain the straightest possible access to the ureteropelvic junction or proximal ureter (Figs 14–19 and 14–20). We then used baskets and graspers in combination with a balloon catheter from below for the stone extraction. Our success with these stones was approximately 66%. However, with experience we later developed a flushing technique that has proved to be quite successful (see Chapter 29).

COMBINATION STONES

There is a complex variety of possible combinations of stones. Each must be approached on an individual basis using the same principles as expounded before. Several examples follow (Figs 14–21 to 14–25). Occasionally, more than one puncture may be required.

CHAPTER 15

Percutaneous Nephrolithotomy: Dilation Techniques

Carol C. Coleman, M.D.

The puncture and dilatation of the nephrostomy tract are crucial steps of renal and ureteral stone extraction. The choice of a puncture site can make the stone removal easy or almost impossible. It can minimize complications or lead to significant bleeding requiring embolization, to colonic perforation, or to hydrothorax formation. Dilation of the tract can be smooth and simple. However, perforation of the renal pelvis with subsequent extravasation, dislodgment of the guide wire leading to loss of the tract, or significant bleeding can occur. Therefore it is essential to know where and how to puncture safely and to know what equipment is available for dilation, how to use it, and when to use it.

ANESTHESIA AND INITIAL DILATION OF THE TRACT

Most of our patients' stone removals are performed with local anesthesia and intravenous narcotics (morphine sulfate and butorphanol tartrate) and sedation. Epidural anesthesia, if well administered, is extremely effective and is becoming more popular. General anesthesia is reserved for potentially difficult cases, such as patients with severe scarring or extreme anxiety and for drug abusers.

After the renal collecting system has been punctured with an 18-gauge needle a 0.035-in. Bentson taper (Cook Inc., Bloomington, Ind.) floppy-tipped guide wire is placed through the cannula. In most cases the guide wire is passed into the distal ureter. This increases the ease and safety of the dilation. The dilators will follow the smooth curve of the wire away from the renal pelvic wall avoiding perforation. In the case with the wire coiled in the renal pelvis, the dilators point perpendicular to the renal pelvis, increasing the chance of perforation (Fig 15–1). If it is impossible to pass the guide wire into the ureter initially the tract can be dilated to an 8 F size, then a curved-tip catheter can be introduced for redirection of the guide wire into the ureter (Fig 15–2). If a ureteral stone is to be extracted the guide wire needs to be coiled in the upper or lower pole of the kidney (Fig 15–3) to avoid spasm and edema of the ureter from the dilation manipulations.

The tract is then further anesthetized from the renal capsule to the skin either through a Chiba needle inserted beside the guide wire or through the original 18-gauge needle with the aid of a Tuohy-Borst side-arm adaptor (Medi-Tech, Watertown, Mass.) (Fig 15–4). If a "skinny" needle is used, fluoroscopic observation of the needle is mandatory because the thin needle may markedly deviate from the tract. For a one-step puncture-di-

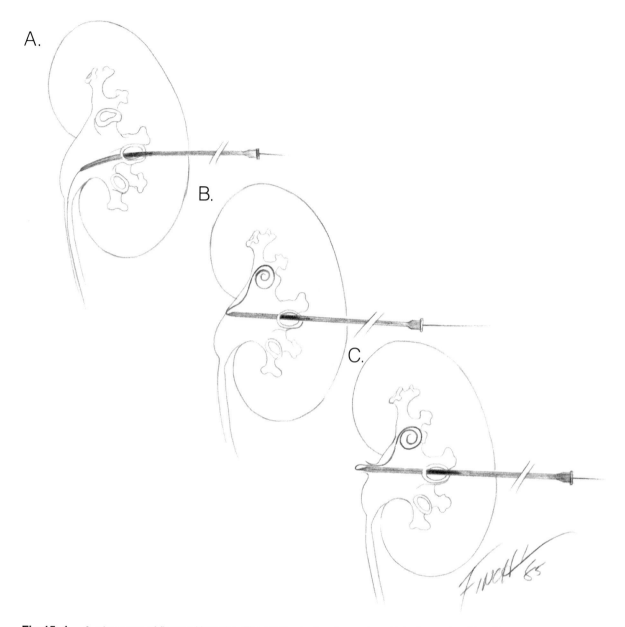

Fig 15–1. **A,** placement of first working wire. The guide wire has been placed into the ureter. The dilator passes easily over the wire curving away from the renal pelvis. **B,** the guide wire in this case is coiled in the upper pole. In this situation the dilators tend not to follow the wire through its acute angulation into the upper pole. Rather, the dilator points perpendicular to the renal pelvis, oftentimes kinking the wire. **C,** because of the kinked wire, the dilator does not easily pass over that segment of wire; therefore, if the dilator is advanced too far into the collecting system the dilator and wire tend to perforate the renal pelvis.

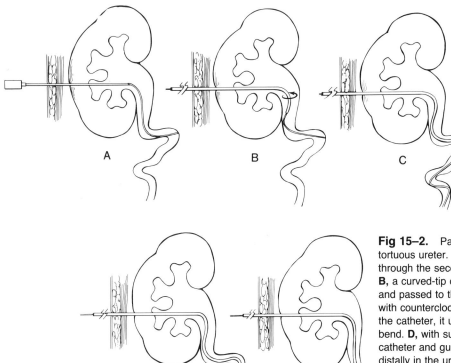

Fig 15–2. Passage of ureteral wire in a tortuous ureter. **A,** the guide wire will not pass through the second bend of the tortuous ureter. **B,** a curved-tip catheter is placed over the guide and passed to the first curve of the ureter. **C,** with counterclockwise or clockwise rotation of the catheter, it usually will advance into the next bend. **D,** with successive manipulations, the catheter and guide wire are advanced further distally in the ureter. **E,** finally, unless encased with tumor or fibrosis, the ureter will straighten, making subsequent placement of catheters and wires easier.

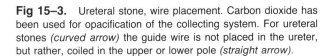

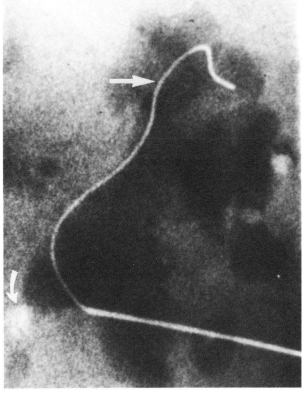

Fig 15–3. Ureteral stone, wire placement. Carbon dioxide has been used for opacification of the collecting system. For ureteral stones *(curved arrow)* the guide wire is not placed in the ureter, but rather, coiled in the upper or lower pole *(straight arrow)*.

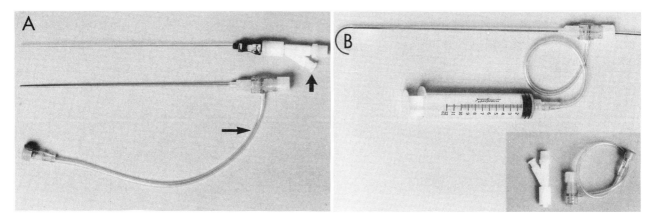

Fig 15–4. **A,** Tuohy-Borst adaptor with a long side-arm for injection *(long arrow).* Plastic side-arm fitting (Cook Inc., Bloomington, Ind.) with a short side-arm *(short arrow).* **B,** the guide wire has been placed through the diaphragm of the adaptor and 18-gauge needle. The local anesthetic can be injected through the side port around the guide wire into the tract.

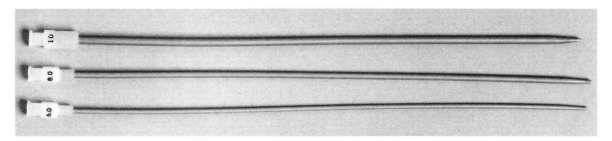

Fig 15–5. Initial dilation: 6, 8, and 10 F dilators can be used for the early tract dilatation before the balloon or semirigid dilators are used.

latation stone extraction procedure, 20 to 30 ml of 1% lidocaine without epinephrine is used.

The tract is enlarged with 6, 8, and 10 F dilators (Fig 15–5). At this time if it previously was not possible to pass the guide wire into the ureter a 7 F curved tipped catheter is passed over the wire and manipulated into the ureter.

When the initial working guide wire is a Bentson taper, care must be taken to assure the distal 10 cm is in the collecting system. Attempts to pass dilators over the floppy segment outside of the kidney often will result in kinking.

If during the dilation the wire kinks, it must be replaced, for subsequent catheter advancement will be impeded and buckling may occur. Once buckling occurs the dilatation becomes fraught with persistent buckling and failure of dilation. If during this process the guide wire within the kidney gradually backs out and there is danger of losing the wire and the tract, a 5 F catheter can be passed over the remaining wire and advanced into the collecting system. Then the guide can be exchanged and a long segment of wire repositioned in the ureter. If the 5 F catheter cannot be ad-

vanced, a small, 4 or 5 F, Teflon (stiff) dilator generally can then be passed over the guide wire into the calyx (Fig 15–6). If the initial dilation is difficult because of scarring or tough fascial layers, the new working wire should have a .038-in. diameter.

Recently a new wire has been introduced, the Amplatz stiffener wire (Cook Inc., Bloomington, Ind.), which comes in a .038- or .035-in. diameter. The wire has a floppy distal tip; however, it is quite stiff proximally, therefore enhancing the ease of dilation. The wire is particularly useful in preventing or overcoming buckling. Others have used a movable-core guide with relatively good success.

THE SAFETY GUIDE WIRE

The introduction of a second guide wire is extremely important. A second wire that will become the new working wire (.038-in.) is always placed, generally before final tract dilation is performed. The original wire (.035-in.) becomes the

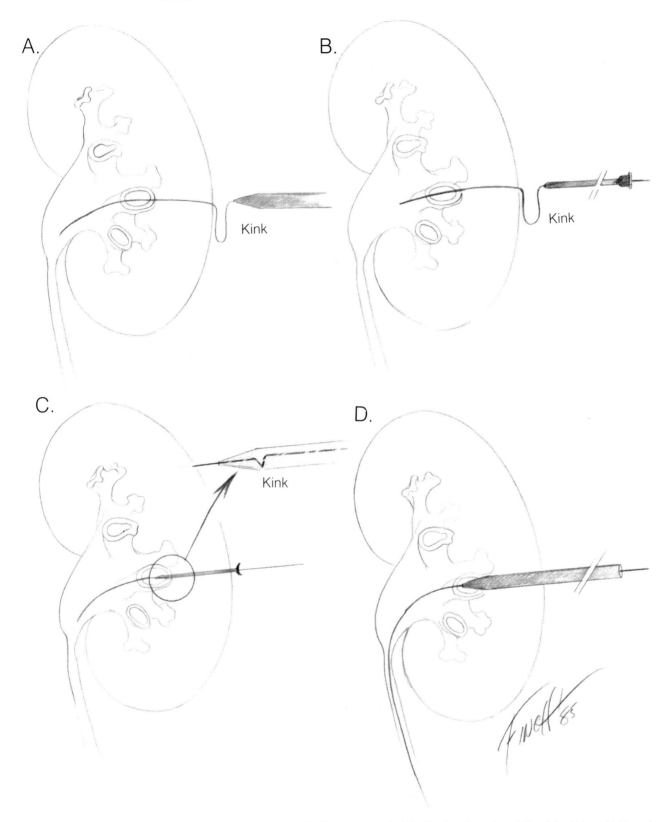

Fig 15–6. If the guide wire is too thin for the dilation or the floppy segment of the Bentson taper is outside of the kidney, kinking of the guide can occur **(A).** If kinking occurs, the wire must be exchanged, otherwise buckling of the catheter and loss of the guide wire may occur. If there is only a short segment of working wire left within the kidney, a 5 F catheter can be manipulated over the wire **(B).** If this fails, a stiff Teflon dilator, 4 or 5 F **(C),** can be advanced into the collecting system over the kink. Then a new guide wire can be placed with its distal end far into the ureter and dilation completed **(D).**

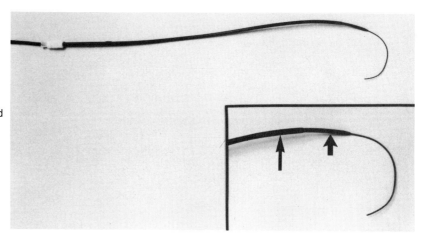

Fig 15–7. From the Amplatz renal dilator set: the 8 F working catheter *(short arrow)* and 10 F two-wire introducer *(long arrow)* are coaxially mounted over a guide wire.

safety guide wire in case the working wire is accidentally pulled out or if the Teflon sheath must be removed with the stone during extraction. This second wire can be inserted through an 8.5 F thin-walled Formocath (Becton Dickinson, Rutherford, N.J.) placed over the first working wire, or through a Safetywire introducer (Cook Urological-VPI, Spencer, Ind.) or through the 10 F sheath included in the Amplatz renal dilator set (Cook Inc., Bloomington, Ind.) (Figs 15–7 to 15–9). By far the most rapid and least expensive technique is the Amplatz double-wire introducer (Cook Inc.,

Bloomington, Ind.) which also serves as a dilator system. The 6, 8, and 10 F vascular dilators are no longer needed and the second guide wire is introduced in one step. The system consists of a 6 F inner Teflon catheter and a coaxial long, tapered 6 to 12 F dilator (Fig 15–10,A). The tract is dilated in one step to a 12 F size, the 6 F catheter is removed and the second guide is introduced through the 6 to 12 F dilator (Fig 15–10,B). A 5 F catheter is placed over the safety wire and sutured to the skin (Fig 15–11). It is not sufficient to suture the guide wire to the skin as a Teflon-coated wire can easily slip through the suture.

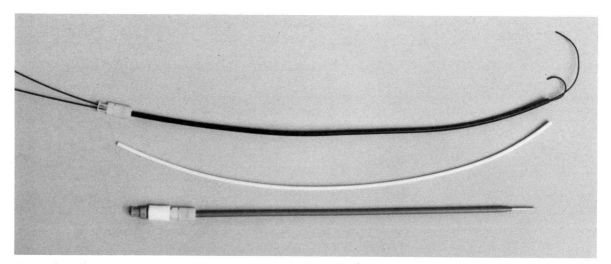

Fig 15–8. Two wire introducers. The 10 F, two-wire introducer from the Amplatz renal dilator set with two wires passed through its lumen *(top).* An 8.5 F, thin-wall Formocath will accept two .038-in. wires *(center).* Two-wire introducer set from Cook Urological *(bottom).*

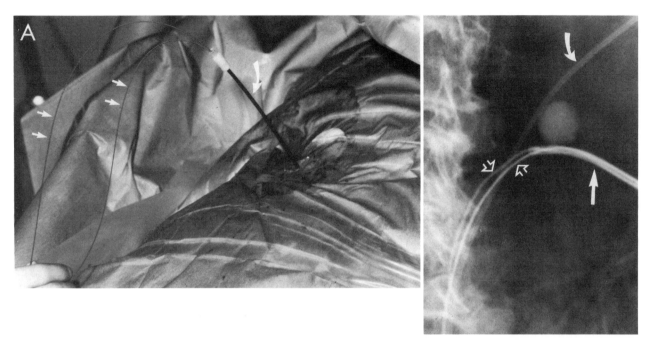

Fig 15–9. **A,** 10 F two-wire introducer sheath from the Amplatz renal dilator set *(curved arrow)*. Two wires have been placed into the kidney *(straight arrows)*. **B,** fluoroscopic view of the two-wire introducer *(straight arrow)* and two wires *(open arrows)* in the ureter. Curved arrow points to the ureteral catheter.

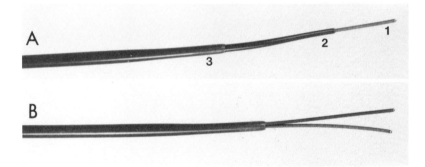

Fig 15–10. Amplatz double-wire introducer set. **A,** (1) Amplatz stiffener guide wire; (2) 6 F Teflon dilator; and (3) 6 to 12 F long tapered coaxial Teflon dilator. **B,** 6 F Teflon dilator has been removed and a second guide wire has been introduced through the 6 to 12 F long tapered dilator. Thus, the second wire can be introduced in one step.

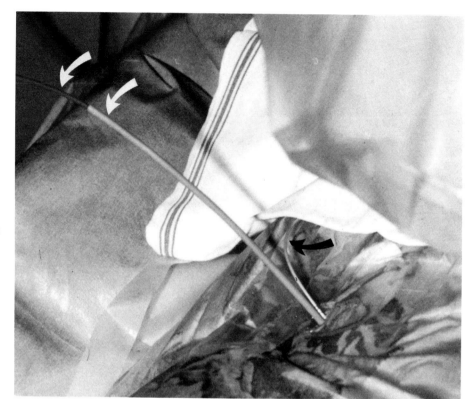

Fig 15–11. The safety guide wire has been covered with a 5 F catheter and sutured to the skin *(black arrow)*. Dilation is in progress with the 12 F coaxial dilator over the 8 F Teflon working catheter *(white arrows)*.

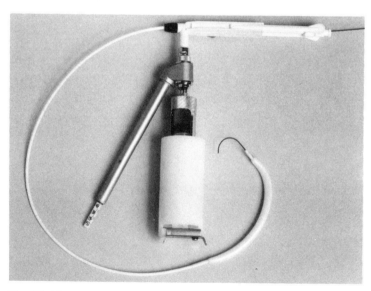

Fig 15–12. Inflated balloon catheter with a pressure gauge and Amplatz inflation device (Cook Inc., Bloomington, Ind.). The helix facilitates inflations to high pressures.

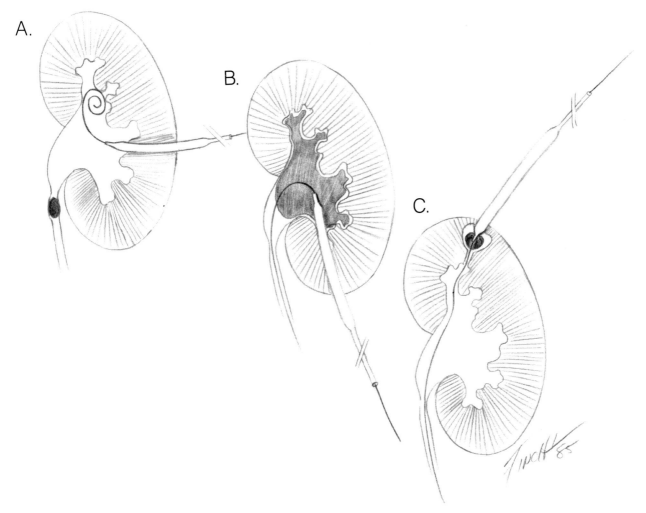

Fig 5–13. Balloon catheter, special uses. **A,** for ureteral stones, in which case the guide wire is not placed in the ureter but rather is curled in the renal pelvis or an infundibulum, the balloon catheter follows the wire easily without potential for perforation, which can occur with rigid dilators. **B,** staghorn calculi can occupy the majority of the space of the renal collecting system. The balloon catheter is easier to manipulate in this reduced area than are the large semirigid dilators. **C,** for diverticular stones, in which case, again, the space for equipment manipulation is limited, the balloon catheter is the easiest dilating system to use.

DILATION WITH BALLOON CATHETERS

The principal advantages of dilating a tract with the balloon catheter are speed and reduced trauma to the tissues and, therefore, less bleeding and reduced pain for the patient (Fig 15–12). The balloon catheter is also easier to use in curved tracts as with lower-pole punctures, and anterior calyceal punctures. It is also particularly useful in situations where there is little room for instrumentation as in staghorn and diverticula calculi (Fig 15–13). Depending on the length of the tract, one or two balloon inflations will enlarge the entire tract to a 30 F (10-mm balloon) size if desired. The principal disadvantage of the technique is cost. The balloon catheters are expensive and generally cannot be reused. There are some that are reusable, but are limited in the number of times they can be utilized. Also there are occasional failures caused by tenacious fascia or scarring from previous surgery.

Equipment

In patients who have not had previous renal surgery, pressures of 4 to 5 atmospheres usually are enough to dilate a nephrostomy tract. However, in patients who have had surgery much higher pres-

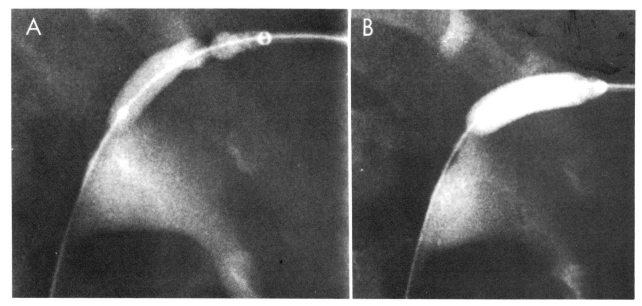

Fig 15–14. Balloon catheter in a nephrostomy tract. **A,** the "waist" indicates incomplete dilatation. **B,** with increasing pressure and time, resolution of the waist indicates successful dilatation.

sures may be needed for dilation. The Olbert balloon catheter (Surgimed, Oakland, N.J.), the Cook Enforcer (Cook Inc., Bloomington, Ind.), the PE Plus (U.S.C.I., Billerica, Mass.), the Tract Master balloon dilation catheter (Medi-Tech, Watertown, Mass.), and the Diaflex nephrostomy dilatation catheter (American Edwards, Ervine, Calif.) take higher pressures, 12, 10, 15, 15, and 17 atmospheres, respectively, and are usually used for nephrostomy tract dilatation. A 10- to 12-cm balloon is used as it can dilate all or most of the tract from a single placement.

Technique

The nephrostomy tract needs to be predilated to a 10 to 12 F size before a balloon catheter will eas-ily pass over the working wire. After the second wire has been placed, the skin incision is enlarged to 1.0 to 1.5 cm and the subcutaneous tissues spread with a curved clamp.

The balloon catheter is then advanced until the most distal radiopaque marker is seen fluoroscopically inside the collecting system. The balloon is inflated with a 30% solution of contrast medium either with the help of an inflation device or with a 5-cc syringe, if the former is not available. As the balloon is inflated, a "waist" will appear when it passes through the renal capsule, posterior renal fascia, or lumbodorsal fascia (Fig 15–14,A). As the pressure is increased the waist disappears usually within one minute (Fig 15–14,B). If necessary, the balloon can be pulled back to dilate the remainder of the tract.

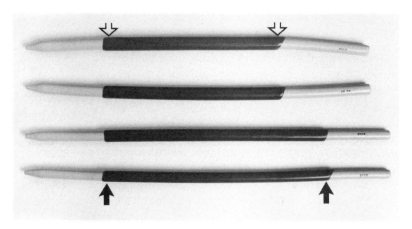

Fig 15–15. Amplatz dilators, 24, 26, 28, and 30 F, with their Teflon sheaths. The sets come with short, 15-cm *(open arrows)* or long, 19-cm *(closed arrows)* sheaths.

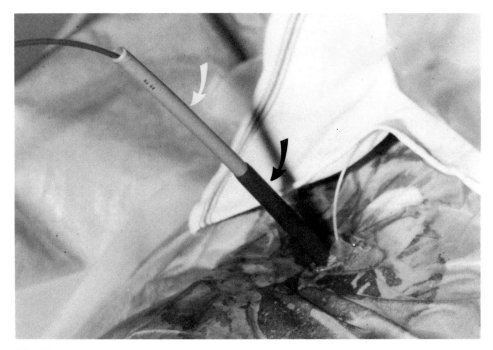

Fig 15–16. The 28 F dilator *(white arrow)* and its Teflon sheath *(black arrow)* have been placed into the kidney.

The balloon is withdrawn and a 26 F or 28 F Amplatz renal dilator with a snugly fitted Teflon sheath (Figs 15–15 and 15–16) are advanced over their 8 F guiding catheter and working guide wire until the tip of the sheath is seen to lie within the collecting system (Fig 15–17). The dilator, guiding catheter, and working wire are then removed, leaving the Teflon sheath in place beside the safety wire for instrument passage or flushing (Fig 15–18). There are new backloading systems in which either a 30 F sheath is backloaded on a balloon catheter and is passed over the inflated bal-

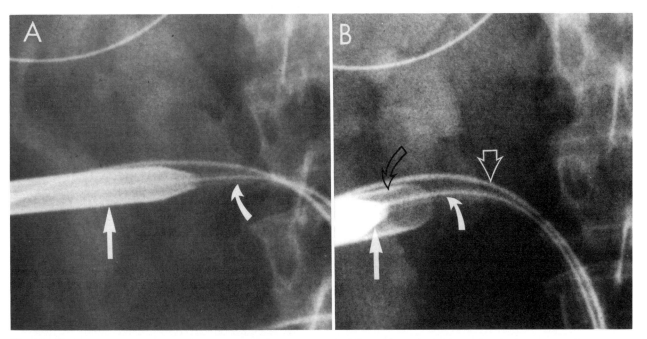

Fig 15–17. **A,** fluoroscopic image of the dilator *(straight arrow)* and guiding catheter *(curved arrow)* in the renal pelvis. **B,** the Teflon sheath *(open black arrow)* has been placed. The dilator *(straight arrow)* is being withdrawn over the 8 F catheter *(curved arrow)*. The safety wire *(open white arrow)* is adjacent to the working wire.

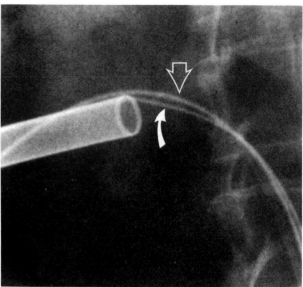

Fig 15–18. The dilator and 8 F catheter have been removed. The sheath, working wire *(curved arrow)* and safety wire *(open arrow)* remain in place.

loon or a dilator and 30 F sheath are backloaded on the balloon catheter and passed over the deflated balloon and the tract. This can shorten the dilation process by one step.

If large tracts are required, as for the removal of a 1-cm stone, the 30 F Amplatz renal dilator and sheath can be placed. Otherwise if an ultrasonic lithotriptor is to be used a 26 F sheath is needed for the Wolf lithotriptor and a 28 F sheath is needed for the Storz lithotriptor.

SEMIRIGID DILATORS

The semirigid coaxial dilators should be used in the patient with a previous history of renal surgery and in cases where the balloon has failed. The coaxial dilators exert more force than bal-

loons and are excellent for tough fascial layers and scarring. The main disadvantage is increased trauma to the tissue, which may produce pain if the local anesthesia is imperfect. There can also be more bleeding, which can interfere with the stone removal.

Equipment

There are several semirigid systems available, the VPI fascial dilators (Cook Urological-VPI, Spencer, Ind.) (Fig 15–19) and the Amplatz renal dilators (Cook Inc., Bloomington, Ind.) (Fig 15–20), which are a modification of a previously described dilating system,[1] and dilating systems produced by other companies copying the Amplatz set. The VPI fascial dilators can be used with their irrigation nephrostomy cannula (Figs 15–21 and 15–22).

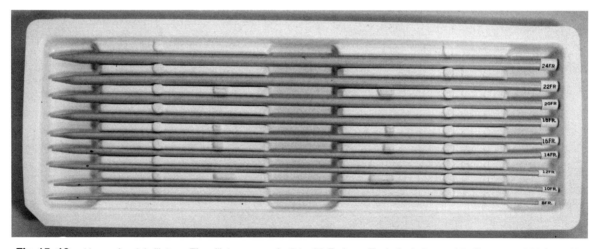

Fig 15–19. Vance fascial dilators. The dilators come in 8 to 24 F sizes. Each tip is tapered to fit over a .038-in. guide wire.

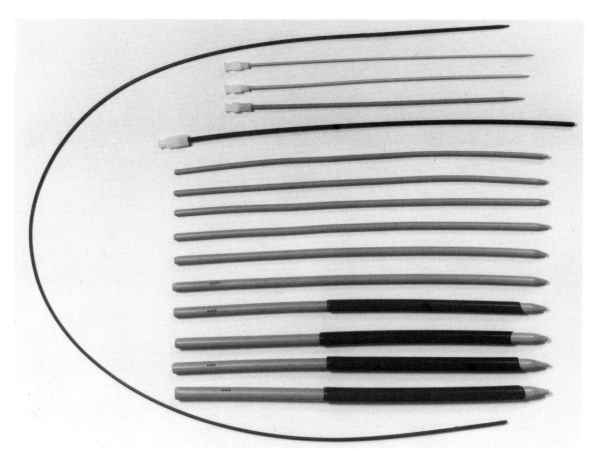

Fig 15–20. Amplatz renal dilators. The set includes 6, 8, and 10 F initial dilators, a 10 F two-wire introducer, an 8 F working catheter, 12 to 30 F coaxial dilators, and Teflon sheaths to fit the 24, 26, 28, and 30 F dilators.

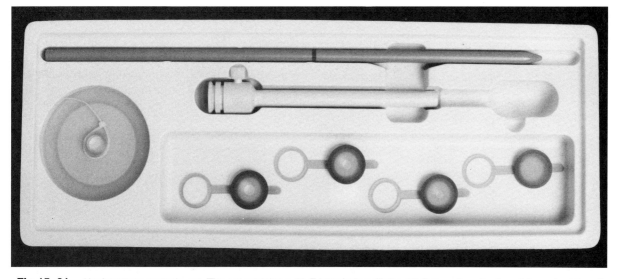

Fig 15–21. Nephrostomy cannula set. The set contains a 28 F introducing dilator, 34 F cannula, retention disk, and septas of 16, 20, and 24 F sizes made to accept various types of scopes and one solid septum.

Cook Urological also produces a Rutner nephroscopy adaptor set (Fig 15–23). Both the cannula and nephroscopy adaptor can be used to maintain a dry field.

Technique

The VPI fascial dilators range in size from 8 to 24 F. Larger dilators up to 36 F are available. Each tapers to fit snugly around an 0.038-in. guide wire. Holding the wire taut, each is passed sequentially with a twisting motion over the wire into the intrarenal collecting system. The disadvantage of this system is that the dilators do not pass easily over the wire that makes a curved path. This can cause kinking of the wire, usually in the renal pelvis. When this occurs the tip of the dilator can easily perforate the renal pelvis (Fig 15–24). The plastic cannula with a side port for suction can be introduced over a 28 F dilator for endoscopic manipulations. Suction applied through the side port helps maintain a dry field.

When the Amplatz renal dilators are used, the 8 F guiding Teflon dilator is advanced over the working wire into the ureter, where it remains throughout the dilation procedure. Progressively larger dilators are coaxially introduced over the 8 F catheter from a 10 F size up to a 30 F size, if needed. The dilators are advanced slowly with a rotating motion to facilitate dilation and decrease trauma to the tissues, until the tip enters the collecting system. The advantage of this system over the VPI fascial dilators is that the 8 F working catheter is larger and stiffer than an isolated wire and is, therefore, less prone to buckling, and the larger coaxial catheters pass easier through a curved course (Fig 15–25). The dilators are supplied with snugly fitting radiopaque Teflon sheaths from sizes 24 to 30 F, which are useful for the introduction of rigid scopes and are used for aspiration and flushing removal techniques. The nephrostomy tract is dilated to 2 F sizes larger than needed, e.g., 30 F if a 28 F Teflon sheath is

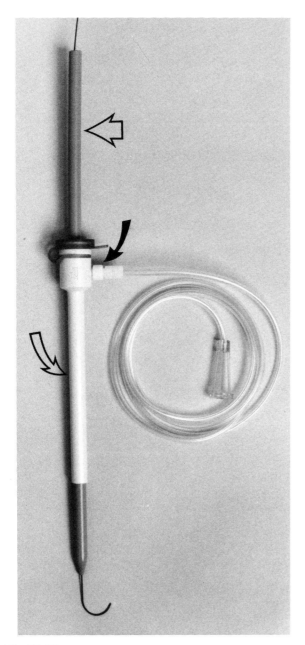

Fig 15–22. The 34 F cannula *(open curved arrow)* fits snugly over the 28 F introducing dilator *(open straight arrow)*. The side port *(curved closed arrow)* allows for drainage of the irrigation fluid, maintaining a relatively dry field.

Fig 15–24. Fascial dilators. These dilators do not follow the course of the curved guide wire easily and may kink the wire **(A)**. Then, as the dilator is advanced it continues in a straight line pushing against the pelvic wall **(B)**. If this is not recognized, the dilator and wire will perforate the renal pelvic wall **(C)**.

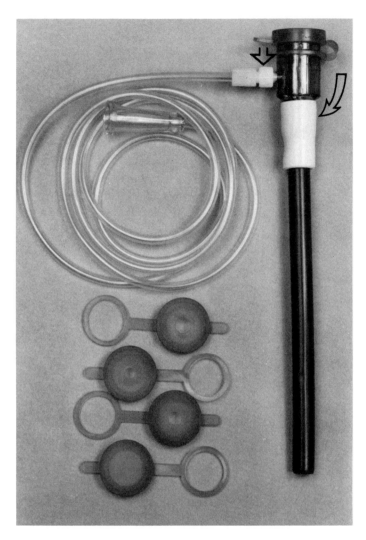

Fig 15–23. Rutner nephroscopy adaptor. The connecting sleeve *(curved arrow)* comes in two sizes, one to fit over the 24 and 26 F Teflon sheaths and one to fit over the 28 and 30 F Teflon sheaths. The side port *(straight arrow)* allows for the egress of irrigation fluid from the kidney through the tubing in order to keep a dry field. There are three septas (16, 20, and 24 F sizes) used for the passage of different sized cystoscopes, and one solid septum.

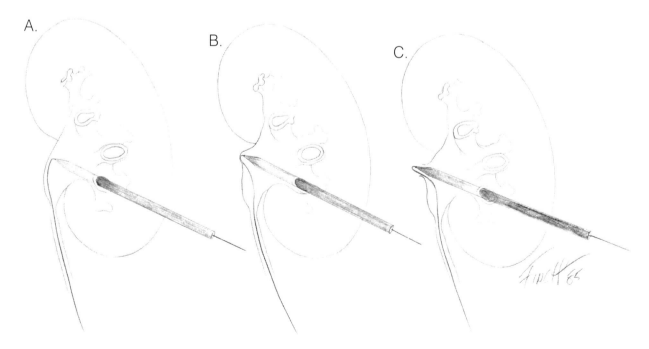

Fig 15–25. Amplatz renal dilator. Because of the added stiffness and thickness of the 8 F working Teflon catheter, the large dilators traverse the curve of the wire and catheter into the ureter easier than with an isolated wire and dilator. Perforation is less likely with this system.

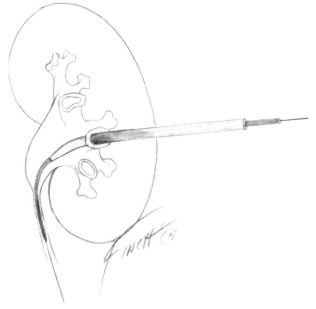

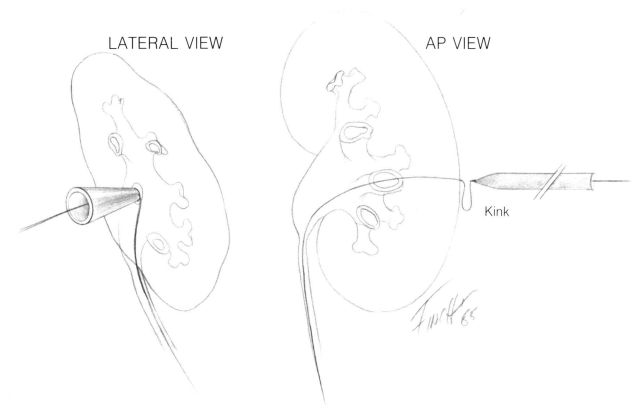

LATERAL VIEW   AP VIEW

Kink

Fig 15–26. Oblique fluoroscopy to demonstrate the full length of the dilators and working wire. **A,** lateral view: the dilator is foreshortened, the exact relationship of the dilator, wire, and kidney are not known. **B,** anteroposterior view: the wire is actually kinked and is covered by the shaft of the dilator in this view.

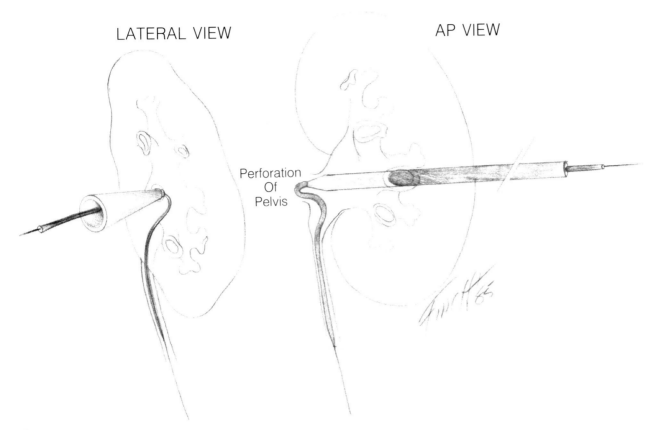

Fig 15–27. **A,** lateral view: again, the shaft of the dilator is foreshortened and the depth of the dilator is unknown. **B,** anteroposterior view: dilator, guiding catheter, and wire have actually perforated the renal pelvis, but could not be seen on the en face view.

to be used. The larger tract makes it easier to place the working Teflon sheath.

The dilation should be monitored fluoroscopically to assure proper placement of the dilators into the collecting system, and to prevent excessive advancement of the dilator with subsequent perforation. Oblique fluoroscopy, perpendicular to the dilators and guide wire is needed in order to see their entire length. The exact depth of the dilator is then known and any possible kinking, buckling, or perforation is not covered up by the catheter shafts (Figs 15–26 and 15–27).

The Teflon sheath has a blunt and a beveled end. If flushing techniques are to be used for stone removal the beveled end of the sheath is used. The purpose of the beveled tip is to allow orientation of the Teflon sheath toward the stone for flushing and aspiration. For instruments used inside the kidney the blunt end is introduced, as the beveled edge may interfere with the endoscopic vision.

The advantage of using the Teflon sheath instead of the cystoscopic sheath is that it remains in the tract at all times, thus affording tamponade to any bleeding vessels in the tract and preventing large amounts of irrigation fluid from dissecting into the retroperitoneum. It also allows for multiple passes of the cystoscope without replacing the working sheath into the tract each time. For drainage tube placement, the catheter can be easily passed through the sheath into the collecting system. Tube placement can be otherwise difficult through a fresh tract. The Teflon sleeve can be simply removed over the drainage tube or cut off if using a Foley-type catheter.

RIGID DILATORS

Metal coaxial dilators (Karl-Storz, Culver City, Calif.) are used chiefly for dilating scarred or otherwise fibrotic tissue. We avoid using these dilators despite their effectiveness because of the ease with which they can perforate the renal pelvis.

Equipment

The metal dilator set is composed of a long, 8 F dilator and 12, 15, 18, 21, 24, and 27 F shorter coaxial dilators. They are designed so that each di-

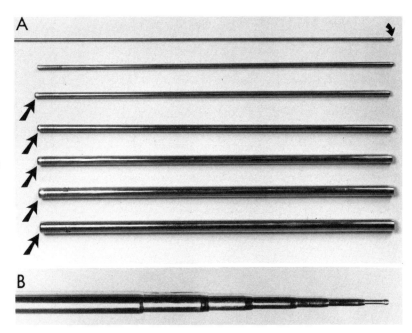

Fig 15–28. **A,** metal coaxial dilators. Dilators come in sizes 8, 12, 15, 18, 21, 24, and 27 F. At the distal end of the long 8 F dilator is a metal bead *(curved arrow).* This prevents the forward motion of the 12 F dilator, which is tapered to 8 F at its distal end. The proximal ends of the 15, 18, 21, 24, and 27 F dilators are tapered *(straight arrows)* to prevent forward motion of their tips beyond the next smaller dilator tip. **B,** metal dilators coaxially mounted, one on the other. They are very rigid and good for dilating tough scars. However, because of their rigidity they also have the potential to easily perforate the renal pelvis.

lator passes only to the tip of the 8 F dilator (Fig 15–28) and not beyond.

Technique

An 8 F metal cannula is first passed over the working guide wire. It has a stop at its distal end to control the forward motion of the next larger dilator (12 F). Each dilator then is successively passed one over the other until the 27 F size is reached. The proximal ends of the 15, 18, 21, 24, and 27 F sizes are tapered to prevent the larger dilator tip from passing beyond the next smaller dilator tip. It is important to pass each dilator sequentially. If one dilator is missed, trauma and tearing of the tissues will occur and the dilator will pass beyond the tip of the previous dilator and can perforate the pelvis. Over the 24 F metal dilator, the sheath of the ultrasonic lithotriptor or the Amplatz renal dilator can be inserted.

DISCUSSION

Other methods of using existing equipment to dilate nephrostomy tracts have been described. For example, Mazzeo et al.[2] used exchanges of progressively larger Foley catheters, but this method required days or even weeks. Modified filiform catheters and followers have also been used.[3, 4] At first we used dilation methods requiring a few days. This was before the advent of the Teflon sheath, which compresses the tract and conse-

quently minimizes bleeding. Previously, procedures were only performed through so-called mature tracts (fibrin-covered), which took four to five days. However, we found that the tracts could be dilated immediately to larger sizes for stone removal or other procedures without increasing the frequency of complications.[1, 4, 5] This method creates a considerable savings in time, money, and duration of hospitalization. Balloon dilation is particularly suitable for the single-step stone removal, as it causes less bleeding and is more comfortable for the patient than the semirigid and rigid coaxial dilators. However, in each case the techniques must be chosen in light of the medical history and the patient's anatomy and pain tolerance level.

REFERENCES

1. Rusnak B.W., Castaneda-Zuniga W.R., Kotula F., et al.: Improved dilator system for percutaneous nephrostomies. *Radiology* 144:174, 1982.
2. Mazzeo V.P., Pollack H.M., Banner M.P.: Techniques for percutaneous dilatation of nephrostomy tracts. *Radiology* 144:175–176, 1982.
3. Ware S.: Dilatation of percutaneous nephrostomy tracts. *Urology* 19:311, 1982.
4. Clayman R.V., Castaneda-Zuniga W.R., Hunter D.W., et al.: Rapid balloon dilatation of the nephrostomy track for nephrostolithotomy. *Radiology* 147:884–885, 1983.
5. Coleman C.C., Kimura Y., Castaneda-Zuniga W.R., et al.: Dilatation of nephrostomy tracts for percutaneous renal stone removal. *Semin. Interventional Radiol.* 1:50–55, 1984.

CHAPTER 16

Percutaneous Nephrolithotomy: Special Puncture Techniques

Antony T. Young, M.D.

A high success rate for the percutaneous extraction of upper urinary tract calculi requires an aggressive but thoughtful approach from the radiologist. Choosing the optimal entry point into the collecting system and then planning a safe access to this site are two of the most important yet frequently neglected aspects of this challenging field. Failure at this planning stage may prejudice the entire procedure and necessitate a new nephrostomy placement.

Most renal stones can be removed using a single-access tract below the 12th rib. However, in certain situations, such as the presence of multiple calculi, a large staghorn calculus, or where there is unfavorable anatomy of the pelvicalyceal system, special puncture techniques are required. These techniques are discussed in this chapter.

INTERCOSTAL NEPHROSTOMY PUNCTURE

Nephrostomy punctures above the 12th rib remain controversial, yet many protagonists of the technique consider it an invaluable addition to the arsenal of the interventionist. If all stones of all comers are to be amenable to percutaneous extraction, then the use of this access route is mandatory for some stones (Fig 16–1) and preferable in others. Complications have been infrequent, and no death has been reported to date.

Indications

Intercostal punctures (through the 11th, and, rarely, the 10th intercostal space) provide access to those calyces that lie above the 12th rib.

During quiet respiration, the upper-pole calyces of most kidneys lie above the lower costal margin. Sometimes the middle- and, rarely, the lower-pole calyces do likewise. Such calyces may often be approached from below the 12th rib by cephalad angulation of the nephrostomy needle. However, this is at the expense of a longer tract, and may create a difficult angle for the passage of instruments from the working sheath, which points cephalad, down to the renal pelvis, lower-pole calyx, or ureter. For a solitary calyceal stone, this is not necessarily a major factor, but when there are multiple stones, or when access to the pelvis or ureter is required, such an approach may be prohibitive.

A direct intercostal puncture obviates the cephalad angulation, and therefore traces a path more along the long axis of the kidney. This leads to an acceptable obtuse angle into the renal pelvis and ureter (Fig 16–2).

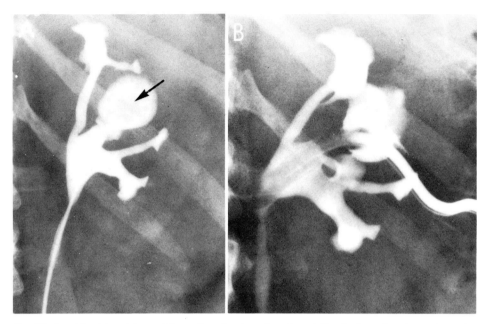

Fig 16–1. Mandatory intercostal puncture for stone in calyceal diverticulum. **A,** retrograde pyelo-gram reveals stone *(arrow)* in upper-pole calyceal diverticulum, overlying the 11th rib. **B,** following stone removal, a nephrostogram through the large-bore nephrostomy tube demonstrates the inter-costal approach. The catheter stents the narrow "neck" of the diverticulum.

Anatomy

The posterior aspect of the diaphragm attaches to the distal ends of the 11th and 12th ribs. Between the end of the 12th rib and the spine, it attaches to the muscles of the posterior abdominal wall at the lateral and medial arcuate ligaments. The diaphragm is therefore traversed by all intercostal nephrostomy punctures, and possibly by some punctures beneath the 12th rib.

The inferior extent of the posterior pleural recess is known to be variable (Fig 16–3). However, it is likely that most intercostal punctures traverse the pleurae. Intercostal punctures to the lower pole of the kidney have been found to be associated with fewer pleural complications than those to the upper pole. This suggests that the pleural cavity does not extend so far down when the entire kidney is positioned high up beneath the ribs. Fusion of pleural surfaces, with partial obliteration of the posterior recess, has been postulated in explanation (Fig 16–4).

The position of the inferior lung edge varies with the phase of respiration, body habitus, and the presence of disease states such as emphysema. However, healthy persons are able to inflate their lungs on deep inspiration so that the posterior pleural recess is totally filled. Intercostal punctures, therefore, have the potential for piercing the lung.

Technique

The general technique is the same as the standard technique outlined previously. However, certain precautions must be observed.

1. The position of the inferior lung edge must be visualized during the puncture, to avoid violation by the needle. The only practical way of achieving this is by fluoroscopy tangential to the needle. This requires a C-arm, or biplane fluoroscopy. It is recommended that the puncture be made during steady, quiet breathing or suspended breathing in expiration (Fig 16–5).

2. The needle is passed through the lower half of the intercostal space to avoid laceration of the intercostal vessels above. The rib below is also avoided to minimize irritation of the periosteum by the subsequent percutaneous nephrostomy tube (Fig 16–6).

3. Particular care should be taken not to make the skin puncture site too lateral. The maximum lateral angulation should be no more than 30 de-

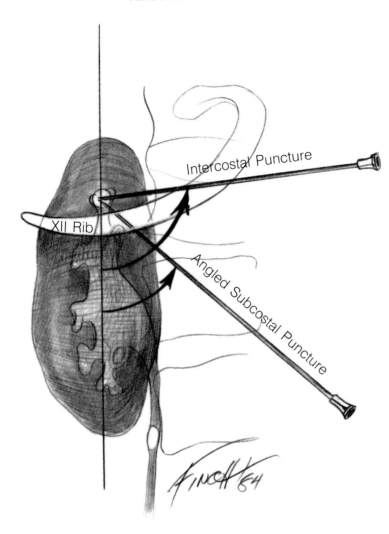

Fig 16–2. Advantage of intercostal puncture. Approaching an upper-pole calyx from beneath the 12th rib may require substantial cephalad angulation, which creates a difficult acute angle between the nephrostomy tract and the renal pelvis and ureter. This may preclude the passage of rigid instruments. An intercostal puncture creates a more favorable obtuse angle, which then allows instruments to reach the remainder of the collecting system and ureter.

grees from the sagittal plane. Further angulation increases the risk of trauma to the spleen, liver, and colon.

4. When the dermatotomy is extended to allow passage of the dilators, care should be taken not to transect the intercostal artery. Sliding the blade into the tissues parallel to the ribs, and against the inferior edge of the guide wire is a useful precaution. Placement of a nephrostomy needle over the wire before passage of the blade provides a more rigid guide for the blade.

5. Insertion of a working sheath well into the collecting system is mandatory during all endoscopic procedures to allow free exit of irrigant from the kidney and thus minimize the risk of hydrothorax (Fig 16–7).

6. Periodic fluoroscopy of the chest should be performed during the procedure, and an expiratory chest roentgenogram is taken at the end of the procedure to detect fluid or air within the pleural cavity.

7. The use of a self-retaining nephrostomy catheter, such as a Foley catheter, following the procedure is recommended. Premature loss of the nephrostomy tube may be more likely, as a result of respiratory motion of the ribs, and is potentially of more consequence than with subcostal approaches, due to the risk of pneumothorax or extravasation of urine into the pleural cavity once the "plug" has been pulled from the tract.

Contraindications

1. Severe respiratory disease is a contraindication because of the possibility of serious and irreversible respiratory embarrassment from a pneumothorax or hydrothorax.

2. Intercostal approaches violate a natural barrier to the spread of infection. Such approaches should be avoided when puncture is made into a septic kidney. Empyema is a potential consequence.

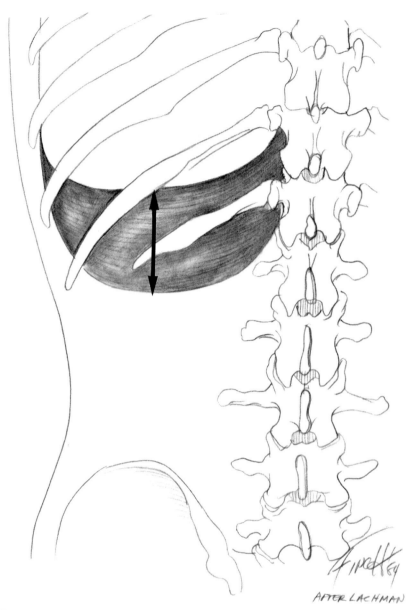

Fig 16–3. Variability of the posterior pleural recess. The shaded area indicates the range of variability of the posterior-inferior pleural reflection.

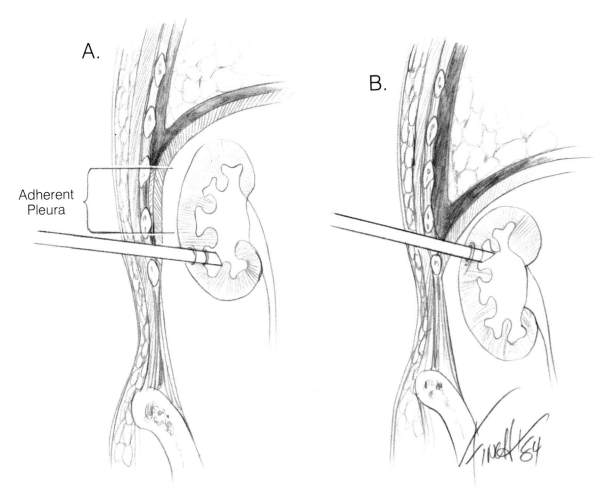

Fig 16–4.   Variation of inferior pleural recess with position of kidney. **A,** when a kidney is placed so high that the lower pole calyx lies above the 12th rib, the upward displacement of the diaphragm leads to adherence of the apposing pleural surfaces and obliteration of part of the posterior pleural recess. **B,** intercostal approaches to the upper pole are associated with a higher incidence of pleural effusion and pneumothorax, because the tract usually crosses the posterior pleural recess.

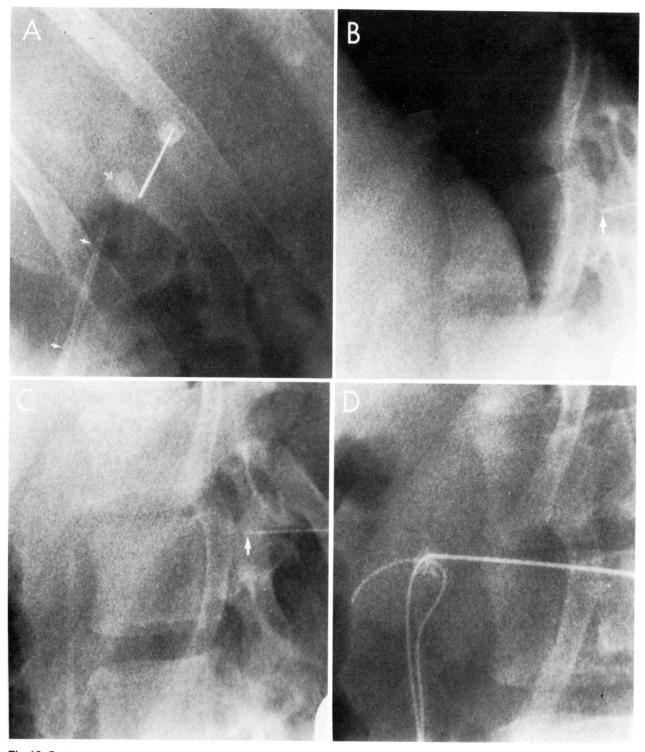

Fig 16–5. Intercostal punctures, avoiding the lung. **A,** a 22-gauge needle marks the intended puncture site above the 12th rib, directly onto the upper-pole calyceal stone *(large arrow)*. Retrograde catheter is present *(small arrows)*. **B,** lateral imaging during inspiration shows the needle posteriorly *(arrow)*. The posterior-inferior lung extends well below the intended path of the needle. **C,** in expiration, the lung is well out of the way of the needle *(arrow)*. **D,** definitive puncture is made during expiration, thus avoiding the lung. A guide wire has been coiled in the renal pelvis.

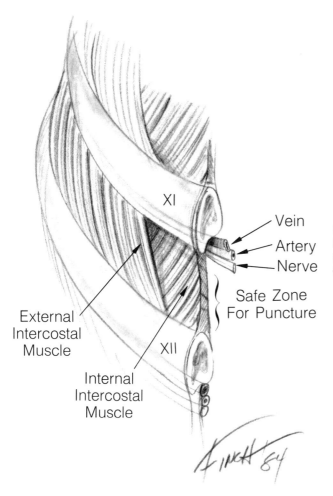

Fig 16–6. Safe intercostal puncture zone. The puncture should be made in the lower half of the intercostal space in order to avoid puncture of the vessels by the nephrostomy needle and scalpel during extension of the dermatotomy.

Complications

Accumulation of Pleural Fluid

Minimal accumulations of pleural fluid, following intercostal punctures, occur in approximately 25% of cases. These are seldom more than "blunting" of the posterior costophrenic angle on the chest roentgenogram, and are of no consequence. Larger effusions have occurred in fewer than 10% of our patients and are usually due to the irrigation fluid flowing from the nephroscope, through the tract, and into the pleural cavity. This may be avoided by using a "working" sheath, which decompresses the collecting system.

Hemothorax from laceration of an intercostal or renal vessel is a potential cause of pleural fluid. In our experience the hemorrhage is usually manifested at the puncture site, and once this is tamponaded with a sheath or nephrostomy tube, it ceases to be a problem. However, although we have not experienced hemothorax in this situation, it remains a possibility. The maintenance of a second "safety" wire in the collecting system at all times ensures access for a large nephrostomy tube or balloon catheter to provide tamponade if hemorrhage is encountered.

Pneumothorax

It is perhaps surprising that pneumothorax is not a common complication from intercostal approaches to the kidney. In our experience of approximately 50 such procedures, it has never occurred. However, it has been experienced by others.

There are two possible mechanisms for pneumothorax during intercostal nephrostomies.

1. The passage of air through the tract to the pleural cavity: this would most likely occur either during the procedure, particularly during exchange of catheters or dilators, or several days later at the time of removal of the final percutaneous nephrostomy tube. The fact that this is not a common occurrence suggests that the tissues seal around the catheters and dilators during the procedure, preventing the inflow of air, and that the established nephrostomy tract has lost its continuity with the pleural cavity, presumably by adherence of the pleurae.

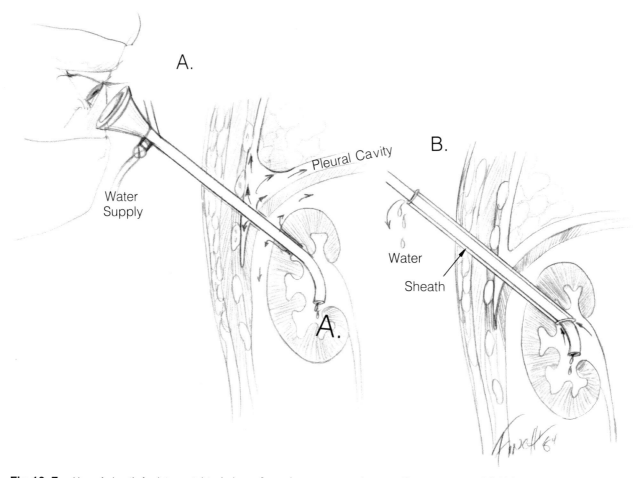

Fig 16–7. Use of sheath for intercostal technique. **A,** nephroscopes require a continuous stream of fluid for adequate vision. In the absence of a working sheath, this fluid percolates through the soft tissue tract into the perinephric space and pleural cavity. **B,** the use of a sheath allows free exit of fluid, decompressing the kidney and minimizing pleural accumulations.

2. Laceration of the lung: experience with lung biopsy suggests a definite risk of pneumothorax caused by needle passage through the lung. We have observed the inferior lung edge to extend beyond a projected nephrostomy tract through the 11th intercostal space, on full inspiration (see Fig 16–5) although never on quiet breathing. Fluoroscopy tangential to the puncture site is necessary in order to determine the position of the lung edge. If this is close to the tract, then puncture should be made on suspended expiration.

Laceration of Adjacent Organs

The spleen and liver are superolateral relations of the kidney, and are therefore at risk during all approaches to the upper pole above or below the 12th rib. The risk is reduced by limiting the lateral angulation of the needle to 30° as outlined above.

DOUBLE PUNCTURES

Indications

In some situations, for example, in the presence of staghorn or multiple calculi, or when the initial nephrostomy has been inappropriately placed, more than one nephrostomy tract is necessary to completely remove stones (Figs 16–8 and 16–9).

Whereas a flexible nephroscope is usually able to reach all parts of the collecting system, the

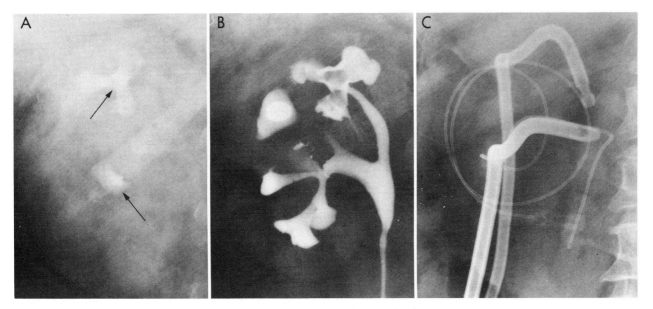

Fig 16–8. Mandatory double puncture. **A,** "scout" film reveals two branched calculi within the right kidney *(arrows)*. **B,** retrograde nephrostogram shows duplex collecting system with one stone in each division, requiring a double puncture. **C,** following successful stone removal, two nephrostomy tubes are present with a 5 F "safety" catheter in the proximal ureter.

graspers that pass through these instruments are quite small, and inadequate for stones much larger than 5 mm. The electrohydraulic probe that passes through the port of a flexible scope may be utilized for larger stones. However, such devices are falling from favor because they are time-consuming to use, potentially traumatic to the kidney, and result in multiple large fragments, which then have to be removed separately with graspers.

Stones over 6 mm in size are now generally removed with rigid endoscopic instruments, either the ultrasonic lithotriptor or the larger graspers that pass through the rigid nephroscopes.

However, there are limitations as to how much of the collecting system is accessible to rigid instruments, from any given entry point. Often it is the middle pole that is inaccessible from an upper or lower approach. In these situations a second nephrostomy puncture may be indicated.

The placement of more than one nephrostomy tube into a kidney also allows continuous infusion of stone-dissolving agents when appropriate.

Advantages and Disadvantages

The double-puncture technique presumably carries with it twice the risk for complications as does a single nephrostomy puncture. However, using the double-puncture technique, stones that would be otherwise inaccessible may be removed.

Methods

Simultaneous Puncture

In some centers, particularly those where the radiologic and urologic stages of the procedure are performed separately, more than one nephrostomy tract may be created by the radiologist at the first sitting. The second nephrostomy tract may then be dilated in the urologic suite if access using the first nephrostomy tract proves inadequate.

However, it is often difficult to predict how much of the collecting system is reachable from any one approach, even using rigid instruments. The experienced urologist may be able to torque a rigid nephroscope around much of the pelvicalyceal system, and remove stones that were first considered inaccessible.

Therefore, it is our opinion that the creation of a second tract at the initial sitting doubles the risk of complications from what may prove to be an unnecessary intervention.

Sequential Puncture

Using this technique, establishment of a second nephrostomy tract is performed only after as much stone as possible has been removed using the initial access. The second nephrostomy is then made into the most suitable calyx for removal of the remainder of the stone.

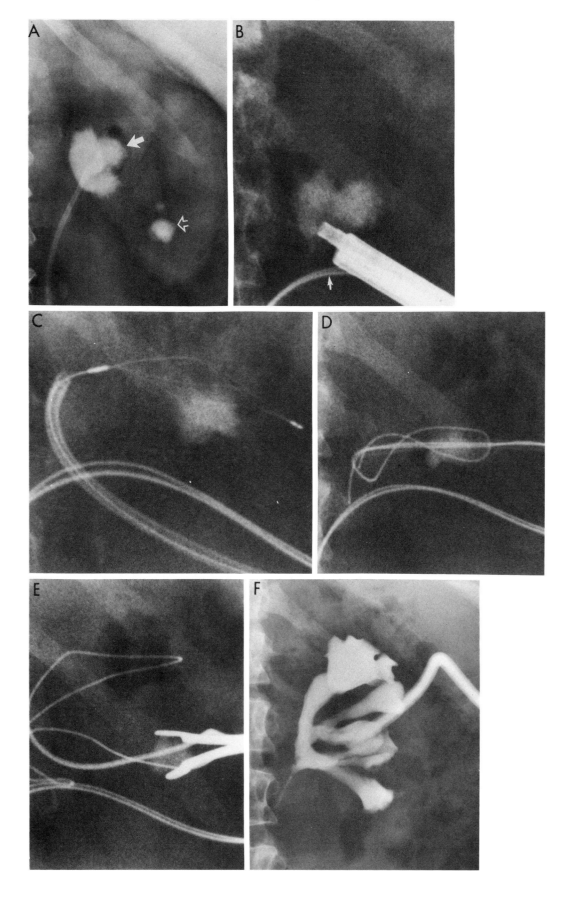

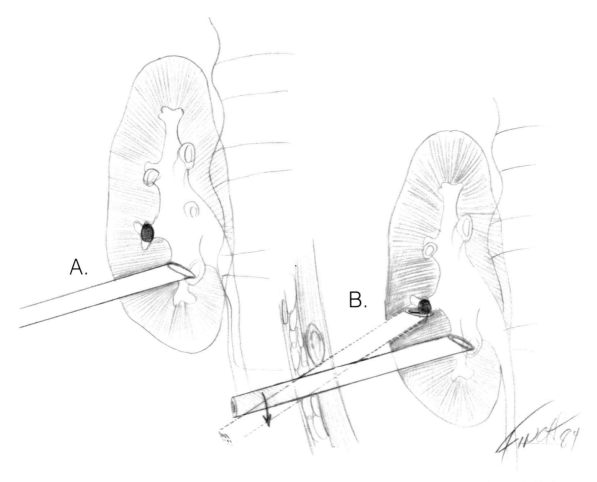

Fig 16–10. Y-Puncture technique. **A,** a stone depicted in a posterior middle-pole calyx may not be reachable from a lower-pole tract. **B,** the Amplatz sheath is withdrawn, and a fresh tract is created as a branch off of the original tract. Following dilation the sheath is reinserted through this fresh tract, directly onto the middle calyx, which contains the stone. Both sites have been entered by a single puncture in the skin.

Fig 16–9. Double puncture for moving fragment. **A,** "scout" film shows large branched stone in renal pelvis *(solid arrow)* and two smaller stones in lower pole *(open arrow).* **B,** a nephrostomy sheath has been placed via the lower pole, the two smaller stones have been removed and the pelvic stone is being fragmented with the ultrasonic lithotriptor. Two "safety" wires *(arrow)* have been passed down the ureter. **C,** a fragment of the large branched stone has shifted into a middle-pole calyx, but cannot be grasped with a flexible nephroscope or basket. **D,** a second puncture (above the 12th rib) has been performed. A 10 F sheath has been inserted in order to pass a second guide wire in the new tract (two guide wires remain through the original tract also). **E,** after dilation to 28 F, the fragment is removed using a Randall forceps (inserted over one of the wires). **F,** follow-up nephrostogram (through new tract) after removal of original nephrostomy tube shows the difficult anatomy of this kidney.

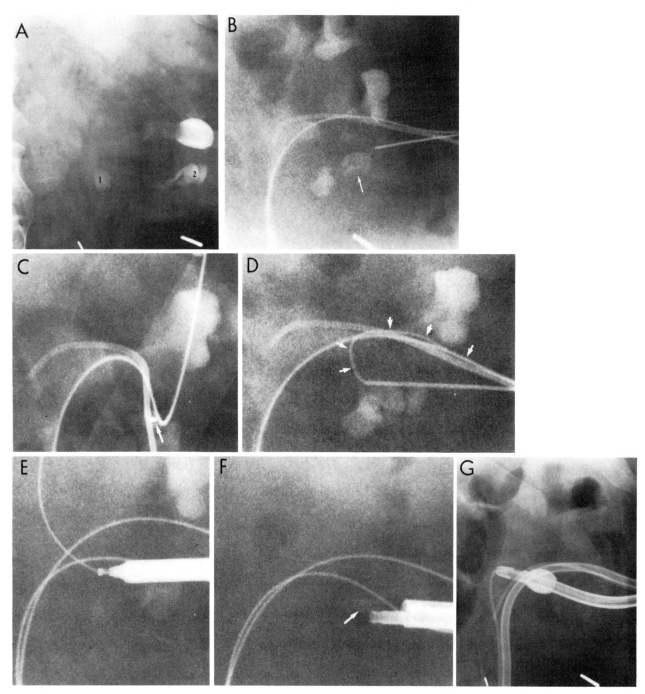

Fig 16–11.   Y-Puncture technique. **A,** patient has a nephrostomy catheter entering the middle-pole calyx, with a residual stone at the ureteropelvic junction (1) and in the lower-pole calyx (2). Ureteropelvic junction stone is removed using this approach, but lower pole cannot be reached. **B,** nephrostomy needle is passed partway down the tract and then angled down onto the lower pole stone *(arrow)*. **C,** use of a C-arm allows accurate "down-the-barrel" aiming of the needle onto the retained calculus *(arrow)*. Needle is seen as a dot *(arrow)* projected over the residual stone. **D,** once the needle has reached the calyx, a guide wire is passed, and may be pulled through the original tract *(small arrows* indicate the new guide wire). **E,** a second guide wire is passed (one enters the ureter, the other is in the upper pole). The "Y" tract is then dilated (metal dilators had to be used due to postoperative fibrosis). **F,** residual calculus *(arrow)* is removed using ultrasonic lithotripsy. **G,** following successful stone removal, two wide-bore catheters are present as well as two 5 F "safety" catheters. One of the large catheters stents the stenotic ureteropelvic junction.

The technique is the same as in the standard nephrostomy technique, with the following modifications:

1. The pelvicalyceal system is opacified using a nephrostomy catheter through the initial tract. Positive or negative contrast may be used.

2. Once the puncture is made, a guide wire is passed and either coiled in the collecting system, passed down the ureter, or pulled from the initial tract using endoscopic graspers or a snare.

3. A second "safety" wire should still be passed as in the standard technique because the ability to rapidly reestablish access through the fresh tract is mandatory should severe bleeding occur.

4. The presence of two nephrostomy tracts allows the use of a circle nephrostomy tube following stone extraction. However, this is not necessary, and in most circumstances two nephrostomy tubes are placed. They are removed separately as appropriate.

THE Y-PUNCTURE

The Y-puncture is an elegant variation of the double-puncture technique, as described above. However, instead of two completely separate nephrostomy tracts, the end result is a Y-shaped tract. The long limb of the "Y" represents the original tract, and the short limb the fresh tract that branches off to enter a different calyx (Fig 16–10).

The only real advantage of the Y-puncture over the double-puncture technique is that it spares the patient a second skin wound. The risk of vascular complications to the kidney is probably similar using either technique, as each entails two holes in the renal parenchyma.

Indications

The indications for a Y-puncture are the same as those of the double puncture, except that the targeted calyx should be adjacent or at least close to the entry point of the original nephrostomy. The Y-puncture is commonly performed into the calyx of the same group as the initial puncture, although a Y-puncture can also be performed into a calyx of an adjacent group (for example, a Y-puncture branching off an upper or lower pole tract, to enter a middle calyx).

Technique (Fig 16–11)

1. The pelvicalyceal system is opacified through a catheter entering the preexisting nephrostomy tract.

2. The 18-gauge needle is passed partway down the established tract, and is then angulated off this tract to aim at an adjacent part of the collecting system (Fig 16–11,B). If the initial tract is recent, it is sometimes helpful to pass the needle down the tract over a guide wire to avoid premature deviation into the soft tissues. If the existing tract is well established (three or more days old) the nephrostomy needle can be inserted down the hole, without a guide wire.

3. "Down-the-barrel" imaging of the needle using a C-arm is highly recommended for an accurate aim (Fig 16–11,C).

4. Once the needle has pierced the pelvicalyceal system, a guide wire is passed, and as in the double-puncture technique, may be coiled in the renal pelvis, passed down the ureter, or brought out the long limb of the Y-tract (Fig 16–11,D).

5. Passage of a second "safety" wire is again mandatory to ensure access once the working wire is removed.

6. Dilation is performed using sequential fascial dilators or a balloon catheter in the standard manner (Fig 16–11,E).

7. At the completion of the procedure, a nephrostomy tube, 20 to 24 F in size, and a 5 F "safety" catheter are left in the fresh limb of the Y-puncture tract for stenting the parenchymal wound. If there is a possibility that the original tract may be used for access at a later date, then a nephrostomy tube should be placed through the long limb of the "Y," also. This tube may be anywhere from 5 to 24 F (Fig 16–11,G).

THE "NEEDLE-PUSH"

The "needle-push" is a technique used for pushing a stone out of an inaccessible calyx into the renal pelvis from where it can be removed (Fig 16–12).

It is employed mainly for stones in posterior calyces, because with these calyces, the direction of the push is along the axis of the infundibulum, and therefore the stone is more likely to be dislodged.

Technique

1. Careful fluoroscopy is essential to evaluate the anatomy and to ensure that a "push" is practicable.

2. An 18-gauge nephrostomy needle is passed directly onto the stone (Fig 16–13,B) using the same

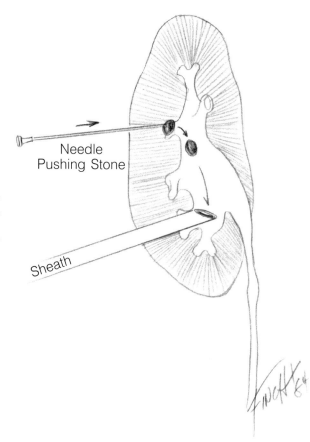

Fig 16–12. "Needle-push" technique. The upper-pole posterior calyceal stone may not be reachable from a middle- or lower-pole approach. An 18-gauge needle is passed directly onto the stone, pushing it from the calyx into the renal pelvis from where it may be removed.

technique and precautions as in the standard and double-puncture techniques.

3. When the needle impinges on the stone it is gently advanced in an attempt to push the stone from the calyx into the renal pelvis, from where it may be grasped (Fig 16–13,C).

4. If this should fail, rapid flushing with 5 ml of saline may be undertaken in an effort to move the stone.

5. If the stone is lodged firmly in the calyx, a guide wire is passed out of the needle into the calyx and advanced into the renal pelvis. The technique is then converted to a double puncture. The stone may then be removed via the new, second tract.

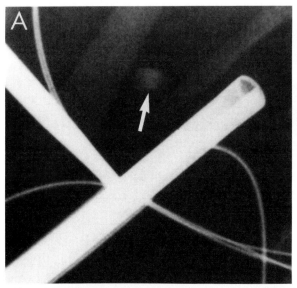

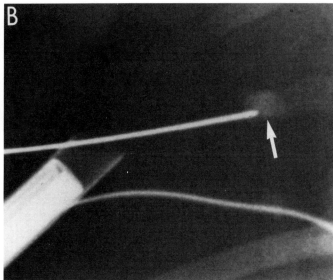

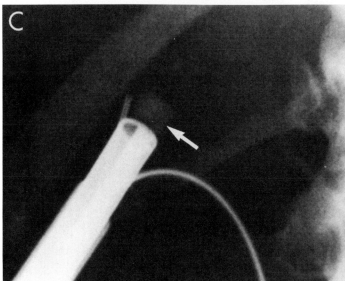

Fig 16–13. Example of "needle-push technique." **A,** from a lower-pole approach, the rigid nephroscope cannot reach a residual calculus *(large arrow)* lodged in a posterior upper-pole calyx. Calculus was too large to be grasped using a flexible nephroscope. **B,** an 18-gauge nephrostomy needle has been passed directly onto the calculus, which was pushed into the renal pelvis. **C,** calculus is now reachable using the rigid nephroscope, and is being removed with ultrasonic lithotripsy.

CHAPTER 17

Percutaneous Nephrolithotomy: Removal Techniques Under Fluoroscopic Control

Wilfrido R. Castañeda-Zuñiga, M.D.

STONE REMOVAL UNDER FLUOROSCOPIC GUIDANCE

Stone extraction under fluoroscopic control has the advantage of being simple and rapid if successful. It is limited to stones smaller than 1 cm and best suitable for free-floating stones in the renal pelvis.

The technique has the drawback that three-dimensional visualization is not feasible; consequently, manipulation of instruments under fluoroscopic control tends to be more traumatic and bleeding frequently occurs. In this regard, the fluoroscopic techniques are inferior to the stone extraction maneuvers under direct vision, except for the flushing techniques, which are atraumatic.

For stone extraction under fluoroscopic control oblique or lateral fluoroscopic observation is mandatory.

Technique

The puncture is made in a proper location, allowing easy access to the stone (similar to the endoscopic approach) (see Chapter 28).

The stone is measured and an Amplatz sheath slightly larger than the stone is inserted, to allow extraction or flushing out of the stone.

On some occasions, the outside of the stone may be partially nonopaque, with consequent underestimation of its size. Under those circumstances, the Teflon sheath has to be removed simultaneously with the calculus, and the stone is pulled through the renal parenchyma. The drawback of this maneuver is the possibility of losing the stone at the level of the renal capsule or in the soft tissues.

Various instruments described below can be introduced through various-sized catheters, which are either preformed or steerable.

Flushing and Aspiration

Free-floating stones in the renal pelvis, smaller than the Teflon sheath, can be simply aspirated. Aspiration of fluid, blood clots and stones from the renal pelvis is difficult because the renal pelvis collapses if negative pressure is applied. This technique is only successful if the renal pelvis is large, since a considerable amount of liquid is required to fill the Teflon sheath. If the renal pelvis is too small, the stones may be aspirated into the sheath but they cannot be delivered into the syringe because the renal pelvis will collapse. Consequently, a combination of simultaneous flushing and aspiration is necessary. The flushing

A.

B.

C.

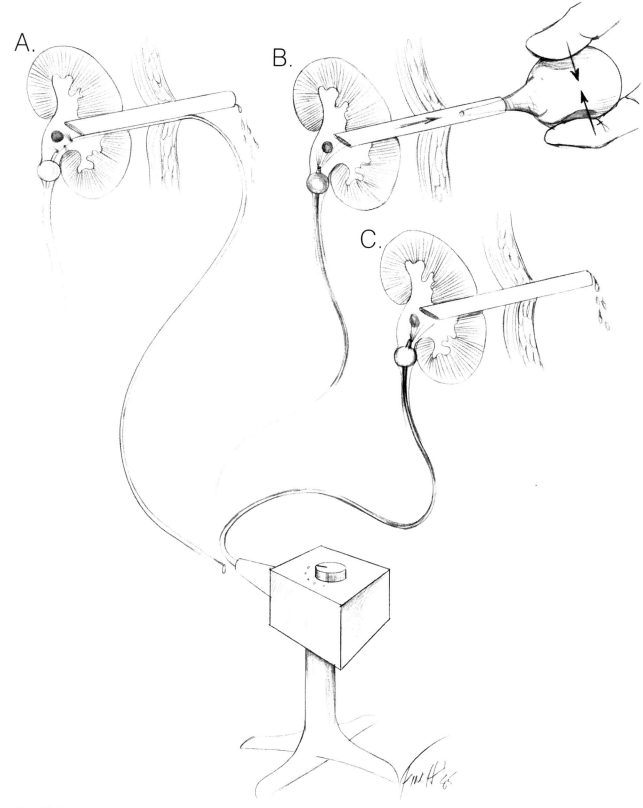

Fig 17–1. Diagrammatic representation of flushing techniques. **A,** an end-occluded balloon catheter has been passed alongside the Teflon sheath to obstruct the ureteropelvic junction (UPJ) and flush proximally into the renal pelvis. The bevel of the Teflon sheath has been turned to point in the direction of the retained stone. **B,** an end-hole occlusion balloon catheter has been advanced in a retrograde fashion to block the UPJ and allow for flushing of the retained stone. Simultaneously, suction is applied to the end of the Teflon sheath. **C,** alternatively, the Teflon sheath can be left open for free drainage of the irrigating fluid, which is injected with a power injector.

technique is particularly useful for the removal of stones less than 1 cm and stone fragments following fragmentation. All safe flushing maneuvers require the insertion of a large Teflon sheath serving as a vent and a second catheter in the collecting system in order to deliver contrast medium or gas. Although it is possible to introduce a second catheter alongside the Teflon sheath (Fig 17–1,A) it is by far better to introduce a catheter in retrograde fashion into the ureter for flushing (Fig 17–1,B and C). This has the great advantage that stone fragments cannot enter the ureter, from where they are difficult to remove.

A large Teflon sheath is introduced into the renal pelvis and the bevel of the sheath is rotated toward the retained stones. Proper position of the sheath is verified with oblique or lateral fluoroscopy.

The Teflon sheath is filled with contrast medium. In spite of proper position, there is usually no filling of the renal pelvis due to the presence of blood clots. An attempt can be made to aspirate the blood clots, but it may be necessary to make them small enough that they can be aspirated into the teflon sheath. Fragmentation of the blood clots is simply accomplished by using a guide wire or a basket.

After the blood clots have been aspirated, the renal pelvis will fill readily if contrast medium is instilled into the Teflon sheath.

A 100-cc syringe filled with contrast medium is connected to the retrograde catheter and the contrast medium is injected at a rate of 15 to 20 ml/second using a power injector. Simultaneously, an assistant aspirates the contrast medium with a manual syringe, which is attached by polyvinyl tubing to the Teflon sheath.

It is of paramount importance that the entire procedure be carried out under careful fluoroscopic guidance since the injection has to be stopped immediately if overdistension of the renal pelvis occurs. Otherwise the renal pelvis or ureter may rupture. However, when there is free flow of contrast medium, the technique has been atraumatic and safe in our hands. One hundred milliliters of contrast medium is usually adequate to deliver the stone into the polyvinyl tubing. Once blood clots or stones are seen in the polyvinyl tubing, the clamp is immediately applied to the tubing, which is detached from the Teflon sheath. Blood clots are carefully examined since stones may be entrapped in coagula. As a matter of fact, the presence of blood clots is very beneficial for the delivery of stones.

Removal of Ureteral Stones by Flushing

Retained stones, particularly in the upper ureter, are removed in identical fashion. The retrograde catheter is placed immediately beneath the stone in order to maximize the jet effect. The rapid delivery of contrast medium or CO_2 also causes some dilation of the ureter similar to that seen in the Rutner balloon catheter technique. It is this dilation of the ureter and the positive jet of contrast medium directed toward the stone that make this technique successful in a high percentage of cases.

Simultaneously with the flushing, negative pressure is applied to the Teflon sheath by a syringe. As with the flushing of pelvic stones, the entire procedure is carried out under careful fluoroscopic guidance and the injector is immediately stopped if overdistension of the ureter should occur. In our opinion, however, the ureter was found to be very distensible and there was always enough room between the stone and the ureteral mucosa to provide passage of the contrast medium. One technical problem has been the recoil of the ureteral catheter into the bladder. It is therefore advisable to firmly secure a preferably stiffer ureteral catheter and start with a slower injection rate of 5 to 10 ml/second. Whenever possible, at least a 7 F end-hole catheter should be used.

A variation of the flushing techniques can be used for the extraction of stones from calyces. A 24 to 26 F red rubber tube is modified by cutting its tip at a slanted angle, to provide a large surface area for suctioning. Over a previously placed angiographic catheter the rubber tube is advanced into the calyx (Fig 17–2) and the bevel is applied against the stone. Forceful aspiration will in some cases force the stone against the tip of the rubber tube, which is then carefully pulled back into the Teflon sheath.

Grasping Techniques

The grasping techniques can be divided in three groups, depending on the instrument used for removal: (1) baskets, (2) flexible forceps, and (3) rigid forceps.

Baskets

The use of baskets is a well-established fluoroscopic technique for the removal of stones from the lower ureter. Baskets are relatively atraumatic, flexible instruments. They work well for

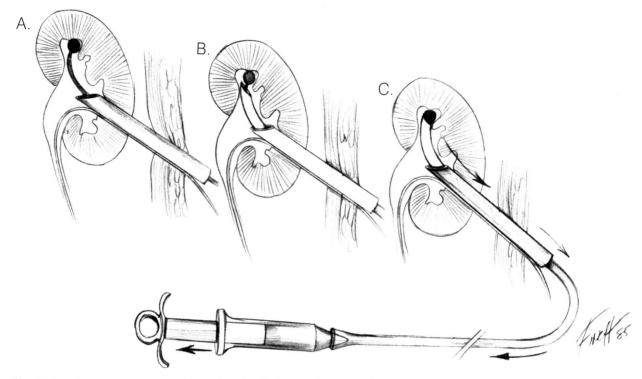

Fig 17–2. Diagrammatic representation of suction techniques for calyceal stones. **A,** an angiographic catheter has been passed through the Teflon sheath and positioned next to the retained calyceal stone. **B,** the modified red rubber tube is advanced over the angiographic catheter and the bevel end is pointed toward the stone. **C,** by applying suction with a syringe to the external end of the red rubber tube the stone is forcefully aspirated against the bevel end of the red rubber tube, which is then slowly withdrawn.

the extraction of stones from the lower ureter, but they are less successful for the extraction of stones from the upper ureter (for reasons unknown) and they are least useful for the extraction of pelvic stones. In the ureter, the space is limited and the stone tends to be forced into the basket. On the other hand, in the large renal pelvis the stones rest on the floor of the pelvis and commonly do not enter the basket. Furthermore, stones are commonly entrapped in blood clots. Specially designed baskets have been devised to overcome this drawback.

Several types of baskets are commercially available:

• Three- and four-wire removable helical design without flexible tip (Fig 17–3,C).
• Three-, four-, or five-wire removable helical basket with a flexible tip (Fig 17–3,D and F).
• Rutner balloon-basket with a flexible tip (Fig 17–3,A).
• Amplatz through-and-through ureteral basket (Fig 17–3,G).

• Davis loop (Fig 17–3,B and H).
• Hawkins basket (Fig 17–4).

In spite of the construction of numerous extracting devices, the failure rate of extracting stones from the upper ureter remains high. This is very likely due to irritation of the mucosa and partial impaction of the stone in the edematous mucosa. Baskets may not open completely and the wires of the baskets may not entrap the stone. Consequently, dilation of the ureter and forceful spreading of the baskets may be successful.

Since even the passage of guide wires beyond the stone may irritate the mucosa and cause lateral displacement of the stone, we have elected not to pass any instruments, to avoid mucosal edema. The first attempt to retrieve a ureteral stone is the delivery into the renal pelvis by a jet of carbon dioxide or contrast medium. This atraumatic flushing technique has proved more successful than the manipulation by the extracting devices.

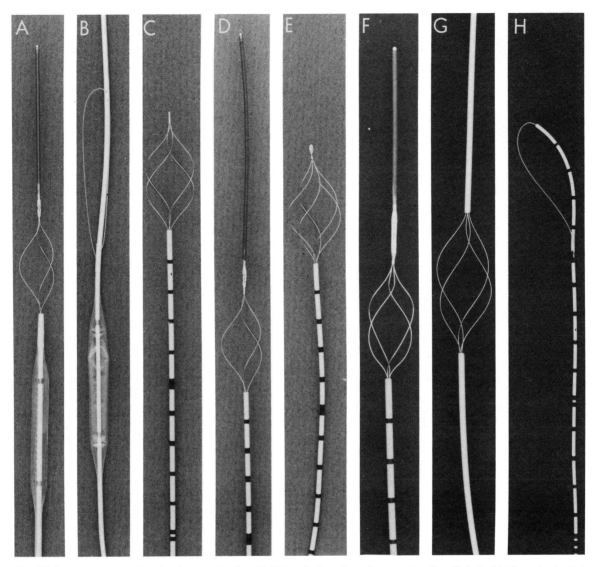

Fig 17–3. **A,** Rutner balloon-basket combination. **B,** Rutner ballon–Davis loop combination. **C,** helicoidal four-wire basket without a floppy tip. **D,** helicoidal three-wire basket with a long floppy tip. **E,** helicoidal five-wire basket without a floppy tip. **F,** helicoidal four-wire basket with a flexible tip. **G,** Amplatz ureteral basket. **H,** Davis loop.

Baskets should be designed so that they can be removed from the guiding catheter. By doing so the guiding catheter is inserted first over a guide wire, the guide wire is removed, and the basket is introduced through the guiding catheter.

Unfortunately, many commercially available baskets cannot be removed from the catheter; consequently, the basket that is mounted with the catheter has to be passed through a Teflon sheath. Manipulation of baskets is facilitated by introduction through a steerable catheter. By doing so, baskets can be easily advanced into the ureter or into the calyceal system.

In the upper ureter, the manipulation of baskets may be quite traumatic, inducing edema of the mucosa. Once this occurs, the stone usually becomes firmly embedded and extraction fails. Because of this, in recent years we have preferred to use the less traumatic flushing technique first in order to deliver the stone into the renal pelvis, from which it can be removed under direct vision or aspirated. Standard baskets are not useful for the entrapment of calyceal stones because the flexible tip prevents entry and a rigid-tipped basket may damage the papilla and induce bleeding during manipulation.

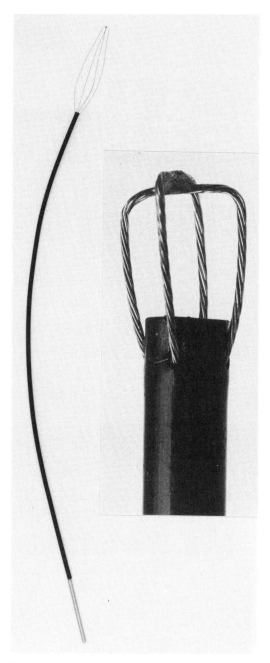

Fig 17–4 Hawkins basket. The basket has been opened by advancing the shaft inside the Teflon tubing. Inset shows the basket in the closed position after pulling back on the shaft.

The Hawkins Basket

This basket is designed in such a fashion that it can be retracted into a Teflon catheter. It can also be extended from the Teflon catheter and is made of braided cable instead of wire (Fig 17–4). The basket is blunt and, consequently, damage is minimized. The basket can also be spread by bracing it against the renal pelvis, facilitating the trapping of pelvic stones (Fig 17–5). By precurving the Teflon tubing, this basket can be used for calyceal stone extraction (Fig 17–6).

For the removal of stones from the ureter, baskets with an attached guide wire are most useful since they can be advanced in relatively atraumatic fashion. Perforation of the ureter during extraction is therefore minimized.

The major technical difficulty with extraction of stones from the ureter is due to mucosal edema and partial compression of the basket by the ureter: in such an instance, the basket cannot open completely and the stone cannot fall into it. Special baskets have been designed that allow active spreading, such as the Amplatz through-and-through basket (see Fig 17–3,G).

The Amplatz basket has long guide wires attached to both ends of the basket. For introduction, a guide wire is first passed into the bladder and the wire is removed cystoscopically (Fig 17–7,A). An 8 F Teflon catheter is advanced over the wire in an antegrade fashion until it exits through the urethral meatus (Fig 17–7,B). The guide wire is exchanged for the Amplatz basket (Fig 17–7,C), which is advanced through the Teflon catheter until it overlaps the stone. The catheter is then withdrawn to a position proximal to the basket and a second Teflon catheter is subsequently advanced in a retrograde fashion over the free end of the basket (Fig 17–7,D). By forward advancement of the Teflon catheters the basket is forced open (Fig 17–7,E) and the stone is entrapped. The entire system is then slowly pulled back into the renal pelvis/Teflon sheath (Fig 17–7,F and G).

Because of the frequent failure of baskets in the upper ureter, Rutner and co-workers combined an angioplasty balloon catheter with a basket (Fig 17–3,A). The 7 F balloon catheter is introduced in a retrograde fashion through the endoscope until the flexible tip of the basket lies beyond the ureteral stone. The balloon is inflated just below the stone in order to dilate the ureter. By dilation of the ureter, entrapment of the stone is facilitated. Once the stone is in the basket, it is withdrawn into the bladder.

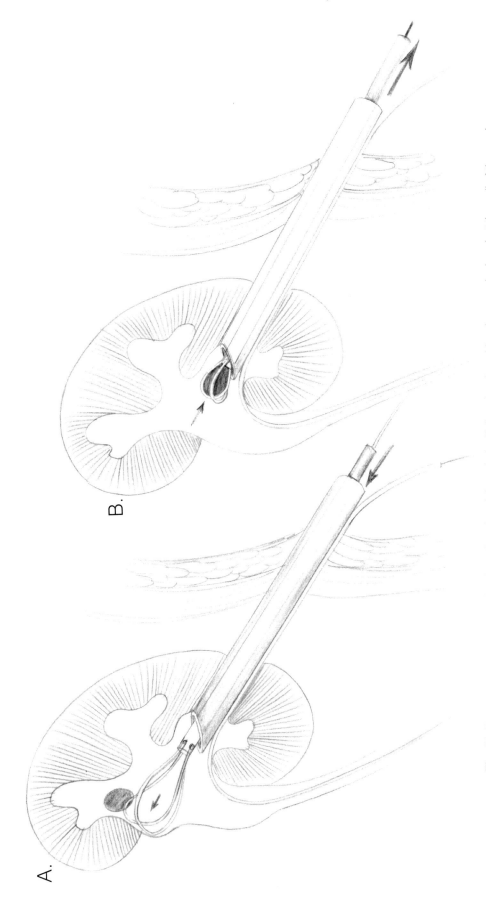

Fig 17–5. A, the Hawkins basket has been introduced through the Teflon sheath and has been pushed against the wall of the renal pelvis to force the wires to open, allowing the stone to be entrapped. **B**, after the stone has been trapped, the wires are pulled back to close the basket, which is removed through the Teflon sheath.

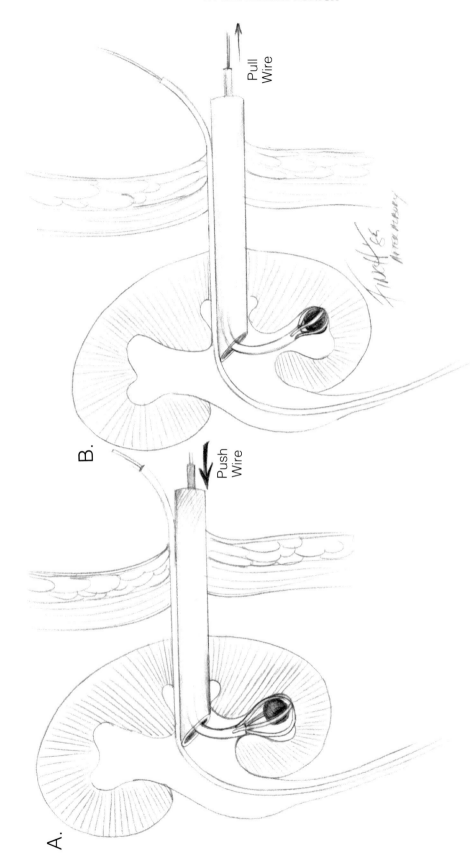

Fig 17–6. Hawkins basket for calyceal stones. **A,** the Teflon tubing has been preshaped to allow for the manipulation of the basket into the calyx with the retained stone. The basket is then opened and the stone is entrapped. **B,** once the stone is trapped, the basket is closed and it is slowly withdrawn.

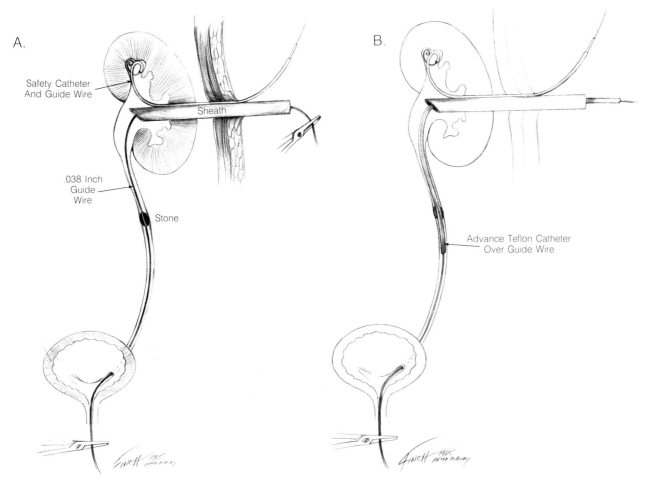

Fig 17–7. Amplatz through-and-through basket technique. **A,** an angiographic guide wire has been passed through the Teflon sheath into the bladder from where it was removed under cystoscopic control. **B,** a Teflon catheter has been advanced over the angiographic guide wire. *(Continued)*

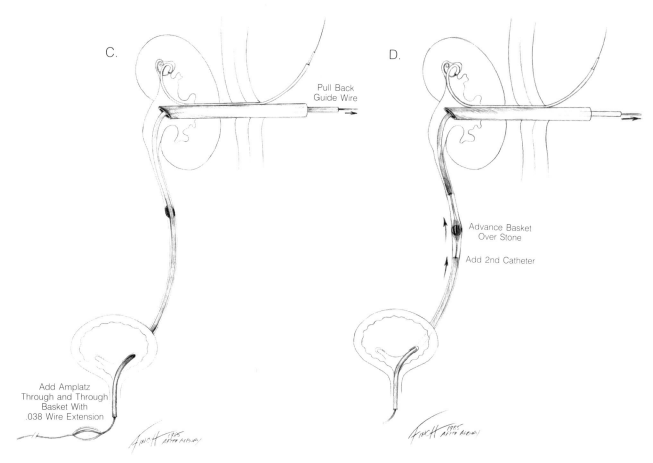

Fig 17–7 (cont.)   **C,** once the Teflon catheter has exited through the urethral meatus, the angiographic guide wire is removed and the through-and-through Amplatz basket is advanced into the Teflon tube. **D,** the basket has been positioned at the level of the stone and a second Teflon catheter has been advanced in a retrograde fashion to a position just distal to the stone, while the first Teflon catheter has been pulled back to a position proximal to the stone. *(Continued)*

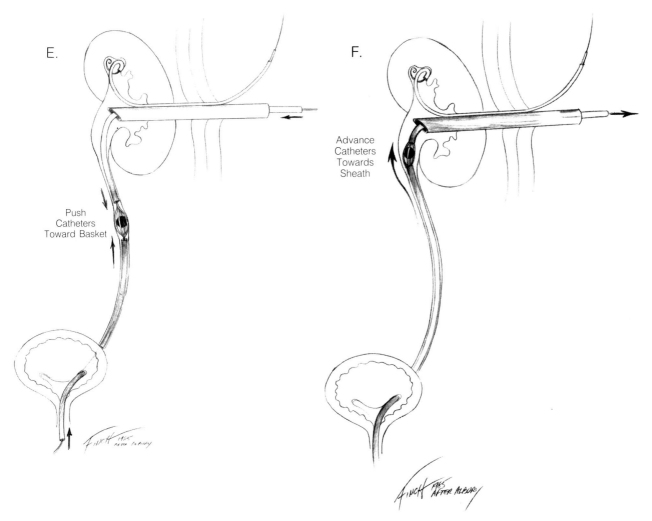

Fig 17–7 (cont.) **E,** by advancing the Teflon catheters over the wires, the basket is forced open entrapping the stone. **F,** after pulling back on both ends of the wires to close the basket, the entire system is slowly withdrawn into the renal pelvis. *(Continued)*

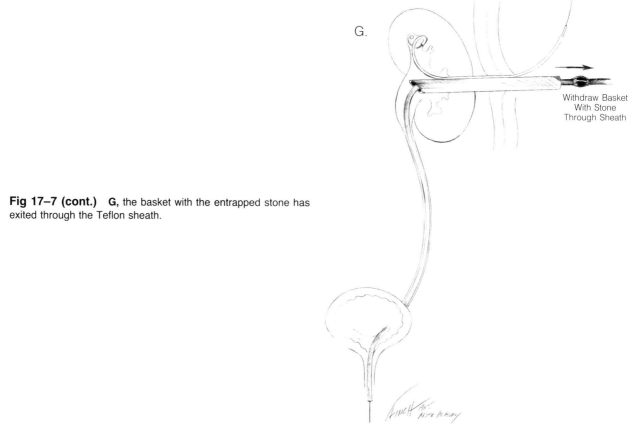

G.

Withdraw Basket
With Stone
Through Sheath

Fig 17–7 (cont.)   G, the basket with the entrapped stone has exited through the Teflon sheath.

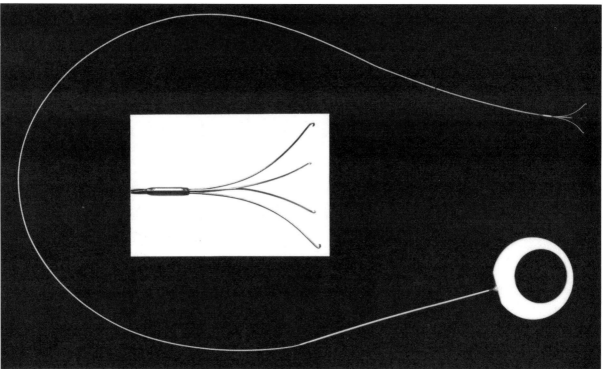

Fig 17–8. Four-prong grasper. The inset shows the hooked end of the wires.

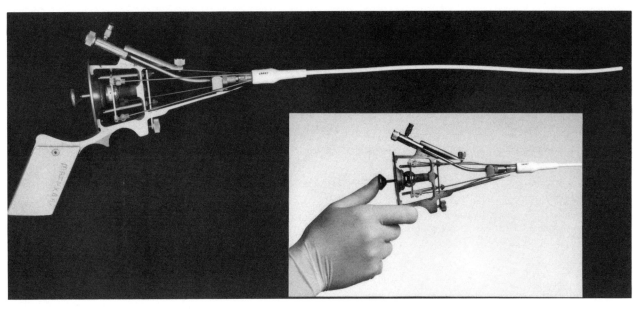

Fig 17–9. Handle for manipulation of steerable catheters. The inset shows the position of the hand during the manipulation of the catheter.

The Davis Loop

The Davis loop stone extractor (see Fig 17–3,B) is commonly used in retrograde fashion. The radiopaque polyvinyl chloride catheter is introduced into the ureter under direct vision and advanced until the nylon monofilament overlies the impacted stone. By pulling on the nylon thread, a catheter loop is formed and the stone may enter the loop. Once entrapped, the stone is gently pulled down into the urinary bladder. The Davis loop is comparatively atraumatic and can also be used through an antegrade nephrostomy tract.

A combination of angioplasty balloon with a Davis loop (see Fig 17–3,H) can also be used to facilitate the removal of impacted stones by predilating the ureter.

The Flexible Three- to Four-Pronged Forceps

Although this instrument has proved useful for endoscopic stone extraction, it should be used with great caution under fluoroscopic control. Since three-dimensional visualization is difficult even with biplane fluoroscopy, the sharp hooks of the grasping forceps (Fig 17–8) can grasp the pelvic mucosa similar to a fishhook. Once caught in the mucosa, the instrument can only be removed by tearing the mucosa, which may induce perforation or bleeding. The forceps can be introduced through a steerable catheter system (Figs 17–9 and 17–10).

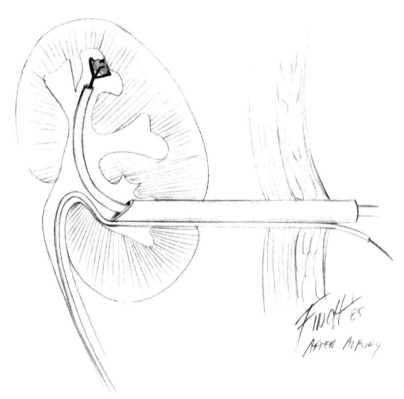

Fig 17–10. A steerable catheter has been passed through the Teflon sheath and manipulated into the calyx, where a retained stone is located. Through the steerable catheter, the four-prong grasper has been passed to trap the stone.

Flexible Alligator Forceps

With this instrument (Fig 17–11) stones up to 4 mm in size may be successfully extracted. Due to the limited opening capability of the forceps, larger stones are usually lost. The flexible 7 F alligator forceps can be introduced through a 13 F steerable catheter (Fig 17–12). The advantage of the flexible alligator forceps is that with the help of the steerable catheter it can be manipulated into remote areas that are not accessible to rigid instruments. This instrument is therefore useful for the extraction of multiple calyceal stones or stone fragments following lithotripsy.

Rigid Forceps

There are three types of rigid forceps that can be used through a percutaneous tract: (1) Randall's forceps, (2) Mazariello-Caprini forceps, and (3) laryngeal biopsy forceps.

The Randall Forceps

The use of a Randall forceps is helpful, particularly for the extraction of stones from the renal pelvis. Successful use of the Randall forceps requires that the tract provides direct access to the stone.

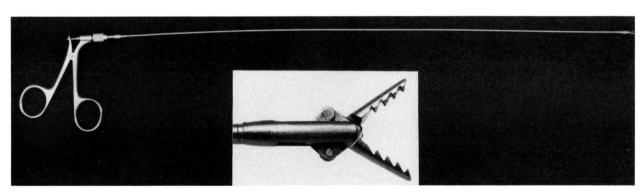

Fig 17–11. Flexible alligator forceps (7 F). The inset shows a close-up of the forceps jaws.

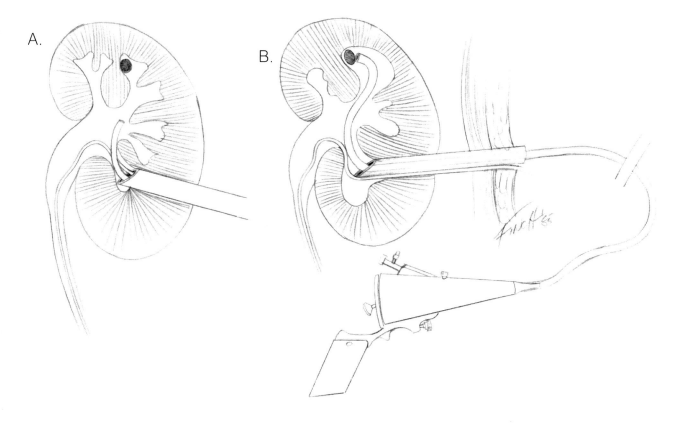

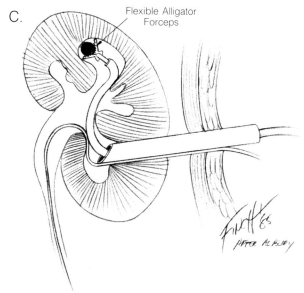

Fig 17–12. Medi-tech steerable catheter technique with flexible alligator forceps. **A,** the 13 F steerable catheter has been advanced through the Teflon sheath. **B,** the tip of the steerable catheter has been positioned in the calyx with the retained stone. **C,** the 7 F flexible alligator forceps has been passed through the steerable catheter and the jaws have been opened to trap the stone.

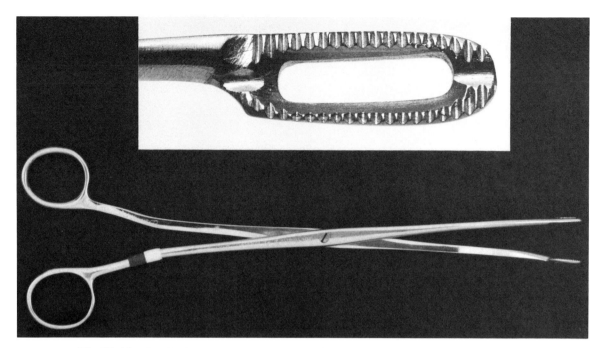

Fig 17–13.   Randall forceps in open position. The inset shows the grooved end of the forceps.

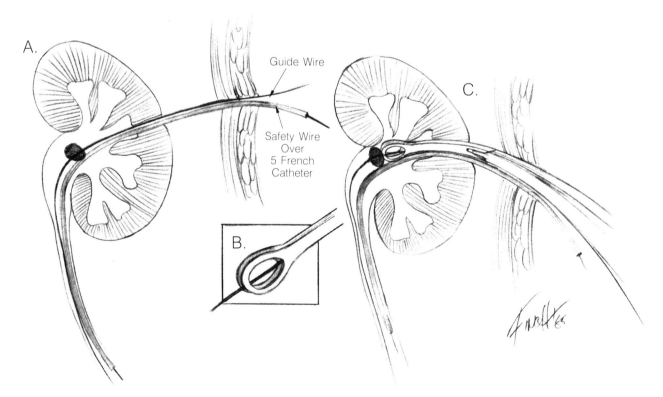

Fig 17–14.   Randall forceps stone extraction technique. **A,** two wires are present within the collecting system. The Teflon sheath has been removed. **B,** the Randall forceps has been closed over the working guide wire. **C,** the Randall forceps has been advanced over the guide wire under fluoroscopic control until in position next to the stone in the anteroposterior plane. **D,** by the use of biplane fluoroscopy, multidirectional fluoroscopy, or by rotating the patient a steep oblique or lateral view of the kidney is obtained to assess the position of the Randall forceps' tip next to the stone. **E,** the working wire has been removed and the forceps has been opened to entrap the stone. **F,** with the stone well wedged within the forceps, the forceps is slowly withdrawn through the tract.

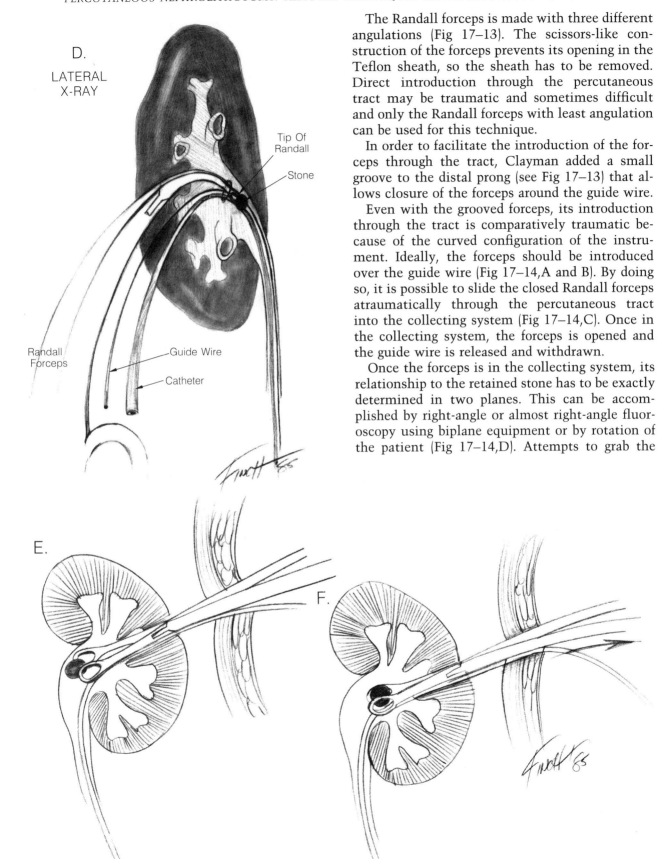

D.
LATERAL
X-RAY

Tip Of
Randall

Stone

Randall
Forceps

Guide Wire

Catheter

E.

F.

The Randall forceps is made with three different angulations (Fig 17–13). The scissors-like construction of the forceps prevents its opening in the Teflon sheath, so the sheath has to be removed. Direct introduction through the percutaneous tract may be traumatic and sometimes difficult and only the Randall forceps with least angulation can be used for this technique.

In order to facilitate the introduction of the forceps through the tract, Clayman added a small groove to the distal prong (see Fig 17–13) that allows closure of the forceps around the guide wire.

Even with the grooved forceps, its introduction through the tract is comparatively traumatic because of the curved configuration of the instrument. Ideally, the forceps should be introduced over the guide wire (Fig 17–14,A and B). By doing so, it is possible to slide the closed Randall forceps atraumatically through the percutaneous tract into the collecting system (Fig 17–14,C). Once in the collecting system, the forceps is opened and the guide wire is released and withdrawn.

Once the forceps is in the collecting system, its relationship to the retained stone has to be exactly determined in two planes. This can be accomplished by right-angle or almost right-angle fluoroscopy using biplane equipment or by rotation of the patient (Fig 17–14,D). Attempts to grab the

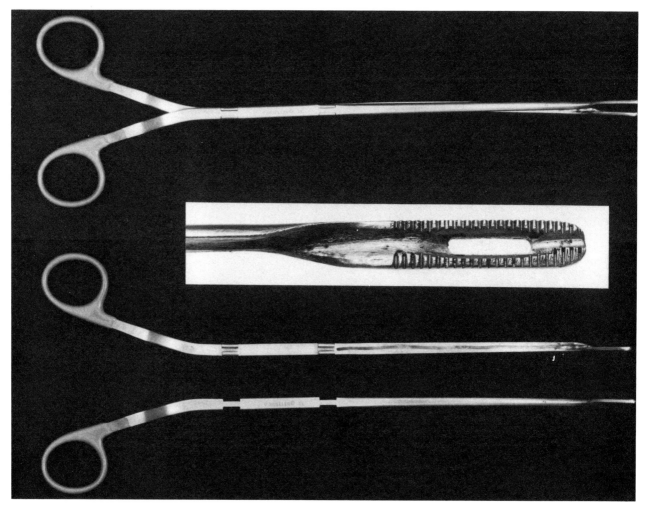

Fig 17–15.　Mazariello-Caprini forceps assembled **(A)** and taken apart **(B)**. The inset shows the grooved end of the forceps for the introduction over the guide wire.

stone after single-plane visualization have usually resulted in bleeding due to damage to the renal pelvis.

Once the proximity of the tip of the forceps to the stone is verified three-dimensionally, the forceps is gently opened and the stone is entrapped (Fig 17–14,E). The stone has to be well-lodged deep in the two prongs of the forceps (Fig 17–14,F); otherwise it may be lost while pulling it through the percutaneous tract.

The disadvantage of the Randall forceps is the necessity of a large nephrostomy tract in order to adequately open the forceps. This is particularly true if the nephrostomy tract is long, as in obese patients. An improvement over the scissors-like Randall forceps is the Mazariello-Caprini forceps (Fig 17–15).

The forceps has an ingenious construction that eliminates the scissors-like hinge, and can be opened in a comparatively small nephrostomy tract. This forceps is available with two curvatures and its introduction can be facilitated by a groove in the prongs that allows passage over the guide wire.

Several retained calyceal stones, free-floating pelvic stones, and stones in the proximal ureter have been successfully removed by us using either the Randall or Mazariello-Caprini forceps.

Even with the grooved forceps, its introduction through the tract is comparatively traumatic because of the curved configuration of the instrument. Ideally, a grasping forceps should be straight, so that it can be introduced through a Teflon sheath. This can be accomplished with the laryngeal biopsy forceps.

The laryngeal biopsy forceps is a straight, rigid forceps that can be introduced through the Teflon sheath, allowing removal of stones smaller than 5 mm (Figs 17–16 and 17–17). The three-dimensional location of the stone in relation to the Tef-

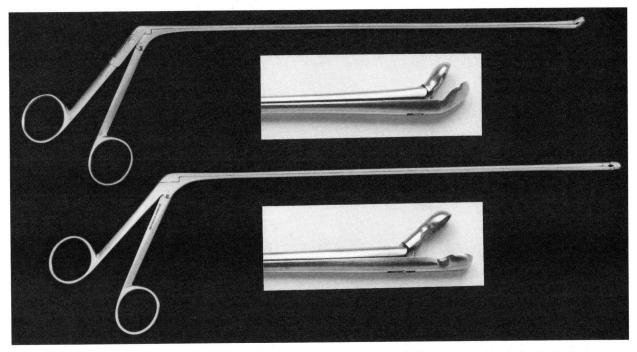

Fig 17–16. Laryngeal biopsy forceps with a slight angulation *(top)* and with a more straight design *(bottom).*

lon sheath is determined by fluoroscopy in two planes prior to manipulation of the instrument. If this important step is omitted, closing of the forceps over the uroendothelium of the renal pelvis may induce severe bleeding. The greater advantage of the laryngeal forceps is the possibility of introducing the instrument and extracting the stone through a Teflon sheath.

Rigid forceps are a very important component of the armamentarium for radiographic stone extraction. The technique's use is limited to stones under 15 mm in diameter and its safe use requires experience, since perforations of the collecting system and severe bleeding may be encountered.

Fragmentation Techniques Under Fluoroscopic Guidance

Stones larger than 1.5 cm in diameter have to be fragmented unless Teflon sheaths of a larger size are used, as has been done successfully at the University of Minnesota; however, the largest commercially available sheath is only 30 F (1 cm) in diameter.

The mechanical fragmentation of stones is only successful with softer stones and usually not successful with hard calcium oxalate stones.

The great disadvantage of mechanical fragmentation is that the resultant fragments are large; this technique has therefore been surpassed by ultrasonic fragmentation, which produces small fragments that are aspirated simultaneously. For fragmentation baskets, the Randall forceps and Mauermeyer stone punch have been used.

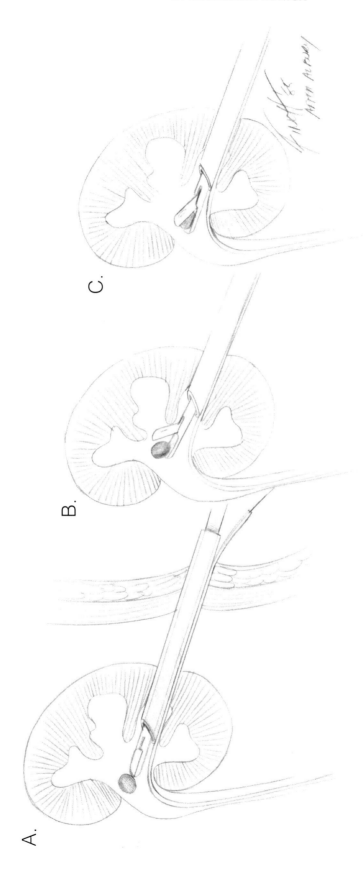

Fig 17–17. Laryngeal forceps stone extraction technique. **A**, the straight laryngeal forceps has been passed through the Teflon sheath into a position next to the stone in the anteroposterior plane. **B**, after demonstrating the position of the forceps next to the stone in the steep oblique or lateral projections, the forceps have been opened and the stone has been entrapped. **C**, with the stone safely trapped, the laryngeal forceps is removed through the Teflon sheath.

CHAPTER 18

Percutaneous Nephrolithotomy: Endoscopic Instruments

Pratap K. Reddy, M.D.

The instruments required for endoscopic stone removal, which are described in this chapter, include the following: (1) Nephroscopes (rigid and flexible), (2) endoscopic accessories (baskets, forceps, and other accessories), and (3) disintegrators (ultrasonic and electrohydraulic lithotriptors).

NEPHROSCOPES

Rigid Nephroscopes

There are three instruments (Storz, Wolf, and ACMI ARN-19) specifically designed for nephroscopy (Fig 18–1). The Storz nephroscope is 26 F in size with a 0-degree wide-angle lens. The Wolf nephroscope is 24 F with a 5-degree lens. Both the Storz and the Wolf nephroscopes are available with a 90- or a 30-degree side-arm viewing system. The ACMI ARN-19 nephroscope is 24 F in size with a 30-degree lens and has a 30-degree side-arm viewing system. All three nephroscopes have a 12 F working port and continuous-flow capabilities. Each nephroscope has an ultrasonic unit that is used for ultrasonic calculus disintegration.

Other instruments (cystoscopes) not primarily designed for the kidney can be used as nephroscopes also (Fig 18–2). The McCarthy cystoscope in particular is used quite frequently for extraction of renal calculi. The smooth beveled tip of this cystoscope can traverse nephrostomy tracts under vision (in cases where a Teflon sheath is not used) and also enables easier access into the calyces. However, there is the potential of perforating the collecting system, as the tip of this instrument extends 1 to 2 cm beyond the angle of view. Many other cystoscopes have curved tips, while the urethrotome has a "cut off" end. Cystoscopes or the direct vision urethrotome can be used to inspect the kidney when nephroscopes are not available, or when the tract is too small to accommodate these nephroscopes.

Flexible Nephroscopes

Flexible fiberoptic instruments were initially used for the common bile duct but are very well suited for use in the renal collecting system. A variety of choledochonephroscopes are available (Olympus, ACMI, and Pentex) (Table 18–1). All are 5 to 6 mm in diameter, and 33 to 37 cm in length, with a 2-mm irrigating instrument port. The proximal shaft is semirigid with a distal 2- to 3-cm flexible tip. A series of interlocking pulley-like structures in the shaft of the scope allow deflection of the tip to a maximum of 220° to 290° in one plane with 110° to 160° being the maximum deflection in one direction. The light is

TABLE 18–1.
Endoscopic Instruments and Accessories

MANUFACTURER	DESCRIPTION AND FEATURES
Rigid nephroscopes	
ACMI	20 F, 24 F McCarthy panendoscope; ARN-19: 24 F nephroscope, 30° lens, 30° side-arm viewing
Storz	26 F nephroscope, 30° and 90° side-arm viewing, 0° fisheye lens
Wolf	24 F nephroscope, 90° side-arm viewing, 5° and 70° lens
Flexible nephroscopes	
ACMI	APN-37: 15 F choledochonephroscope, 37 cm long, 5 F working port, 180° distal tip deflection, both directions
Olympus	CHF 4B: 15 F choledochonephroscope, 33 cm long, 5 F working port, tip deflection 160° up and 90° down
Pentax	15 F choledochonephroscope, 30 cm long, 5 F working port, tip deflection 160° up and 130° down
Lithotriptors	
ACMI	Ultrasonic lithotriptor: 24 F nephroscope, single transducer, generator and disposable probes; 3-kV electrohydraulic lithotriptor with 5 F and 9 F probes.
Storz	Ultrasonic lithotriptor: 26 F nephroscope, single transducer, generator and suction apparatus, disposable oscillating probes
Wolf	Ultrasonic lithotriptor: 24 F nephroscope with 2 sonotrodes, generator and suction apparatus; 8-kV Riwolith 2135 electrohydraulic lithotriptor with 5 F and 9 F probes
Pentax	5-kV electrohydraulic lithotriptor with 5 F and 10 F probes
Endoscopic accessories	
ACMI	6 F, 7 F, 11 F foreign-body forceps; flexible and rigid alligator forceps (11-mm and 6-mm length jaws); 5 F biopsy forceps; 5 F grasping forceps; 5 F rat-tooth grasping forceps; 5 F 4-strand grasping forceps; 5 F Bugbee electrode
Olympus	6 F, 7 F, 10 F foreign-body forceps; 10 F flexible stone-grasping forceps; 5 F biopsy forceps; 5 F grasping forceps; 5 F 2-prong grasper; 5 F washing pipe (Retroject); 5 F retrieval basket
Storz	5 F, 7 F, 9 F flexible alligator grasper; 5 F, 7 F, 9 F flexible biopsy forceps; 3-pronged grasping forceps with channel for electrohydraulic probe; 5 F Dormia stone dislodger; 26 F Mauermeyer kidney stone punch; triradiate stone forceps with telescope; 5 F, 7 F, 10 F foreign-body forceps
Wolf	9 F coagulation-biopsy forceps; 5 F, 7 F, 10 F biopsy forceps; 5.5 F, 4 F Dormia stone basket; 7.5 F rigid stone forceps; 7.5 F rigid stone forceps with fine teeth; 7.5 F rigid stone dislodger with parallel jaws; 9 F stone dislodger, 3-arm
Pentax	5 F biopsy forceps; 5 F crocodile forceps; 5 F 3-pronged grasper; 5 F V-shaped grasping forceps; 5 F retrieval basket
Wolf	5 F helical stone extractors (3-, 4-, 5-wire baskets with flexible tip, occlusive tip, or removable tip); 5 F grasping forceps (55 cm long); 4.5 F loop retrievers; 11 F Hawkins stone basket
Cook	Ureteral catheters: 5-8 F safety wire ureteral catheter (open-ended catheter), 70 cm long, accepts 0.038-in. diameter wire guide; guide wires: straight safety wire guide (for use with safety wire ureteral catheter) 0.038-in. diameter; Teflon-coated straight safety wire guide, 0.038-in. and 0.028-in. diameter; with 1 cm, 3 cm, or 10 cm flexible tip
Van-Tec	Ureteral catheters: 5-8 F open-ended ureteral catheter with 0.038-in. diameter wire guide; guide wires: Teflon-coated, 0.038-in. and 0.028-in. diameter, 150 cm long, 3 cm flexible tip

transmitted through two fiberoptic bundles (noncoherent bundles) and visualization is through a single image-transmitting bundle with coherent bundles (Fig 18–3).

ENDOSCOPIC ACCESSORIES

Endoscopic accessories (Fig 18–4 and Table 18–1) consist of (1) baskets (loops, stone baskets with no tip, and baskets with filiform tip), (2) grasping forceps (flexible forceps, alligator forceps, stone forceps, biopsy forceps, triradiate forceps, and three- and four-pronged graspers), (3) other accessories (forceps with diathermy facility, 4 F and 9 F electrosurgical probes, 26 F kidney stone crusher, and 26 F Mauer-Mayer stone punch).

DISINTEGRATORS

Ultrasonic Lithotriptor

In ultrasonic lithotripsy electrical energy is transformed into ultrasonic energy, which, when applied to a calculus, causes it to disintegrate. Ultrasonic energy is produced by electrically activating a piezoceramic element in the transducer. The acoustic resonators in the transducer then transmit longitudinal vibrations (approximately 23,000

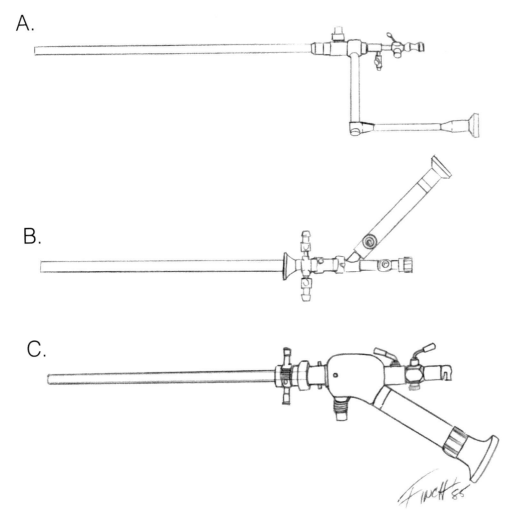

Fig 18–1. Rigid nephroscopes. **A,** Wolf nephroscope (24 F) with 90 degree offset lens. **B,** Storz nephroscope (26 F) with 30 degree offset lens. **C,** ACMI ARN-19 (24 F) with 30 degree offset lens.

to 27,000 cycles/second, that is 23 to 27 kHz) along a long hollow metal probe, the vibrating tip of which when applied to calculus causes it to fragment. These fragments are simultaneously suctioned through the hollow center of the probe and transducer into a collecting chamber (Figs 18–5 and 18–6).

Equipment and Assembly

The ultrasonic equipment consists of the nephroscope, the sonotrode, and the generator (see Fig 18–5). The nephroscope consists of the sheath, which adapts to the offset lens. The lens is offset to allow for the rigid ultrasound probe and other rigid instruments. The sonotrode consists of the metal probe and the transducer (see Fig 18–6). The proximal part of the transducer has two attachments; one is a wire to be plugged into the generator and the other, an open-ended channel, is connected to suction and is in direct continuity with the hollow metal probe. The suction tubing can be connected either to wall suction or to a suctioning device marketed with the equipment.

When the Storz equipment is used, the metal probes have to be tightened with a wrench (provided with the set) to the distal shaft of the transducer. These metal probes need to be replaced when the distal oscillating crown of the probe wears off. With the Wolf equipment the metal probe and the transducer is a fixed unit (sonotrode) and two sonotrodes are provided. Physiologic saline is used for irrigation and delivered to

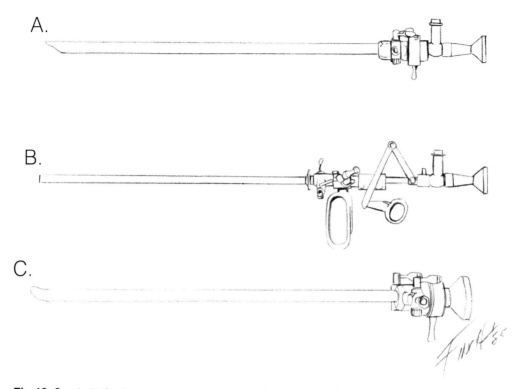

Fig 18–2. **A,** McCarthy panendoscope, 20 and 24 F with 30 and 70 degree lens. **B,** direct vision urethrotome, 21 F, 0 degree lens. **C,** cystoscope (Olympus, ACMI, Storz, Wolf) showing curved tip.

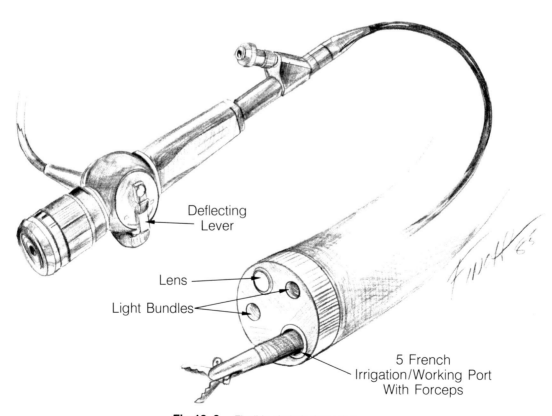

Fig 18–3. Flexible choledochonephroscope.

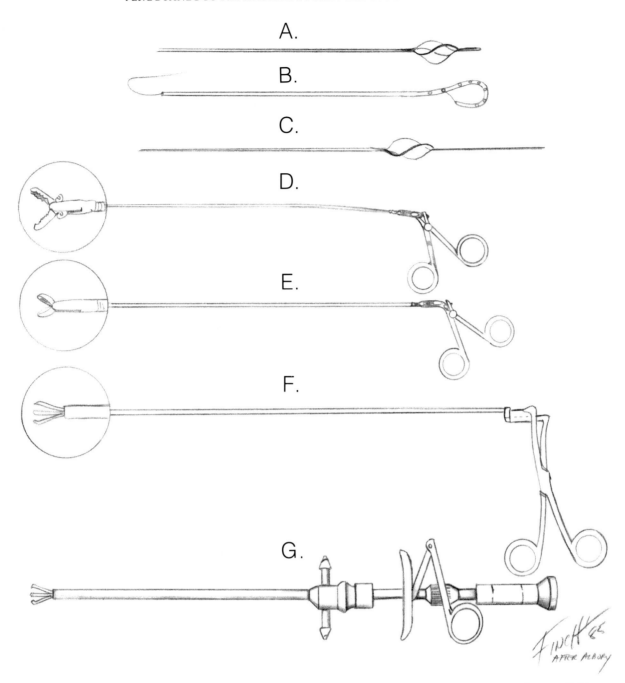

Fig 18–4. **A,** stone basket with no tip. **B,** ureteral snare. **C,** stone basket with filliform tip. **D,** alligator forceps. **E,** biopsy forceps. **F,** three-pronged graspers. **G,** triradiate forceps.

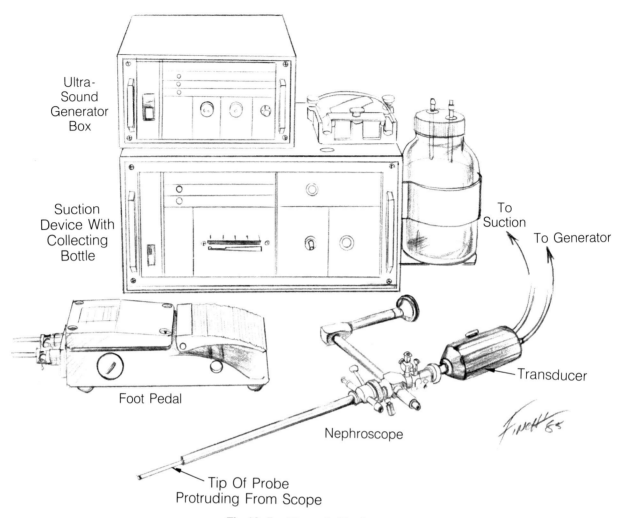

Fig 18–5.   Ultrasonic lithotripter.

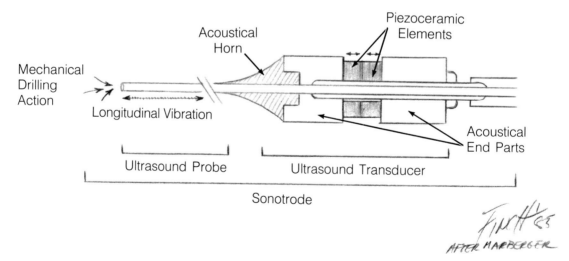

Fig 18–6.   Details of ultrasonic sonotrode.

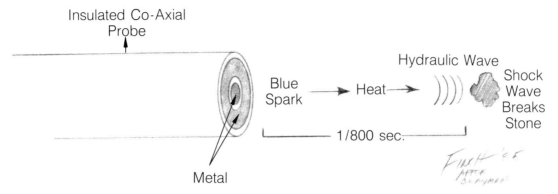

Fig 18–7. Principle of electrohydraulic lithotripsy.

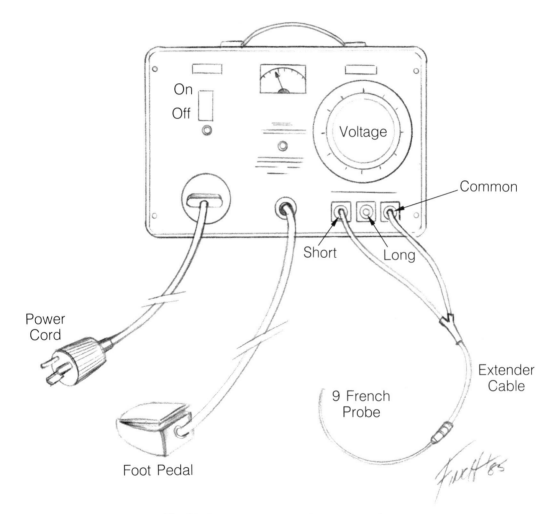

Fig 18–8. Electrohydraulic lithotriptor: overview.

the inflow port of the nephroscope sheath. The outflow channel can be connected to suction to provide for continuous flow.

Caution

When using the suction device it is very important to connect the suction tubing from the transducer in the correct direction (i.e., suction from transducer to the suction bottle). If it is hooked up in the opposite direction, there is a significant risk of air embolism.

Electrohydraulic Lithotriptor

In electrohydraulic lithotripsy, electrical energy is transformed in a fluid medium to hydraulic shock waves sufficient to disintegrate calculi.

An electrical discharge transmitted through an insulated coaxial probe creates a high-voltage spark at the tip of the probes and sets off hydraulic shock waves, the force of which crack the calculi (Fig 18–7).

Equipment and Assembly

The electrohydraulic lithotriptor consists of the generator and the cable, to which is attached the working probe (Fig 18–8). The generator is connected to a power outlet through the power cord and activated by the foot pedal. The power of discharge can be varied by adjusting the voltage (0 to 120 volts, ACMI). Most calculi can be disintegrated between 70 and 100 volts. Also, the discharges per second, short (50 cycles/second) or long (100 cycles/second), can be selected. The cable has two arms, one of which is connected to the common terminal and the other to either the short or long terminal of the generator box. The distal end of the cable connects to the flexible coaxial probes (5, 7, or 9 F). Depressing the foot pedal results in discharge at the tip of the coaxial probe (the Pentax and Wolf equipment work on a similar basis).

The life span of the coaxial probe varies from 15 to 50 seconds. Disintegration of a large calculus (especially bladder) often requires several probes.

CHAPTER 19

Percutaneous Nephrolithotomy: Techniques of Rigid Endoscopy

Pratap K. Reddy, M.D.

After an appropriate size nephrostomy tract is established, endoscopic techniques should precede fluoroscopic techniques of stone removal because endoscopic stone extraction is simple and less traumatic. Fluoroscopic attempts may cause bleeding or clotting, making subsequent endoscopy difficult; if endoscopy is unsuccessful, however, fluoroscopic maneuvers are still possible.

It is easier and preferable to remove calculi with the rigid endoscope rather than the flexible one, because for any given stone, the vision and grasping capabilities of the rigid endoscope are much better (Fig 19–1).

To be able to use the rigid nephroscope, access to the calculus should be relatively straight (Fig 19–2).

After the nephrostomy tract is dilated, removal of calculus is first facilitated by the use of the Teflon sheath. Its advantages include the following: provides repeated access to the collecting system; effects tamponade of the tract, prevents absorption of fluid through tract, prevents buildup of intrarenal pressure from irrigating fluid, and prevents trauma to the tract during stone extraction (Fig 19–3).

Calculi smaller than 1 cm are best removed intact through a Teflon sheath of appropriate size,

using nephroscopes and alligator graspers (7 or 9 F) (Fig 19–4).

However, if the calculus has a larger diameter than 1 cm (greater than 30 F), it still may be possible, depending on the shape of the stone, to extract it intact by rotating the stone in the appropriate axis (Fig 19–5).

Occasionally a stone slightly larger than the internal diameter of the Teflon sheath (the internal diameter of all sheaths is 4 F smaller than the outer measurement) can be removed intact by withdrawing the sheath, the nephroscope, and the stone, together. Of course, the safety catheter stays in place (Fig 19–6).

When removing stone and sheath, one must be prepared to place a nephrostomy tube immediately, because significant bleeding may occur from the tract. Also, on occasion the stone may be trapped at the level of the lumbodorsal fascia (Fig 19–7,A). If this happens, then a single attempt can be made to perform endoscopy of the tract by following the guide wire. If the calculus is visualized, attempts may be made to rotate the stone, grasp it in a different axis, and retrieve it. Alternatively, a larger grasper may be used to secure a better grip on the stone for extraction. If these attempts are unsuccessful then a knife can be advanced alongside the nephroscope to incise the

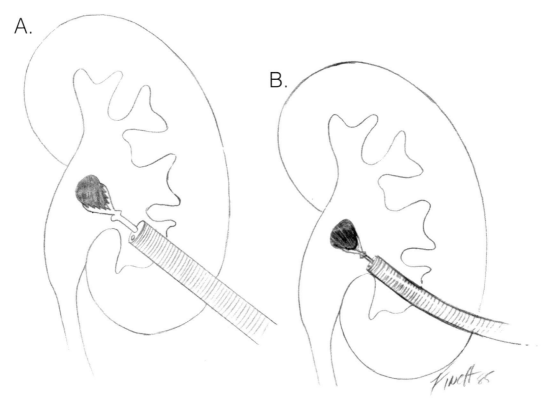

Fig 19–1.   Calculus removal with: rigid nephroscope and grasper **(A)**; flexible nephroscope and grasper **(B)**.

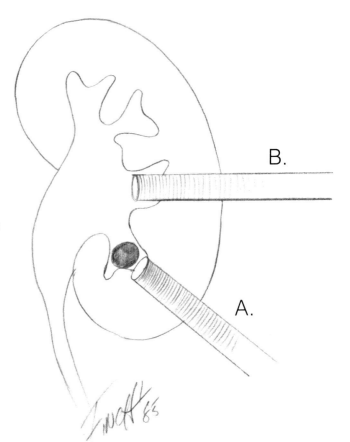

Fig 19–2.   Access to calculus: straight **(A)**; through adjacent calyx **(B)**.

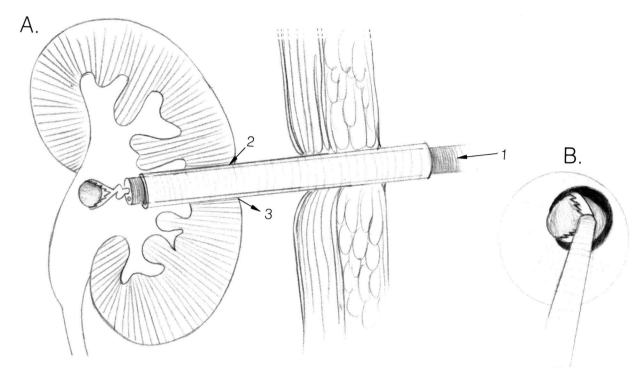

Fig 19–3. **A,** advantages of calculus removal through Teflon sheath: (1) enables repeated access to collecting system; (2) effects tamponades of the tract; and (3) prevents loss of irrigating fluid in retroperitoneum. **B,** end-on view of calculus traumatizing the tract if Teflon sheath is not used.

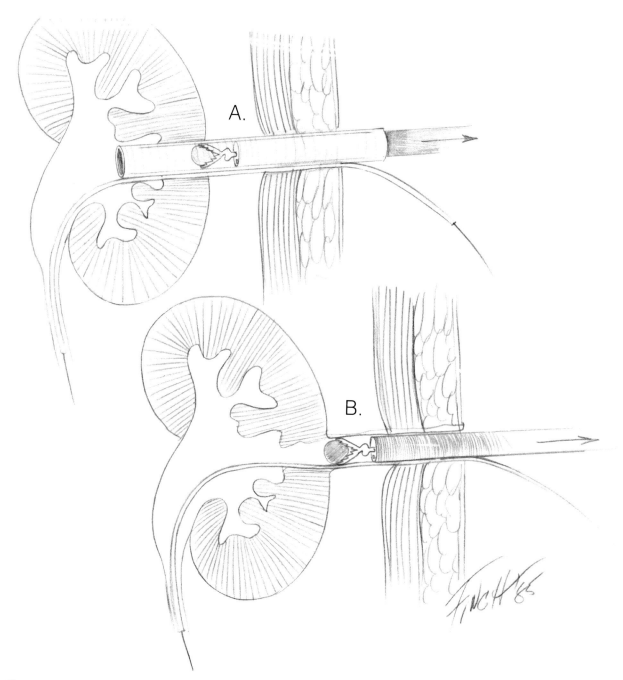

Fig 19–4. Removal of calculus with rigid nephroscope and graspers: through teflon sheath **(A)**; nephrostomy tract without Teflon sheath **(B)**.

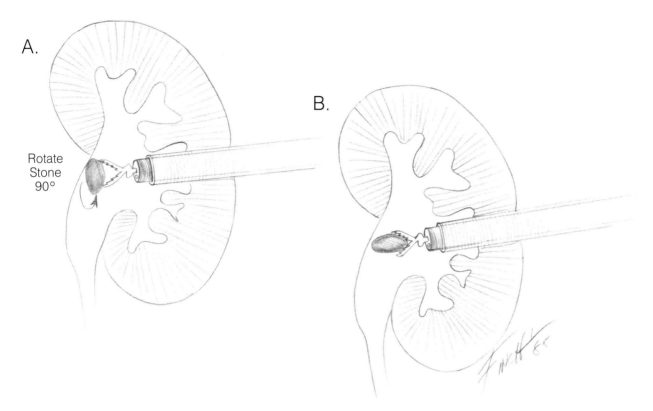

Fig 19–5. Removal of a large calculus by rotating it in the appropriate axis.

fascia (Fig 19–7,B). If endoscopic attempts are unsuccessful, then a Randall or a Mazzariello-Caprini forceps should be used under fluoroscopic control to stretch the fascia and remove the stone (Fig 19–7,C). Persistence of endoscopic attempts to remove the stone can at times lead to further dislodgment of the stone in the retroperitoneum, making subsequent fluoroscopic removal difficult. This also increases the risk of fluid absorption (Fig 19–7,D). Leaving the stone in the tract is an option, though it is disappointing to the patient and the physician and may hinder placement of the nephrostomy tube.

When access to the collecting system is not through the stone-containing calyx or when two calyceal stones are located in different calyces, occasionally the rigid nephroscope can be manipulated into the appropriate calyx. This procedure is more feasible with a large intrarenal pelvis and with kidneys that have not been operated on (Fig 19–8). If this is not possible, then other techniques may be necessary to dislodge the stone into the renal pelvis. These techniques include a variety of purely fluoroscopic maneuvers or intrarenal cutting to gain access.

Sometimes large calculi (about 1.2 cm) can be removed intact by using the triradiate grasper. The prongs of this grasper are strong, affording it better grip on the stone; also, the lens system can be retracted to better accommodate the stone in the sheath (see Chapter 18).

Calculi larger than 1.5 cm are best removed by disintegration using the ultrasonic lithotriptor.

INSERTION OF THE ULTRASONIC NEPHROSCOPE

After the nephrostomy tract is dilated to the appropriate size (28 F for Storz and 26 F for Wolf instruments), the sheath with its tapered hollow obturator is passed over the guide wire into the collecting system (Fig 19–9,A). Alternatively, the nephroscope sheath with appropriate fascia dilator

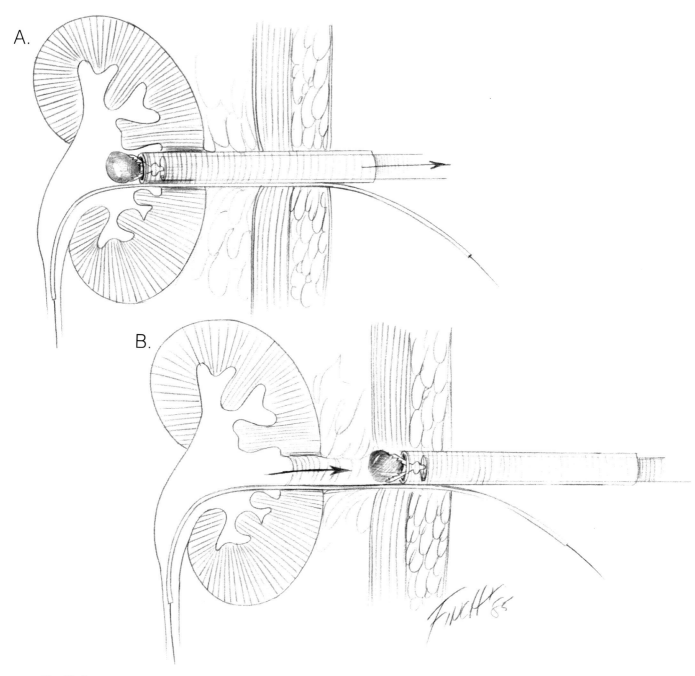

Fig 19–6.   Removal of a calculus slightly larger than the lumen of the Teflon sheath. **A,** calculus snug against the Teflon sheath. **B,** removal of calculus along with the Teflon sheath. The safety catheter remains.

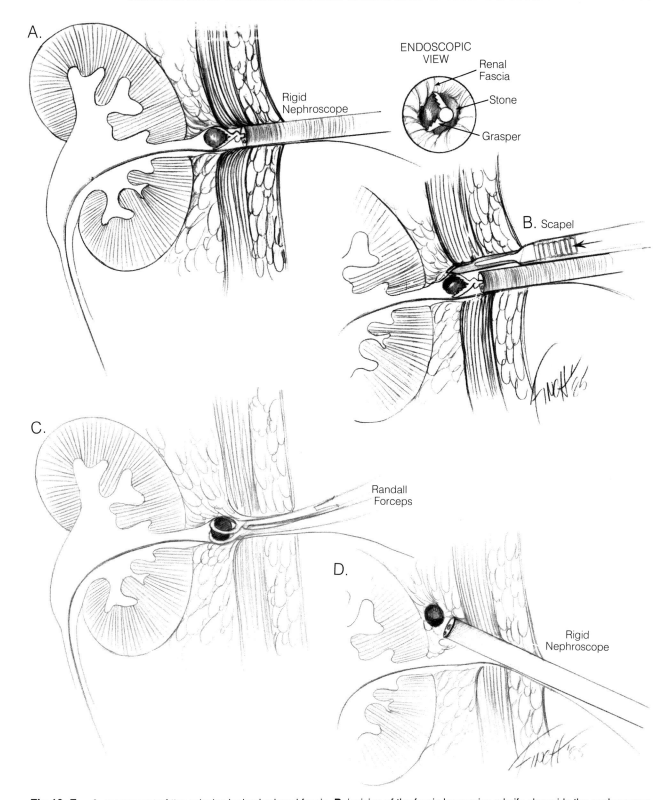

Fig 19–7. **A,** entrapment of the calculus by lumbodorsal fascia. **B,** incision of the fascia by passing a knife alongside the nephroscope. **C,** removal of calculus using Randall forceps. **D,** dislodgment of calculus in the retroperitoneum.

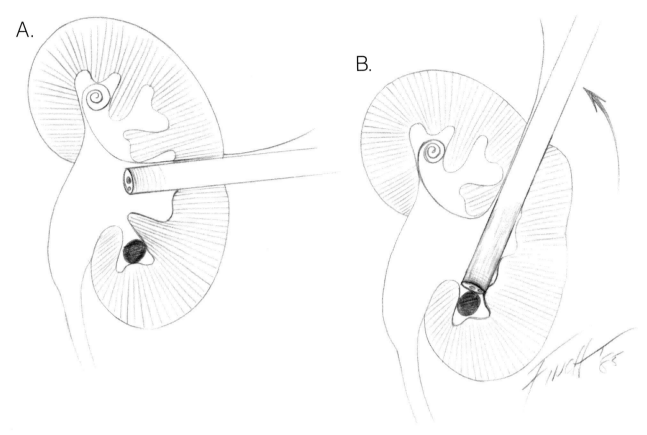

Fig 19–8. **A,** access through an adjacent calyx. **B,** rigid nephroscope successfully manipulated into stone-containing calyx.

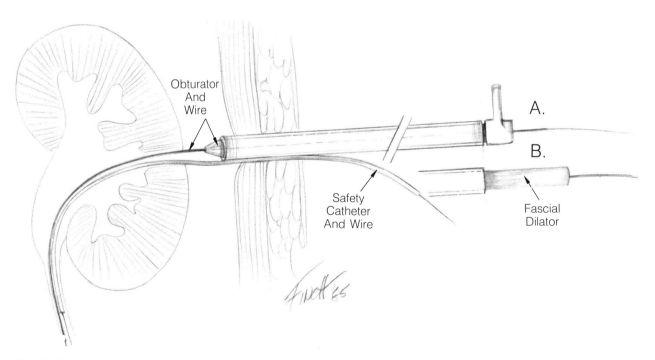

Fig 19–9. Insertion of ultrasonic nephroscope sheath. **A,** using the nephroscope obturator. **B,** using fascial dilator (showing proximal end).

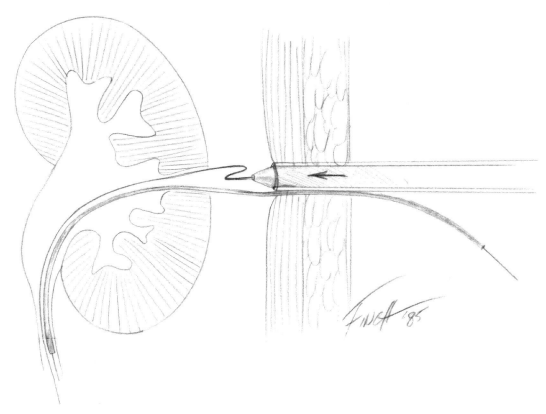

Fig 19–10.   Kinked guide wire. Avoided by keeping the guide wire taut during dilation.

(22 F for Wolf and 24 F for the Storz nephroscope) is passed over the guide wire (Fig 19–9,B). This part of the insertion is done under fluoroscopic control. Care is taken not to kink the guide wire, as this may lead to bleeding and/or false passage. Also, it may require having to change the guide wire (Fig 19–10). The nephroscope sheath and obturator should be passed as a single unit well into the collecting system; otherwise, the tip of the sheath may remain outside the collecting system and further endoscopic advancement (without the obturator) will lead to trauma and bleeding (Fig 19–11). The position of the sheath should be checked with contrast material.

The ultrasonic nephroscope can be used through a Teflon sheath (26 F and 28 F respectively for the Wolf and Storz nephroscopes). This allows for multiple passes of the nephroscope while providing constant tamponade of the tract. It also facilitates nephrostomy tube placement at the end of the procedure. However, use of the Teflon sheath may decrease maneuverability of the nephroscope within the kidney and may prevent adequate distension of the collecting system.

TECHNIQUE OF ULTRASONIC LITHOTRIPSY

Proper Positioning

The sonotrode is held with the right hand and the nephroscope sheath is held with the left hand and the left forearm rests on the patient's body reducing operator fatigue while ensuring a firm grip on the instrument throughout the procedure (Fig 19–12). If the nephroscope sheath is not supported, there is a tendency to plunge the nephroscope sheath deeper than is necessary (due to the weight of the equipment and the operator's body), resulting in renal pelvic perforation.

Visualization

Under fluoroscopic control, the nephroscope usually can be placed in close proximity to the stone. The initial endoscopic view may not be clear due to blood clots. Following suction of these clots, the stone usually is easily visualized. Also, distending the collecting system by clamping the suction tubing improves vision.

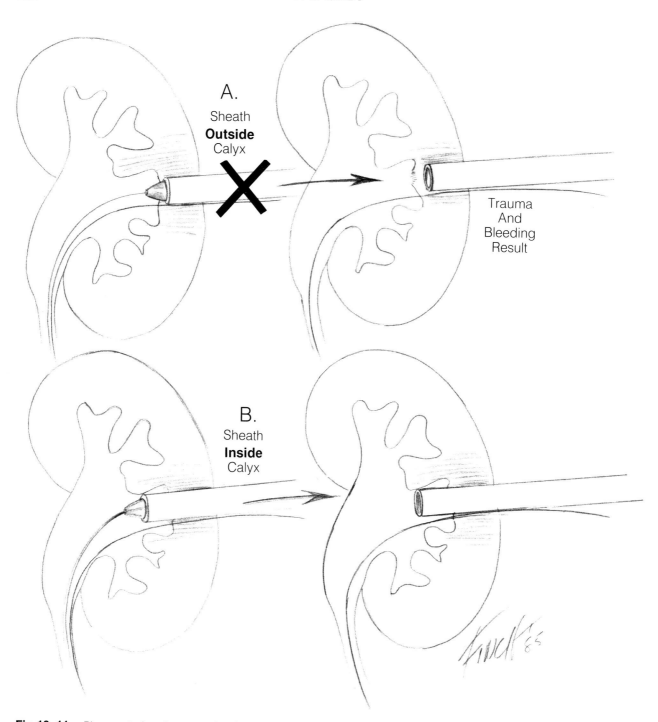

Fig 19–11. Placement of nephroscope sheath under fluoroscopy. **A,** incorrect placement of nephroscope sheath. Removal of obturator leaves the sheath outside the calyx, causing trauma and bleeding when the sheath is further advanced under endoscopy. **B,** correct position of the nephroscope sheath.

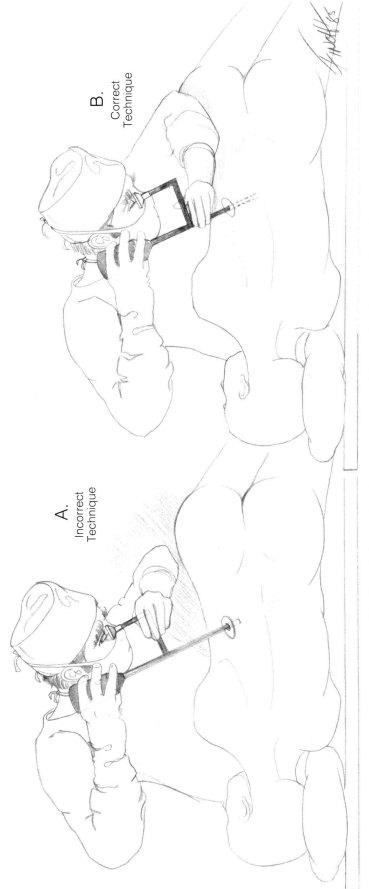

Fig 19–12. Position of the operator during ultrasonic lithotripsy. **A,** incorrect posture causes operator fatigue and tendency to plunge the nephroscope into the kidney due to his weight and the weight of the equipment. **B,** correct position: forearm rests on patient's body; this stabilizes the instrument and increases operator comfort.

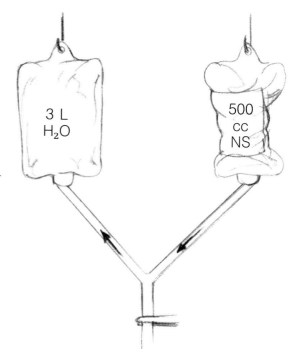

Fig 19–13. Technique of preparing 1/7 normal saline (NS): The contents of normal saline bag are squeezed into the bag containing water.

Disintegration

Introduction of the ultrasonic probe should be under vision because the probe is longer than the nephroscope sheath and blind passage may perforate the renal pelvis. The probe should be in contact with the stone for disintegration. Usually with small stones, the negative force of the suction causes the stone to adhere to the tip. However, larger calculi may need to be pinned against the wall of the renal pelvis. The suction tubing must be clamped to allow expansion of the renal pelvis for clear visualization of the stone. During lithotripsy the irrigant should flow freely to avoid overheating of the probe and the suction tubing should be patent for removal of the disintegrated fragments. Occasionally stone fragments clog the suction tubing; the operator can usually recognize this because vision is impaired or the probe becomes hot.

Disintegration commences along the periphery of the stone, gradually decreasing its size. The particles are suctioned as they disintegrate. When larger fragments break off from the main stone mass they should be immediately pursued and disintegrated with the probe lest they move into an inaccessible calyx. The main stone mass can subsequently be disintegrated.

With care, significant maneuverability can be achieved with the rigid nephroscope. In situations in which the nephroscope cannot be advanced into a stone-containing calyx due to a narrow infundibulum, the probe is advanced into the calyx and the stone disintegrated under fluoroscopic control (Plate 6). This can be done safely, as the ultrasonic probe does not cause damage to the mucosa. Irrespective of the location of the stone following disintegration, it is always important at the end of the procedure to look at the ureteropelvic junction since it is not uncommon to find several small fragments held in position by the occluding ureteral catheters, and these fragments can easily be suctioned out.

TECHNIQUE OF ELECTROHYDRAULIC LITHOTRIPSY

Electrohydraulic lithotripsy is less commonly used than ultrasonic lithotripsy for calculus disintegration.

The essential steps in electrohydraulic lithotripsy are as follows:

1. The irrigating fluid should consist of 1/7 normal saline. Water may be used, but the discharge is suboptimal and in pure electrolyte solution it does not function. An easy way of preparing 3.5 L of 1/7 normal saline is to transfer 500 ml of normal saline to a 3-L bag of water (Fig 19–13).

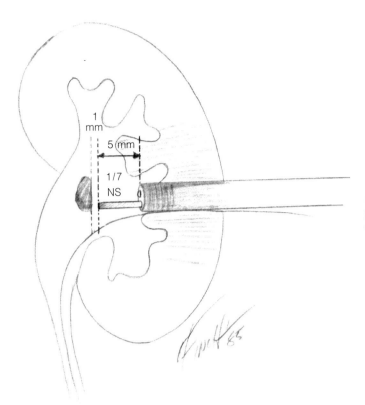

Fig 19–14. Technique of electrohydraulic lithotripsy: The probe is 5 mm from the lens, 1 mm from the stone. Solution of 1/7 normal saline (NS) is used for irrigation.

2. The 7 and 9 F probes are used with the rigid nephroscopes. The 5 F probes fit through the flexible choledochonephroscope. The disintegrating capability proportionally increases with the size of the probe. During disintegration, the tip of the probe should be at least 5 mm from the tip of the lens (to prevent lens damage) and about 1 mm from the calculus (Fig 19–14). The probe should be discharged only under vision, starting at the most irregular area on the stone. Repeated discharges at this particular spot quickly break the stone.

Electrohydraulic lithotripsy should be used to disintegrate larger calculi into one or two smaller pieces, which are subsequently removed with the graspers. Disintegration of the stone into multiple small pieces only makes subsequent removal more difficult.

Drawbacks of Electrohydraulic Lithotripsy

The drawbacks of electrohydraulic lithotripsy are as follows: (1) If the probe is accidentally discharged on the renal pelvic mucosa, perforation or bleeding may ensue. (2) Due to the use of hypotonic solution, absorption of the fluid may lead to hyponatremia and hemolysis. (3) The system does not allow for simultaneous disintegration and removal of stone fragments. Use of the 5 F probe and electrohydraulic lithotripsy is the only available method for disintegration using the flexible choledochonephroscope. However, this maneuver is tedious when trying to disintegrate larger calculi.

CHAPTER 20

Percutaneous Nephrolithotomy: Techniques of Flexible Endoscopy

Pratap K. Reddy, M.D.

Flexible nephroscopy permits adequate visualization of the entire collecting system. However, significant problems exist when trying to retrieve stones greater than 5 mm in diameter. The instrument is most useful for removing stone fragments after lithotripsy or small calculi not in direct line of the nephrostomy tract.

FAMILIARITY WITH THE INSTRUMENT

The instrument is held with the right hand (dominant hand). The left hand steadies the shaft of the scope at the skin level and helps to gently guide the shaft in coordination with manipulations of the right hand (Fig 20–1). The tip of the nephroscope is deflected in one plane by movement of the thumb on the deflecting lever. Deflection in the perpendicular plane is obtained by rotating the wrist and the instrument through 90° (Fig 20–2).

Most instruments have an endoscopic marker at the 12 o'clock position, for orientation (Fig 20–3).

PASSAGE OF THE INSTRUMENT

The flexible nephroscope is ideally used through a Teflon sheath. However, in mature tracts the instrument can be passed under vision, similar to urethroscopy with a cystoscope. Unlike the rigid endoscope, the flexible endoscope is advanced around bends in the tract by deflecting the tip (through the deflecting lever) rather than by bending the shaft of the scope. If resistance is encountered in negotiating the lumen of the tract, it is advisable to retract the scope a centimeter or two and to readvance it under vision. Blind passage of the scope may occasionally be required when traversing a short segment of the nephrostomy tract or a short infundibulum into a calyx (similar to blind passage of the rigid cystoscope through the prostatic urethra).

INTRARENAL ENDOSCOPY

The endoscopist should first have a mental image of the anatomy of the collecting system (Fig 20–4). It is also important to know through which calyx the nephrostomy tract has been established. In the initial stages of nephroscopy it is ideal to follow a set pattern. The nephroscope is advanced into the renal pelvis and guided to the ureteropelvic junction by following either the guide wire or the safety catheter. It is then successfully manipulated into the lower, middle, and upper calyces (Fig 20–5).

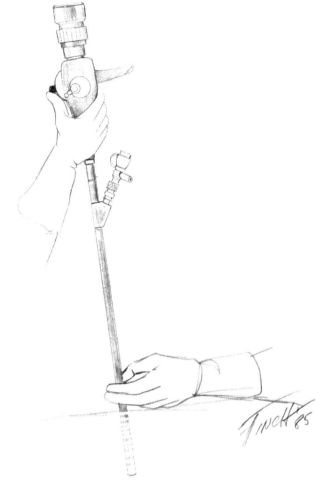

Fig 20–1. Flexible choledochonephroscope: The right hand (dominant) holds the instrument with the thumb on the deflecting lever. The left hand steadies the shaft at the entry site into the body.

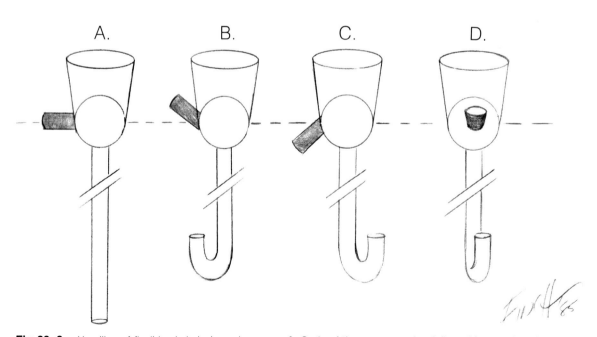

Fig 20–2. Handling of flexible choledochonephroscope. **A–C,** tip of the scope can be deflected in one place by turning the deflecting lever. **D,** deflection in a perpendicular plane is obtained by 90 degree rotation of the instrument.

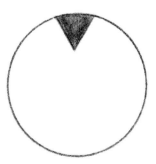

Fig 20–3. Endoscopic marker usually seen through flexible scope at 12 o'clock position for orientation.

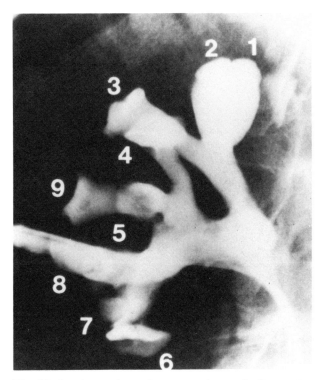

Fig 20–4. Antegrade pyelogram to show collecting system anatomy for endoscopic orientation.

AIDS FOR INTRARENAL ORIENTATION

The ureter is best identified by following the safety catheter. To enter the calyx, the infundibular opening into the renal pelvis is first identified; entering this orifice will lead into the calyx iden-

tified by the papilla (Fig 20–6). If during endoscopy (especially if the renal pelvis is small) it is not possible to visualize the infundibular ostium, then radiopaque contrast can be injected through the flexible nephroscope and the anatomy determined by fluoroscopy. The nephroscope can then be advanced into the desired calyx using fluoroscopic control (Fig 20–7). Alternatively, a guide wire can be placed in the desired calyx under fluoroscopy after which the nephroscope can easily follow this guide wire under vision into the proper calyx. Sometimes an endoscopist may suddenly lose orientation. This can be easily regained by fluoroscopic visualization, with or without injecting a bolus of radiopaque contrast.

CALYCEAL STONE REMOVAL USING GRASPERS

The flexible 5 F alligator grasper works well for retrieving stones. However, due to the small size of the jaws (3 mm) usually only stones 5 mm or less can be removed. Several technical problems can be encountered during stone removal. When the stone is visualized and the grasper is advanced, more often than not the grasper passes alongside the stone. This is because the catheterizing port of the flexible nephroscope is set to one side of the lens (Fig 20–8,A and B). In order to grasp the stone, the nephroscope tip with the grasper jaws opened must be actually deflected onto the stone (Fig 20–8,B and C). Sometimes the endoscopist may find that he can clearly see the jaws of the grasper but that he is still unable to open the jaws. This is because of the construction of the jaws; it is necessary that they be advanced far beyond the tip of the nephroscope before they can be opened (Fig 20–9). As a result, visualization of the stone becomes more difficult; also, attempts at opening the grasper in a small calyx may result in the nephroscope retracting into the renal pelvis, thus totally losing sight of the stone (Fig 20–10). Also, when the stone is securely grasped the scope should be withdrawn into the sheath under vision, lest the stone be dislodged by intervening tissue. Sometimes it may be possible to visualize a stone that is located in a calyx at an acute angle to the nephrostomy tract, yet it may be impossible to pass any instruments through the acute bend in the scope. Forcing the graspers through this bend will only result in damage to the scope (Fig 20–11).

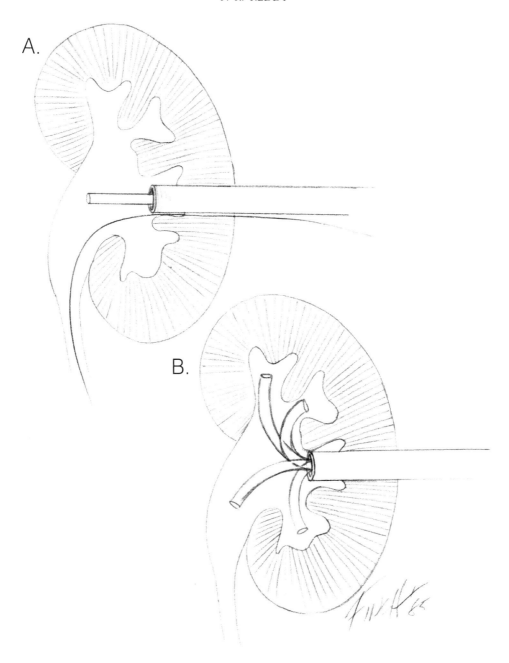

Fig 20–5.   Flexible nephroscopy. **A,** finding the ureteropelvic junction by following the guide wire. **B,** subsequent visualization of the lower, middle, and upper calyces.

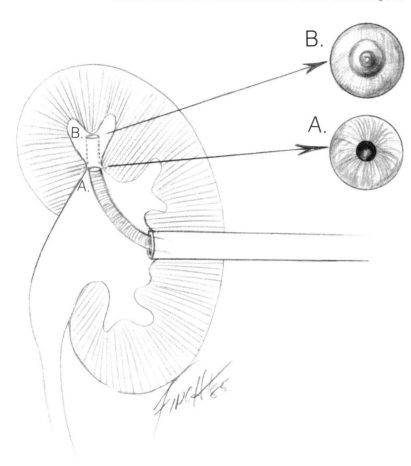

Fig 20–6. Flexible nephroscopy. **A,** appearance of infundibular opening. **B,** calyx identified by the renal papilla.

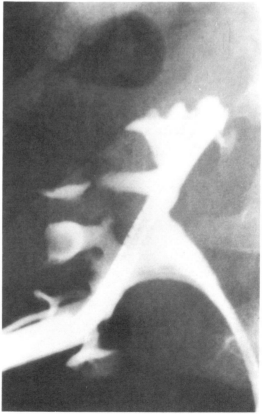

Fig 20–7. X-ray of nephroscope being advanced into calyx under fluoroscopic control.

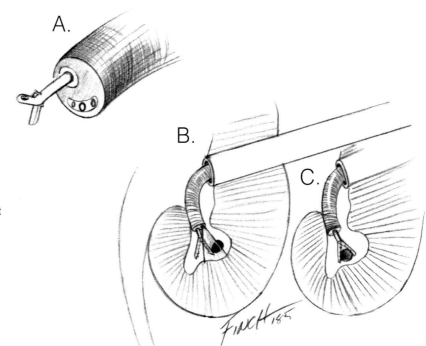

Fig 20–8. Calyceal stone removed with flexible choledochonephroscope and graspers. **A and B,** tip of the flexible choledochonephroscope showing the catheterizing part offset from the lens. **C,** with the jaws of the grasper open alongside the stone the nephroscope must be further deflected to engage the stone.

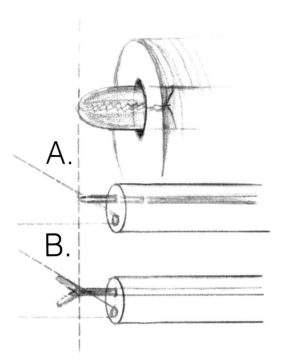

Fig 20–9. **A and B,** tip of the graspers exiting from the flexible choledochonephroscope.

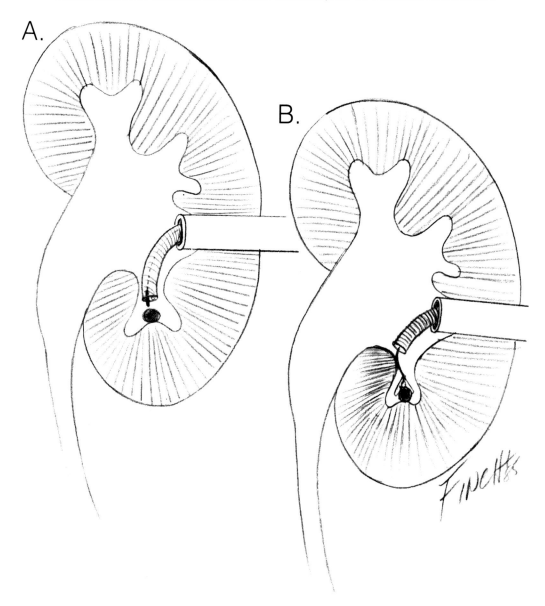

Fig 20–10. **A,** grasper seen but cannot be opened since the jaws are still within the nephroscope. **B,** graspers advanced sufficient to open them results in retraction of the nephroscope and the stone is no longer seen.

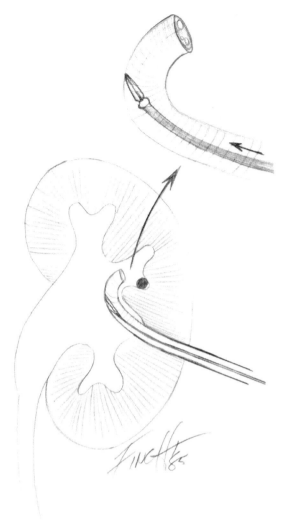

Fig 20–11. Calculus seen with the flexible choledochonephroscope, but graspers cannot be passed through the acute bend.

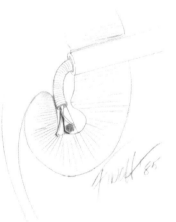

Fig 20–12. Stone retrieval using flexible choledochonephroscope and three-pronged grasper. Note one of the prongs embedded in the calyx.

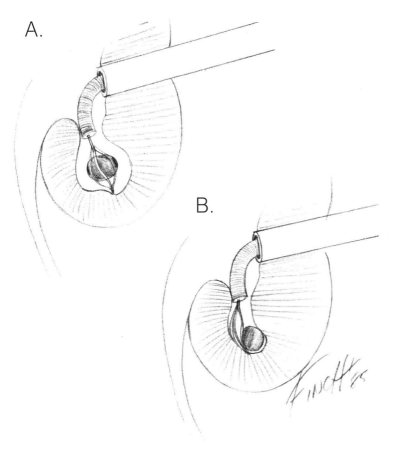

Fig 20–13. Calyceal stone removal using baskets. **A,** dilated calyx enables stone entrapment with basket. **B,** nondilated calyx does not allow basket to open.

STONE RETRIEVAL WITH THREE- AND FOUR-PRONGED GRASPERS

Occasionally the three- and four-pronged graspers may be used for retrieving stones. However, these graspers do not have a strong hold on the stones and there is a greater tendency of losing the stone within the infundibulum. Also, during endoscopy, one or more prongs may not be seen (since the angle of view in water is approximately 25° less than in the air). Hence with this semi-blind grasping and manipulation of the stone, significant bleeding from the urothelium or renal damage can occur (Fig 20–12).

STONE RETRIEVAL USING BASKETS

The nonfiliform-type baskets may be used through the nephroscope to engage stones. Such an instrument is best used in situations in which the calyx is significantly dilated. If the calyx is not dilated, often there is no room for the basket to open. Forceful attempts at opening will result in bleeding or perforation (Fig 20–13).

TECHNIQUES TO DISLODGE THE STONE INTO THE RENAL PELVIS

A number of techniques can be utilized to dislodge a small calyceal stone into the renal pelvis for subsequent removal. A retroflushing catheter can be positioned adjacent to the calyceal stone, either by fluoroscopy or using a flexible nephroscope, and attempts can be made to flush the stone into the renal pelvis. Similarly, a Fogarty balloon can be used to withdraw the stone into the renal pelvis. The flexible tip of the nephroscope can, on occasion, be used as a snare to push the stone into the renal pelvis. Also, a significant length of the guide wire can be coiled around the stone and used as a "lasso" (Fig 20–14).

USE OF THE ELECTROHYDRAULIC PROBE

In selective instances, the 5 F probe of the electrohydraulic lithotriptor can be used to disintegrate large calyceal calculi. However, this is quite time-consuming because the transfer of energy

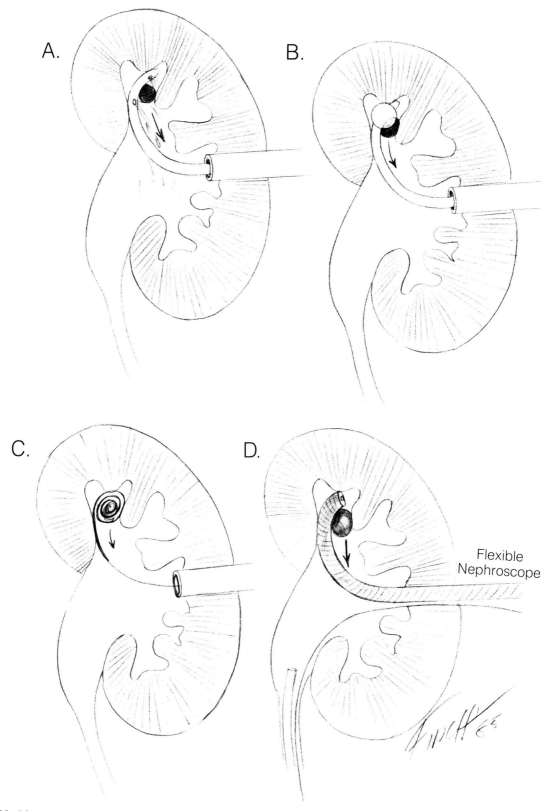

Fig 20–14. Dislodgement of calyceal stone into renal pelvis using retroflushing catheter **(A)**, Fogarty balloon **(B)**, guide wire **(C)**, and flexible choledochonephroscope **(D)**.

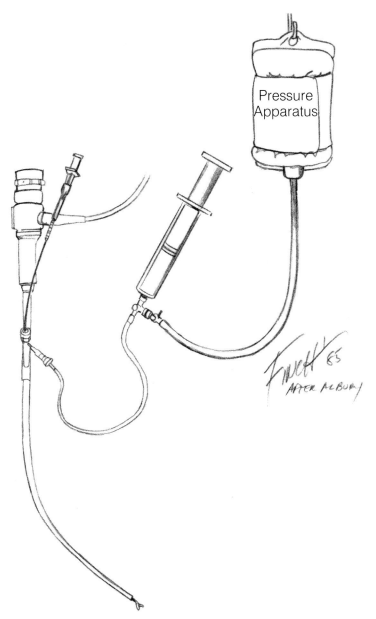

Fig 20–15. Irrigation assembly for flexible nephroscopy. Through the three-way stopcock, fluid can be delivered either through the pressurized bag or by a hand-injected piston syringe for better visualization.

through this small probe is very low, and disintegration can be tedious.

AIDS TO BETTER VISUALIZATION

Flexible endoscopy affords good visualization of the collecting system and the calculus. However, when any manipulative instrument is passed (common channel for irrigation and manipulation) vision is obscured due to a decrease in the flow of the irrigating fluid. This can be improved by increasing the pressure of the fluid delivery system (Fig 20–15). Alternatively, a second catheter can be positioned within the calyx adjacent to the stone and the irrigating fluid can be delivered through this catheter (Fig 20–16).

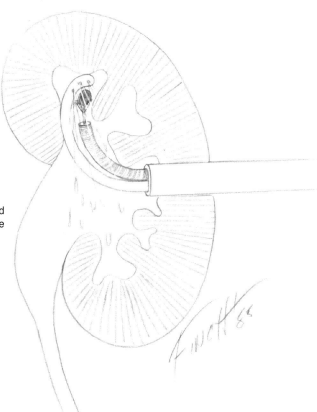

Fig 20–16. Irrigation for flexible nephroscopy. Irrigating fluid delivered through a catheter placed adjacent to the stone in the calyx for better visualization.

CHAPTER 21

Percutaneous Nephrolithotomy: Endoscopic Access and Manipulation

John C. Hulbert, M.D., F.R.C.S.

EVOLUTION OF CONDUIT TECHNOLOGY

The development of the percutaneous approach to the upper urinary tract has been dependent on the evolution of techniques of establishing safe access into the renal collecting system. The initial purpose was purely to aid drainage of the upper urinary tract with the aid of small (8 F) pigtail catheters. Subsequently the tract was dilated, first and tentatively by gradual dilation with urethral dilators or progressively larger nephrostomy tubes over a number of days, and then with increasing expertise by means of specifically designed Teflon dilators that could be passed over a guide wire. This allowed for more rapid dilation with dilators of increasing size up to 30 F. More recently rapid balloon dilation with angioplastic balloon catheters has gained increased acceptance.

Initially the nephrostomy tract was established and dilated a number of days prior to stone manipulation to allow the tract to mature around the nephrostomy tube. As far back as 1941 it had been observed that a blood-free conduit could form around a nephrostomy tube and allow endoscopic inspection of the interior of the kidney (Plate 7). Experience revealed that from two to five days are required for maturation sufficient to allow safe endoscopic instrumentation. This two-stage technique is still useful for those urologists with limited experience in endourology or for those cases likely to be especially difficult.

A one-stage percutaneous nephrolithotomy became a practical possibility as experience was gained and because of the practice of inserting a sheath prior to endoscopy. Although it is possible to insert a rigid instrument down a fresh tract, this technique is only suitable for single, small renal stones. Alternatively, with prior placement of a sheath bleeding will be tamponaded, which allows easier instrumentation of the interior of the collecting system in the acute instance. Also, repeated passage with the instrument can be achieved without trauma to the kidney.

ADVANTAGES AND PRECAUTIONS WHEN USING THE SHEATH

The sheath itself is made of Teflon and comes in sizes varying from 24 F to 30 F (Fig 21–1). The sheath will fit snugly over its respective Teflon dilator (Fig 21–2) and can be slid into the collecting system over the dilator by a firm twisting action on the sheath (Fig 21–3). Care should be taken to ensure that both sheath and dilator are advanced far enough into the collecting system so that the tapered end of the sheath is clear of the renal pa-

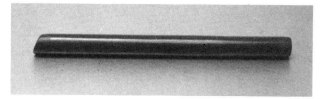

Fig 21–1. Teflon sheath. Note its tapered end.

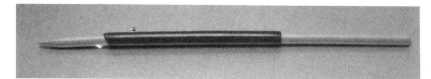

Fig 21–2. Sheath and dilator together.

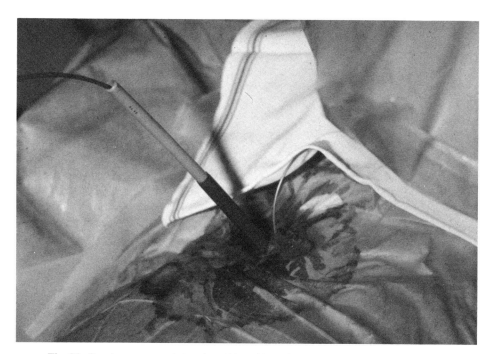

Fig 21–3. Appearance of sheath positioned in patient prior to removal of the dilator.

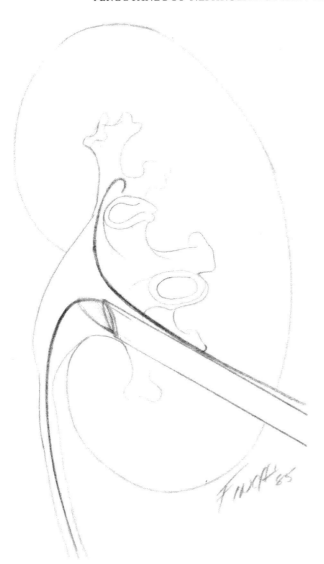

Fig 21–4. Dilator and sheath being advanced into the kidney over a guide wire.

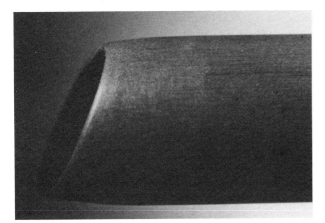

Fig 21–5. End of sheath illustrating its sharp edge and the potential of trauma to the kidney.

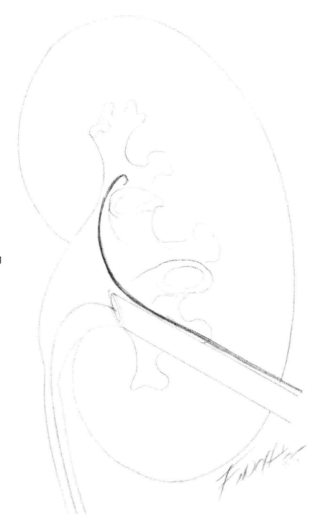

Fig 21–6. Following removal of the dilator, the sheath is sitting comfortably within the collecting system.

renchyma (Fig 21–4). If this precaution is not observed the sharp leading edge of the sheath (Fig 21–5) may cut the parenchyma and cause a significant hemorrhage.

When dilation, which is performed over a guide wire, is complete and the sheath inserted, the dilator is removed (Fig 21–6). The sheath should fit snugly inside the kidney (Plate 8) with a safety catheter having been passed over the safety guide wire alongside the sheath (Plate 9). The sheath is relatively radiolucent (Fig 21–7) and C-arm fluoroscopy will enable views to be obtained directly down the "eye" of the sheath (Fig 21–8). This will enable better appreciation of location and orientation of the stone with respect to the sheath. In addition, contrast can be passed down the sheath to ensure that it is sitting comfortably within the

collecting system and that there is no extravasation (Fig 21–9).

The location of the sheath within the kidney may be of importance. In the case of ureteral stones, the sheath should be advanced to the ureteral pelvic junction to allow the stone to be flushed up into the sheath (Figs 21–10 and 21–11). In those cases in which intrarenal surgery (electrosurgery or cold-knife incision) is anticipated in the region of the ureteropelvic junction or, indeed, if there is a stone located in the upper part of the kidney, then puncture and sheath placement into the upper part of the kidney facilitate intrarenal manipulation (Fig 21–12). For such an angle it may be necessary to transgress the pleural cavity by puncturing between the 11th and 12th ribs (see Chapter 16). In these circumstances the sheath

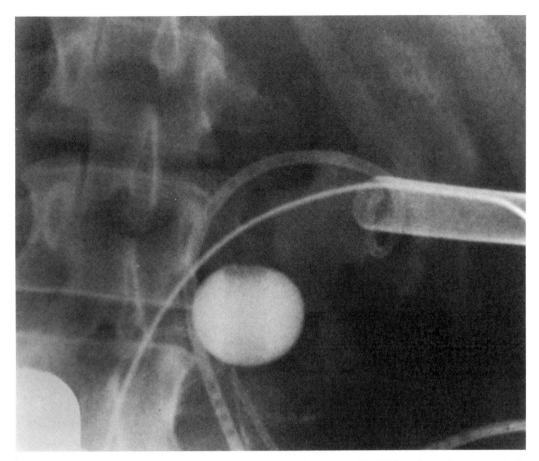

Fig 21–7.   Appearance of sheath on roentgenogram. Note the contrast-filled Foley of a nephrostomy tube in a second tract.

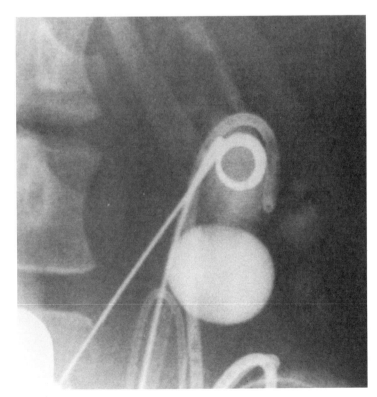

Fig 21–8.   Roentgenographic view directly down lumen of sheath (radiopaque ring) in the kidney as shown in Fig 21–7.

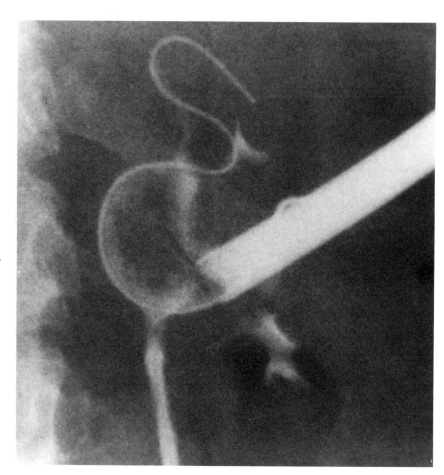

Fig 21–9. Roentgenographic appearance of sheath with contrast injected to confirm its correct position.

has the additional important function of preventing irrigation fluid from diffusing into the pleural cavity.

Visual inspection down the sheath of a freshly dilated tract will initially reveal a "red-out" (Plate 10). A guide wire left in place inside the sheath is a useful landmark (Plate 11). Grasping forceps will remove much of the clot, and the end of the sheath can be seen quite clearly in contact with the urothelium, which is inclined to be erythematous (Plate 12). The sheath will allow an endoscopic instrument to be passed gently and repeatedly in and out of the kidney without exacerbating hemorrhage or unduly disturbing the kidney (Plates 13 and 14). Small stones can be simply removed with suitable grasping forceps (Plates 15–17). Stones that are too large to be removed intact through the sheath can be either disintegrated by ultrasonic or electrohydraulic lithotripsy (Plate 18) or removed by withdrawal of the stone, instrument, and sheath at the same time. In the latter circumstance it is crucial to be prepared for prompt insertion of a nephrostomy tube or even an angiographic balloon catheter, because brisk bleeding may ensue from the abrasive effects of the stone in the nephrostomy tract (see Chapter 19). A significant increase in vascular complications has been noted following the simultaneous, intact removal of large stones and sheath.

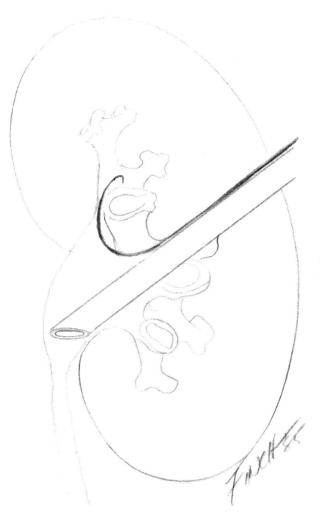

Fig 21–10.   The tapered end of the sheath is positioned over the ureteropelvic junction after puncture through a middle calyx. This will facilitate the removal of ureteral stones by retrograde flushing.

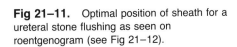

Fig 21–11.   Optimal position of sheath for a ureteral stone flushing as seen on roentgenogram (see Fig 21–12).

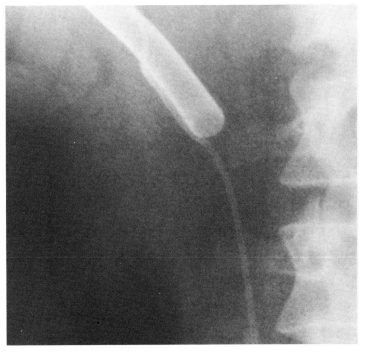

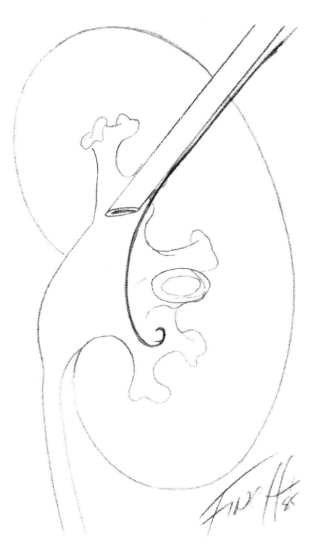

Fig 21–12. Puncture into the upper part of the kidney is preferable for stones in the upper part of the kidney and for intrarenal surgery in the region of the ureteropelvic junction.

CHAPTER 22

Percutaneous Nephrolithotomy: Drainage After Stone Removal

David W. Hunter, M.D.

Following percutaneous stone removal, the catheters that are left in the patient serve three functions: the first is to drain the collecting system, the second is to provide tamponade of the tract, and the third is to preserve access to the kidney in case either further procedures are necessary or complications, especially bleeding, should arise.

Almost all patients at the University of Minnesota have tract creations and stone removal performed in a single sitting. In these large (24 to 34 F) freshly dilated tracts, we prefer to use large (18 to 28 F) catheters to tamponade the tract and reduce bleeding complications. If it is obvious that a future procedure will be necessary, a catheter should be placed that is within 2 to 4 F of the size of the sheath or instrument that will be used in the next sitting. If no more procedures are planned, the size of the drainage catheter depends on the amount of bleeding. If the procedure has been easy, with minimal bleeding, we have used a catheter as small as 16 to 18 F, even if the external diameter of the working sheath was as large as 28 or 34 F.

In most patients a simple red rubber catheter is adequate (Fig 22–1). It is available in a variety of sizes and has a smooth external surface, which facilitates its introduction through what is often an irregular tract. The rubber material is firm enough so that it is easy to create an end hole and extra side holes, but soft enough to negotiate "corners" in the collecting system and be comfortable for the patient. It has a large lumen, which allows free outflow of urine, clots, and any residual tiny stone fragments. To place a Red Robinson through a tract from which the working sheath has been removed, a stiffener such as a dilator or an angiographic catheter is often useful (Fig 22–2). If the working sheath is still in place, introduction of the drainage catheter is even easier. Indeed, even a non–end-hole catheter such as a Malecot (Fig 22–3) can be used without difficulty. However, we prefer to place any drainage catheter over a guide wire to ensure that it will be inside the collecting system.

The drainage catheter tip is usually placed into the renal pelvis (Fig 22–4). In some cases, however, this would mean that only a short length of catheter would be intrarenal. In order to have a

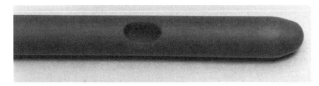

Fig 22–1. Red Robinson catheter tip.

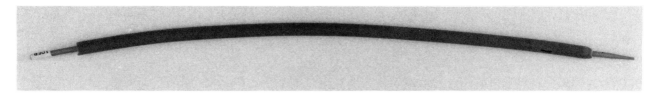

Fig 22–2.   10 F fascial dilator used as a stiffener in placing Red Robinson catheter through tract from which the working sheath has been removed.

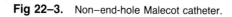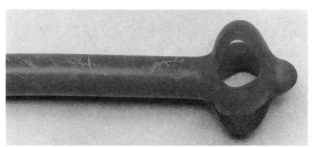

Fig 22–3.   Non–end-hole Malecot catheter.

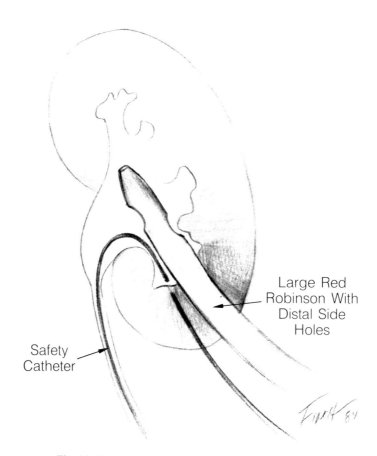

Large Red
Robinson With
Distal Side
Holes

Safety
Catheter

Fig 22–4.   Drainage catheter tip, placed in renal pelvis.

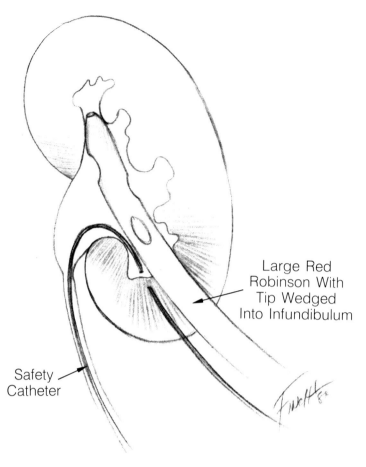

Fig 22–5. Catheter tip placed in upper pole calyx to prevent side holes from being outside of collecting system.

Large Red Robinson With Tip Wedged Into Infundibulum

Safety Catheter

more secure tract in such cases, and to prevent the side holes from being outside the collecting system, the tip of the catheter can be placed into a remote calyx (Fig 22–5). A nephrostogram must then be performed to ensure that the side holes are draining the whole collecting system and that the catheter itself is not causing any obstruction.

In certain patients, a Foley or Council catheter is used (Fig 22–6). In patients who have moderate or severe bleeding, the balloon is used to tamponade the bleeding site. In obese patients, the balloon is used to prevent catheter dislodgment, which is very common if a nonretention catheter is used. In patients with an intercostal (11th or 12th rib) puncture, a balloon catheter is also used to prevent catheter dislodgment secondary to rib motion with respiration.

Balloon catheters do have some slight disadvan-

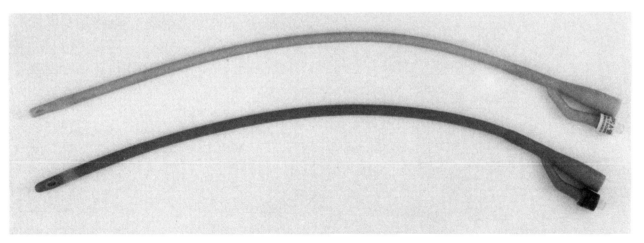

Fig 22–6. Foley *(top)* and Council *(bottom)* catheters.

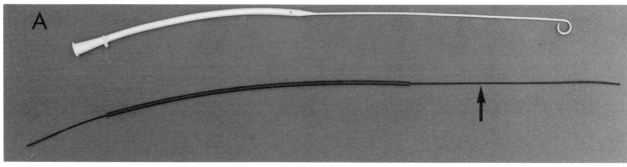

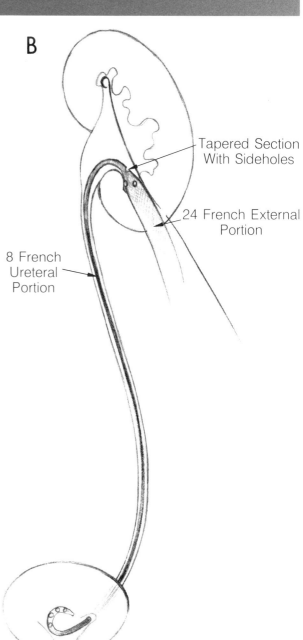

Tapered Section
With Sideholes

24 French External
Portion

8 French
Ureteral
Portion

Fig 22–7. **A,** the black Teflon stiffener *(arrow)* fits inside of the catheter making it much easier to pass it over the guide wire. The stiffener passes over a 0.038-in. guide wire. **B,** 24 F Amplatz tapered catheter placed with sideholes in renal pelvis and 8 F tapered segment with pigtail tip in the bladder.

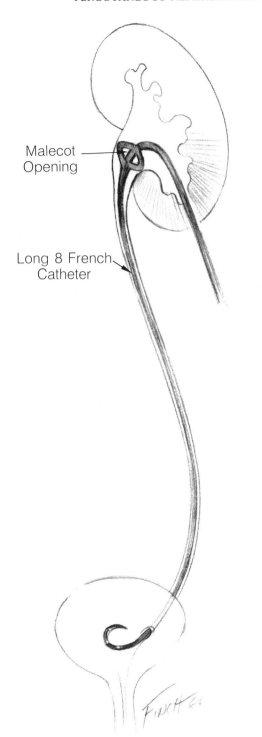

Malecot Opening

Long 8 French Catheter

Fig 22–8. 8 F Castaneda's Malecot internal-external drainage catheter, which is placed across traumatized region when Amplatz catheter is removed.

tages. The balloon adds to the catheter profile and can make it difficult to introduce the catheter through the tract. The balloon may deflate and then dislodge. And, there is risk of overdistending and even rupturing a portion of the collecting system.

Following the removal of a stone from the ureter or ureteropelvic junction, it is often desirable to stent the traumatized ureter and simultaneously tamponade the large percutaneous tract. A new catheter from Cook Inc. (Bloomington, Ind.) developed by Kurt Amplatz, M.D., has a 24 F portion that extends from the renal pelvis to the outside of the patient, and an 8 F portion that extends from the renal pelvis to the bladder (Figs 22–7,A and B). Both the pigtail in the bladder and the tapered connecting portion in the renal pelvis have side holes so that internal drainage is possible. The 24 F external catheter is quite stiff and is therefore only suitable for short-term use. When performing the final nephrostogram prior to catheter removal, the catheter must be pulled back so that the pigtail portion is in the renal pelvis. The 24 F and tapered portions are cut off, and the injection done through a connector. Alternatively, the Amplatz catheter can be replaced over a guide wire by another catheter prior to the nephrostogram.

If ureteral trauma has been severe, the ureter is stented for two or three weeks. An 8 or 10 F internal-external drainage catheter is placed across the traumatized region when the Amplatz drainage catheter is removed (Fig 22–8).

After any drainage catheter has been placed, a nephrostogram is performed to make sure that the catheter tip and the side holes are within the collecting system and to see if there is any extravasation. Especially during the removal of multiple, large, or staghorn calculi, perforation of the collecting system is not uncommon. This usually occurs in the renal pelvis (Fig 22–9). As long as the drainage catheter is clearly inside the collecting system, the false pass will usually heal within 24 hours (Fig 22–10). If any portion of the catheter extends through the false pass it will not heal at all. In such cases the catheter can either be repositioned or a smaller catheter placed in a position remote from the false pass, but still within the collecting system.

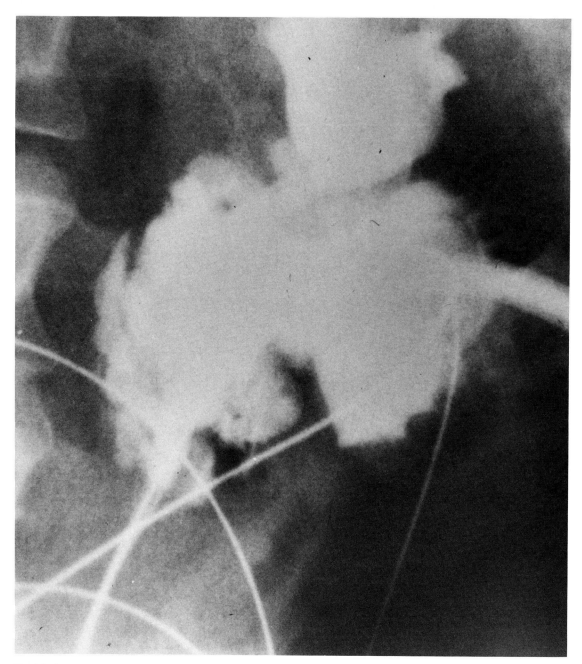

Fig 22–9. Roentgenogram showing massive extravasation of contrast medium. An Amplatz tapered catheter is placed across the tract with the tip into the ureter.

Although the large drainage catheter serves as the primary means by which access to the kidney is maintained, the safety catheter is available to reestablish access if the larger catheter should become dislodged. The safety catheter can therefore be of critical importance, and careful attention should be paid to ensure that it is securely positioned, preferably with its tip in the distal ureter (Fig 22–11). (The sequence for removing the safety catheter and larger drainage catheters is discussed in Chapter 23.)

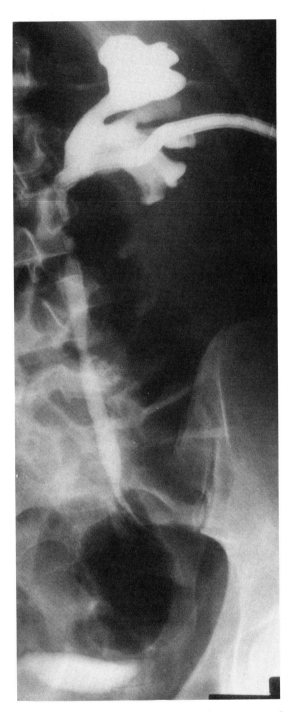

Fig 22–10.—Follow up nephrostogram 24 hours post nephro-stolithotomy shows no evidence of extravasation. The Amplatz catheter was replaced by a red rubber tube.

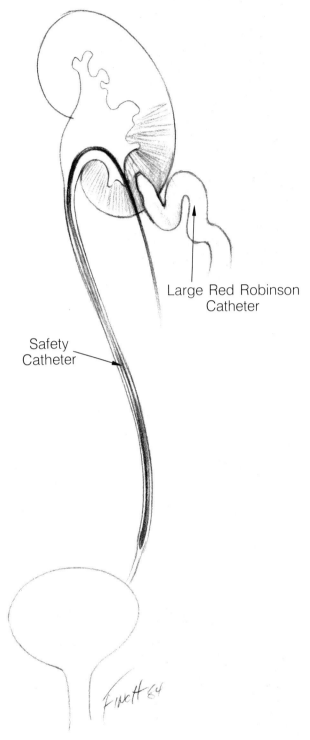

Fig 22–11. Safety catheter positioned with tip in distal ureter. The tip of the red rubber catheter slipped back into the tract.

CHAPTER 23

Tube Care After Percutaneous Nephrolithotomy

Betty Dale, R.N.

INITIAL TUBE MANAGEMENT

Successful percutaneous stone removal requires careful management of the catheters that are in the kidney, ureter, and bladder. Although the sequence of events from the beginning of the first catheter placement to the completion of the stone removal may vary from institution to institution, the number and type of tubes are fairly consistent. In most cases, a patient can expect to have a Foley catheter to prevent the bladder from overdistension, a ureteral catheter to prevent stone fragments from descending into the ureter, a nephrostomy tube through which the stones are removed, and a "safety catheter" to maintain the tract in the event that the nephrostomy tube is dislodged (Fig 23–1). Commonly, the ureteral catheter is removed at the end of the procedure and the patient returns to the ward with a Foley catheter, a nephrostomy tube, and sometimes a safety catheter.

Immediate postoperative care involves accurate monitoring of the patient's vital signs and urine volumes. Sometimes a designated output per catheter is ordered, such as 30 ml/hour from the Foley catheter and 15 ml/hour from the nephrostomy tube. It is important to remember, however, that the total urine output is usually more important than the tube from which it emerges. Factors such as ureteral edema or spasm, the position of the

tube, or the influence of gravity may determine which tube will drain the greater amount of urine. All tubes must be securely taped in place so that adequate drainage can be maintained and the possibility of tube dislodgment can be diminished (Fig 23–2).

For the first 24 hours, urine output should be monitored every one to two hours. Observe the tubing for kinks or twisting that may obstruct the flow of urine. Low urine volumes, particularly when accompanied by pain, can be symptomatic of conditions that may require immediate attention (Fig 23–3). If clots are present, it may be necessary to irrigate the nephrostomy tube with 5 to 10 ml of 0.9% normal saline. Gently instill and draw back the fluid. Forceful irrigation can increase the intrarenal pressure, which may damage the kidney. If there has been intraoperative trauma, however, irrigation may be contraindicated. Other causes of obstruction will require a nephrostogram for accurate diagnosis and management.

The Foley catheter is usually removed on the following day and the patient is able to void normally. An exit urine culture may be indicated to check for a urinary tract infection. The nephrostomy tube and the safety catheter, if present, are left in place until nephrotomograms of the kidney determine that the patient is stone-free. If a ne-

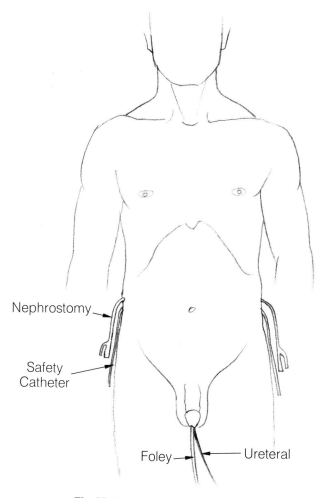

Fig 23–1. Catheter placement sites.

phrostogram shows that there is no extravasation of urine, the nephrostomy tube is removed and the patient is ready for discharge.

While the patient is hospitalized, the nephrostomy dressing should be changed daily. Sterile technique is preferred to prevent possible cross-contamination of infection from or to another patient. It is important that standards be developed and maintained for the removal and reapplication of dressings. If all staff know the same procedure, the chance of accidentally dislodging a tube will be significantly decreased. The equipment needed for the dressing change in a patient with a nephrostomy tube and a safety catheter is as follows:

- Sterile gloves
- Hydrogen peroxide
- Povidone-iodine (Betadine) swabsticks
- Sterile cotton swabs (Q-tips)
- 2-in. Micropore or Dermiclear tape
- Five-package sterile 4x4 gauze sponges

CHANGING THE NEPHROSTOMY DRESSING

Wash hands thoroughly. Use clean gloves when removing the old dressing. Dispose of it as you would other contaminated material. Put on sterile gloves and proceed to clean the site with hydrogen peroxide. Let it dry and then apply povidone-iodine (Betadine) solution. Observe the skin for signs of infection such as redness, swelling, and tenderness. Apply the gauze sponges as described in Figures 23–4 through 23–8. Cover the dressing entirely with three 6-in. pieces of tape. Dermiclear tape is preferable to an occlusive tape, such as adhesive or foam tape. It provides a moisture barrier yet allows the dressing to be observed for signs of bleeding and/or urinary drainage.

If urine leaks around the tube, several options may be tried. Minimal leaking can be controlled by more frequent dressing changes. If, however, the patient and the linen are constantly wet, a temporary ostomy bag can be applied in the manner shown in Figure 23–9. Attach stomahesive to the adhesive disk of the pouch. Cut a hole large enough to accommodate the tube or tubes. Cut a small opening in the upper portion of the pouch and pull the nephrostomy tube through. If a clamped guide wire is still present, it can be left inside the pouch. Cover the opening with a sterile 4x4 gauze sponge and seal with Dermiclear tape. The nephrostomy tube can then be attached to a leg bag (Fig 23–10). This allows the patient to move freely without the discomfort of constant urine-soaked dressings. Urine that leaks around the tube will be collected in the pouch, which can be periodically emptied.

DISCHARGE INSTRUCTIONS

After stone removal, the patient can go home in one of three manners. Ideally, the patient will be stone-free and tube-free. Discharge teaching will focus on changing the dressings over the tube site every other day until all drainage has stopped. Gauze sponges and nonocclusive tape are usually the only supplies needed. A temporary ostomy bag, however, may be needed for the first one to two days until the drainage decreases. A pouch is also a good idea for those patients who have to travel a great distance to get home and cannot change a dressing while in transit.

A patient can also be discharged with one or more clamped tubes in place. These tubes may re-

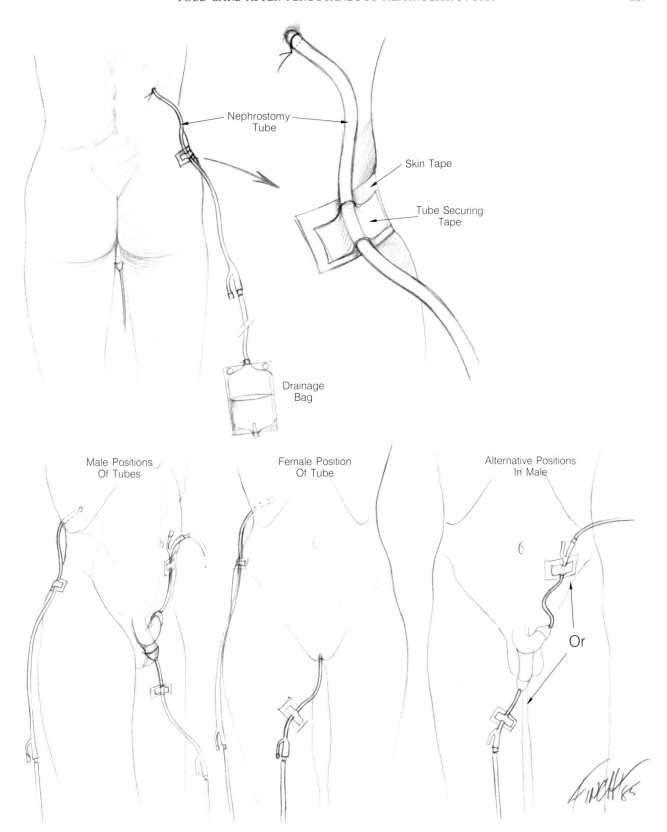

Nephrostomy Tube

Skin Tape

Tube Securing Tape

Drainage Bag

Male Positions Of Tubes

Female Position Of Tube

Alternative Positions In Male

Or

Fig 23–2. Proper securing of tubes.

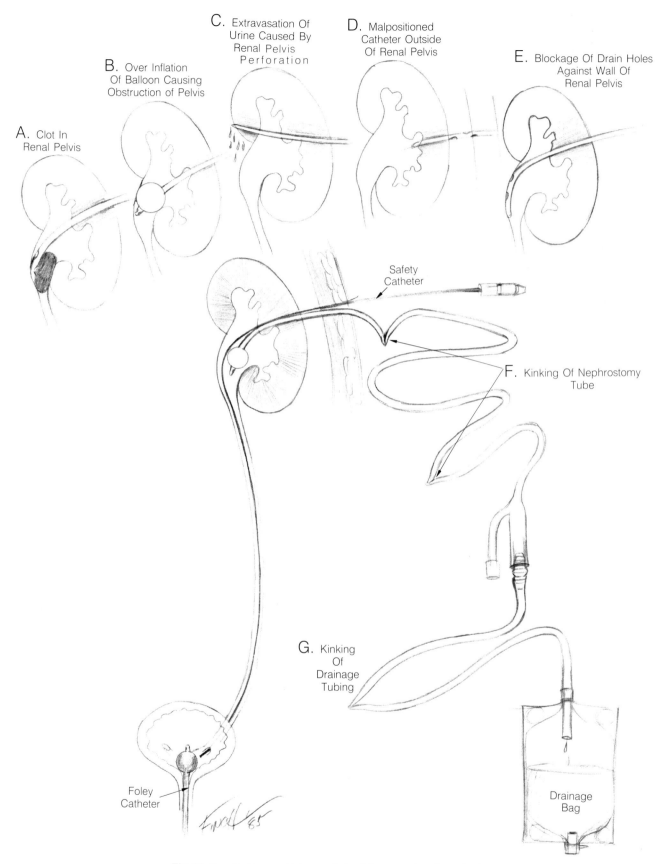

A. Clot In
Renal Pelvis

B. Over Inflation
Of Balloon Causing
Obstruction of Pelvis

C. Extravasation Of
Urine Caused By
Renal Pelvis
Perforation

D. Malpositioned
Catheter Outside
Of Renal Pelvis

E. Blockage Of Drain Holes
Against Wall Of
Renal Pelvis

Safety
Catheter

F. Kinking Of Nephrostomy
Tube

G. Kinking
Of
Drainage
Tubing

Foley
Catheter

Drainage
Bag

Fig 23–3. Problems which can obstruct the normal outflow of urine.

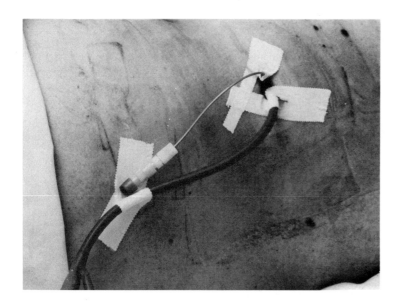

Fig 23–4. Nephrostomy site. Observe for signs of infection around site, for proper securing of tubes, and that tubes are stitched in place.

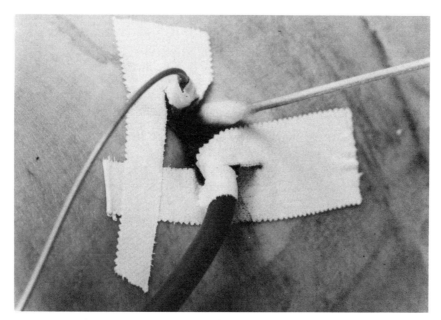

Fig 23–5. Clean around the tubes with hydrogen peroxide. Let dry. Apply povidone-iodine (Betadine) solution to area around tube site.

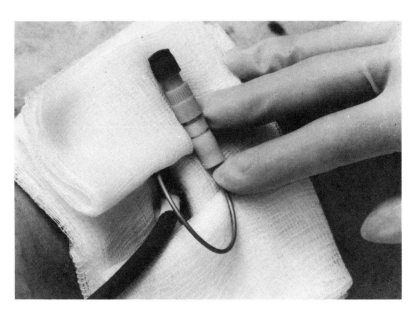

Fig 23–6. Place folded 4 × 4 gauze sponge under tubes to prevent kinking near the skin entry site. Continue to place four folded 4 × 4 gauze sponges in a picture frame fashion around tubes. Place folded edges against the tubes. Coil safety catheter and place on top of 4 × 4 sponges.

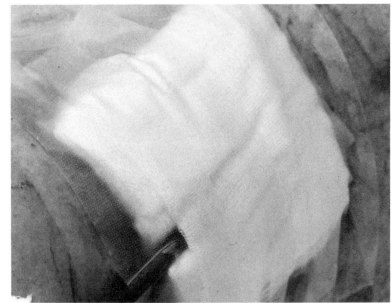

Fig 23–7. Cover the entire dressing with the remaining gauze sponge. Cover the dressing completely with three 6-in. pieces of tape.

main in place up to two weeks and may be removed either in the physician's office or in the hospital, depending on the need of the patient and/or the preference of the physician. It is difficult but not impossible for a patient to be taught to do his own dressing change if a relative or public health nurse is unavailable. The patient is taught to build the dressing from the outside to the inside. On a flat surface overlap three to four pieces of 2-in. Micropore or Dermiclear tape. Place an open 4 × 4 gauze sponge in the center of the tape. Place three folded 4 × 4 gauze sponges in a

picture-frame fashion around the center. Rolled pieces of tape will help hold the folded 4 × 4 sponges in place (see Fig 23–8). After removing the old dressing and cleaning the tube site, the new dressing is applied and secured above the site. A fourth folded gauze sponge is placed under the nephrostomy tube and the remaining lower dressing is secured. Clean technique is used. The patient is taught to carefully wash his hands and to avoid touching the center of the dressing.

The tube should remain clamped at all times but if back pain, fever, and/or chills occur the pa-

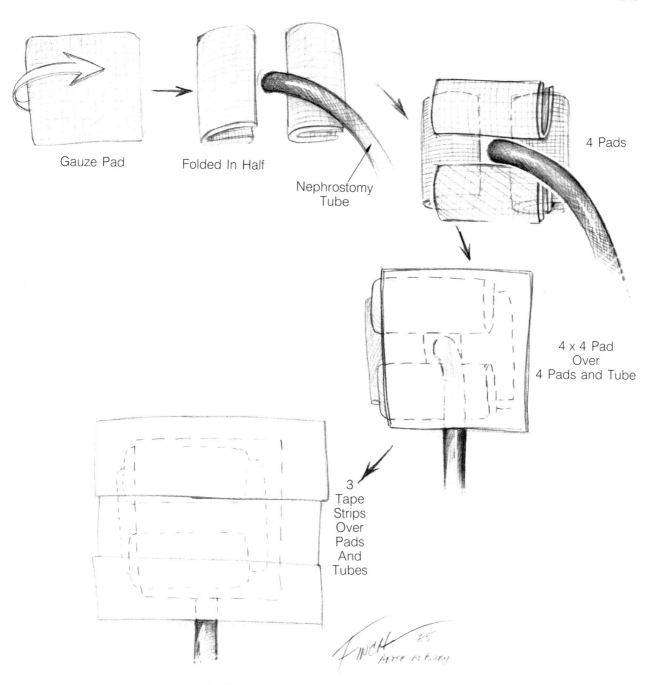

Gauze Pad

Folded In Half

Nephrostomy Tube

4 Pads

4 x 4 Pad Over 4 Pads and Tube

3 Tape Strips Over Pads And Tubes

Fig 23–8. Overview of the sterile dressing change.

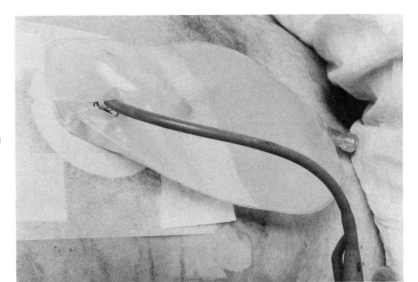

Fig 23–9. Temporary ostomy bag for leaking nephrostomy site.

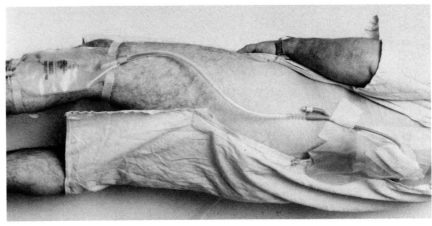

Fig 23–10. Tape nephrostomy tube securely to flank. Attach tube end to a 5-in-1 connector, bubble tubing, and then to leg bag.

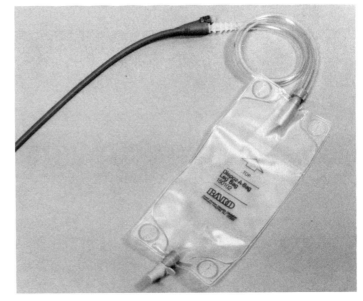

Fig 23–11. Supplies needed to attach a nephrostomy tube to a leg bag: 5-in-1 adapter, bubble tubing, and leg bag.

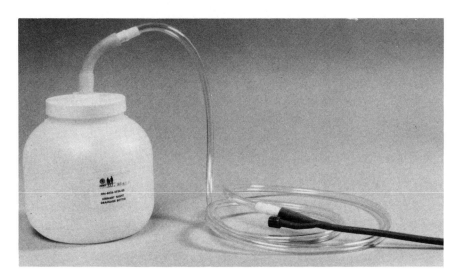

Fig 23–12. Nephrostomy tube attached to the night drainage bottle. Note that the drainage tubing attaches directly to the nephrostomy tube. No 5-in-1 adapter is needed.

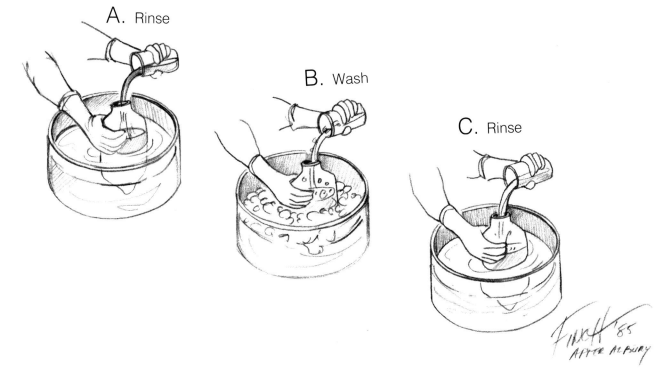

Fig 23–13. Clean equipment before disinfecting it. **A,** rinse used equipment thoroughly. **B,** wash with soap and water. **C,** rinse thoroughly with warm tap water.

tient may need to connect the nephrostomy tube to a drainage system (Fig 23–11). Before the patient leaves the hospital he should be given the necessary equipment and instructed in how to use it. Figure 23–11 illustrates how a nephrostomy tube can be attached to a leg bag. Equipment to be given to the patient includes a 5-in-1 connector, bubble or extension tubing, and a leg bag.

Finally, the patient may be discharged with a nephrostomy tube to continuous straight drain-age. Supplies and instructions are more complicated. The patient must not only be taught how to hook the nephrostomy tube to a leg bag (see Fig 23–11) and to a night-drainage receptacle (Fig 23–12), but he must also be taught to disinfect the equipment (Figs 23–13 through 23–17). All equipment must be cleaned and disinfected before it is reused. Proper instruction prior to the patient's discharge will decrease the possibility of complications, particularly infection.

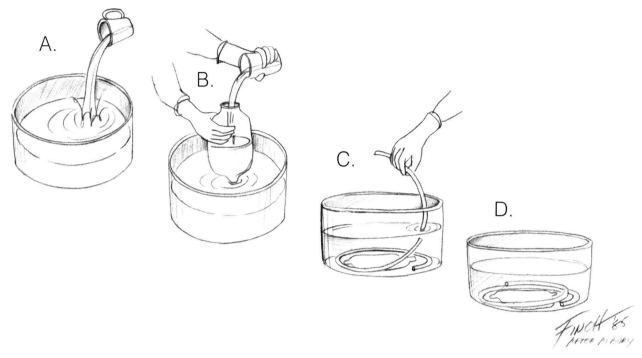

Fig 23–14. Disinfecting reusable equipment. **A,** add ½ cup O-Syl or other disinfectant to 1 gallon of water in a large container. **B,** fill leg bag with solution and place in container. **C,** coil the tubing so that it will fit in the container. **D,** soak for 30 minutes.

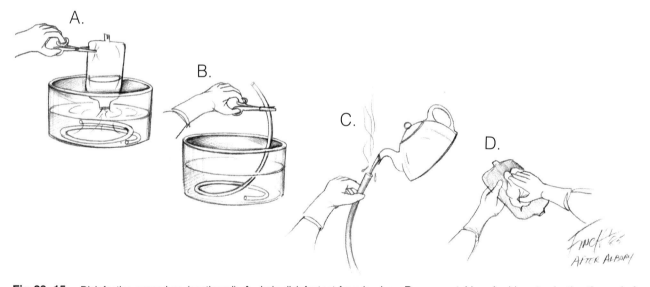

Fig 23–15. Disinfecting procedure (continued). **A,** drain disinfectant from leg bag. **B,** remove tubing. Avoid contaminating the end of the tube. **C,** pour boiled water into tubing and leg bag to rinse well. **D,** wipe outside with dry cloth.

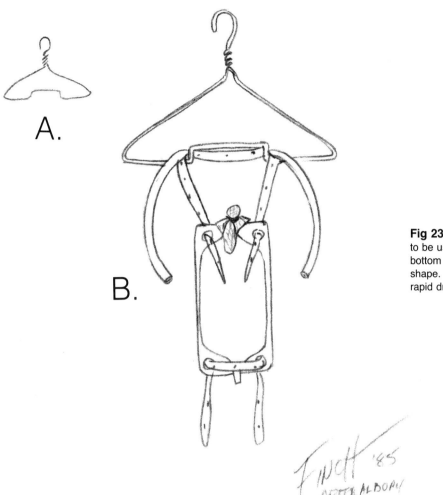

Fig 23–16. Hang equipment to dry if it is not to be used again immediately. **A,** bend the bottom of a coat hanger to form indicated shape. **B,** pull apart sides of bag to allow more rapid drying.

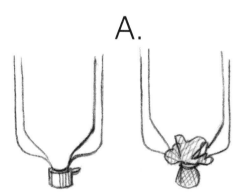

Fig 23–17. Cover all open ends with sterile gauze or disinfected caps.

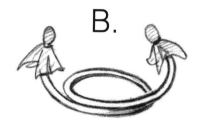

CHAPTER 24

Percutaneous Nephrolithotomy: Complications and Their Management

Paul H. Lange, M.D.

The number of major acute and chronic complications from percutaneous nephrolithotomy has been surprisingly low. These are listed in Table 24–1. Some of them are more theoretical than real, or are very rare. For example, fever to 38.5 C for one to two days is common, but significant persistent infection, pyelonephritis, or perirenal abscesses are extremely unusual. Urinomas significant enough to require drainage are also rare and when they occur they are usually the result of a nephrostomy tube malpositioned such that a drainage hole is outside the kidney. Retroperitoneal hematomas do occur, usually with other more overt signs of hemorrhage. Sometimes these hematomas can cause significant discomfort but generally they are almost always contained and limited by the retroperitoneum. Indeed, as in other types of renal trauma associated with parenchymal injury, the excellent capabilities of the retroperitoneum for tamponade should be appreciated and open surgery for control of bleeding or drainage of a hematoma has rarely been necessary, and should be a procedure of last resort. Certainly, if open surgical intervention is necessary, clot evacuation and drainage should always be accompanied by meticulous control of bleeding; otherwise, hemorrhage will almost certainly continue.

TABLE 24–1.

Complications of Percutaneous Nephrolithotomy

Acute
  Hemorrhage
  Perforation-avulsion
  Urinoma
  Retroperitoneal hematoma
  Fever
  Infection
  Pulmonary complications (e.g., atelectasis-pneumonia, ureteral stricture, pneumohydrothorax)
  Systemic absorption of fluid or air
  Failure to retrieve stone or stone fragments
  Malposition of nephrostomy tube or loss of tract access
  Contrast media reaction
  Abdominal organ puncture
  Temporary ureteropelvic junction or ureteral obstruction
Chronic
  Delayed hemorrhage (e.g., arteriovenous fistula, pseudoaneurysm, vessel erosion by tube)
  Perirenal abscess
  Renal malfunction
  Accelerated recurrent stone formation
  Infundibular, ureteropelvic junction, or ureteral stricture

Absorption of fluid or air is a potentially serious problem and it should be remembered that the renal parenchyma and retroperitoneum have great absorbent capacities. Thus, except for short periods when electrohydraulic lithotripsy or intrarenal electrosurgery are required, the irrigant should always be a physiological solution, such as Ringer's lactate or normal saline. Also, precautions against hypervolemia should be exercised, especially if perforation of the renal collecting system has occurred. During endoscopy, a record of input and output should be kept and if a deficit of greater than 1 L exists, the irrigation should be stopped. Irrigations with stone-dissolving solutions (e.g., Suby's G solution or Renacidin) should not be attempted in the acutely dilated percutaneous tract or infected kidney, and precautions against undue absorption should be observed.

Failure to retrieve the targeted stone is an event that has rarely occurred in our hands. This success is facilitated by the variety of ancillary procedures discussed in this book, including accurate percutaneous puncture, the use of secondary percutaneous tracts (including those above the 12th rib), liberal use of flexible endoscopy, and intrarenal surgery. Retained stone fragments are also undesirable, but their importance is controversial. We attempt to remove all detectable fragments and have been successful in most circumstances (truly stone-free status among our patients is 99%). Others believe that these fragments, if not infected, do not contribute to stone occurrence and are less vigorous in removing them.

In this chapter we review the complications of hemorrhage, perforation-evulsion, surrounding organ perforation, and contrast media allergic reactions.

HEMORRHAGE

From the nature of the procedure itself, this complication cannot ever be completely avoided. Certainly one must get used to some blood flow out of the sheath and onto the drapes. What constitutes an acceptable or worrisome amount is a matter of judgment and experience, but both interventional radiologists and surgeons alike often have to adjust their expectations initially. Yet the severity of hemorrhage can be minimized and usually easily managed. For example, as discussed elsewhere, it is important to enter the kidney in the posterior and, preferably, lower-pole areas whenever possible to lessen the chances of hitting major arteries. Also, inadvertent placement of the tract through an intercostal vessel should be avoided. Thus, tracts should avoid the inferior border of the ribs. Infection and inflammation predispose to bleeding. Whenever possible, severe infection should be treated before percutaneous ne-

phrostomy, but if this is not possible, one should consider draining the collecting system with a small catheter for several days before dilation and manipulation. Also, stone-dissolving irrigants can cause urothelial inflammation and they should be stopped for several days before the percutaneous nephrolithotomy is initiated.

Once dilation is completed the usual bleeding is most often easily controlled with a sheath. However, it is not infrequent for bleeding to increase during endoscopy. Often this is due to mucosal irritation or dislodgment of the tamponading sheath—conditions that are easily corrected or self-limiting. However, careless endoscopy must be avoided; thus the endoscopist must take care not to bend the scope excessively (especially in fixed kidneys, as might occur from previous surgery), and to proceed gently, always under direct vision, within the kidney (Fig 24–1).

If bleeding is initially severe or becomes so (Fig 24–2,A), the dilated tract should be tamponaded for 15 minutes with a dilator, a urethral balloon catheter, or an angioplasty balloon (Figs 24–2,B-D). Bleeding usually decreases significantly with this maneuver and the procedure can either be resumed or (often more advisably) a nephrostomy tube can be placed and the tract allowed to heal for a period of time. If bleeding is especially severe, we often delay the secondary procedure for two weeks, since by that time a mature and much safer access to the kidney will exist. However, if bleeding does not stop sufficiently after this period of time, depending on the physician's judgment and the circumstances, the patient may be returned to his hospital bed with a well-tamponaded tract or immediate percutaneous embolization of a torn vessel(s) may be necessary (Figs 24–2,E-G). For the last maneuver, the patient is turned to the supine position, a selective arteriogram is performed, and the site of bleeding is identified. The method of embolization varies; we often use a Gianterio coil plus absorbable Gelfoam (Figs 24–3,A-C). On very rare occasions (less than 0.3% in our hands) open surgery may be necessary to control bleeding.

Sometimes, on placement of the nephrostomy tube, there is a steady venous flow of blood through or around the tube. This occasionally alarming ooze can be controlled by clamping the nephrostomy tube for a short period of time and/or inflating the balloon on the nephrostomy tube and placing it on mild traction. Though the dilated tract often collapses snugly around the nephrostomy tube if it is only 2 to 4 F sizes less than the dilated tract, getting this sufficiently sized

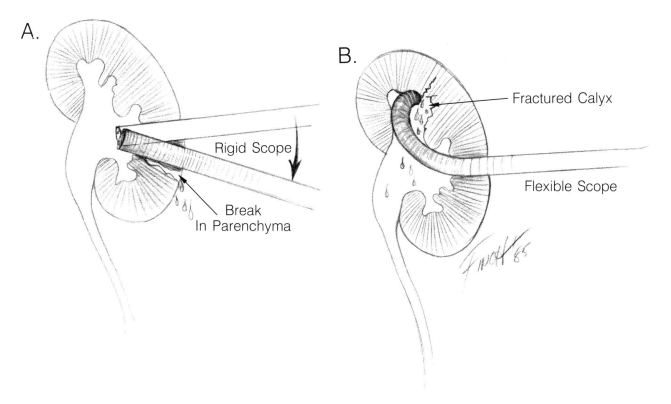

Fig 24–1. Nephroscope injuries. **A,** excessive bleeding from rigid endoscope causing tearing of renal parenchyma. **B,** flexible endoscope causing damage to calyx.

tube positioned correctly may be difficult or not adequate. Recently another catheter (called the Kaye catheter) has become available; it is surrounded by a sausage-shaped balloon and is of sufficiently small size to be easily inserted into the nephrostomy tract, where the balloon is inflated appropriately for very snug tamponade (Fig 24–4).

PERFORATION AVULSION

The ill effects of perforating the renal collecting system during percutaneous nephrostomy are extravasation of contrast media—thereby obscuring radiographic visibility (Fig 24–5), absorption of irrigant solution, anatomical disruption, and loss of percutaneous access. The most common sites of perforation are the perirenal sinus, the renal pelvis, and the ureter (Figs 24–6,A-C). The seriousness of this event is a matter of degree. Minor perforations often occur during the procedure that are

of little consequence other than that the amount of contrast used after discovery of the perforation must be curtailed. At other times, visualization or the degree of disruption requires that the procedure be terminated. The extreme example of perforation is avulsion, which is rare and most often occurs at the ureteropelvic junction or in the ureter.

The initial management of perforation-avulsion is its recognition. Frequent assessment of position and extravasation should be made throughout the procedure. Once this event is recognized as significant, the procedure should be terminated in most cases and drainage and stenting of the renal pelvis and ureter established. This can be done by placing a nephrostomy tube and ureteral stents separately or by placing a drainage stent through the nephrostomy tube (Figs 24–6,E and F). A ureteral catheter can also be used to facilitate drainage. Using these maneuvers, a perirenal abscess or urinoma occurs rarely.

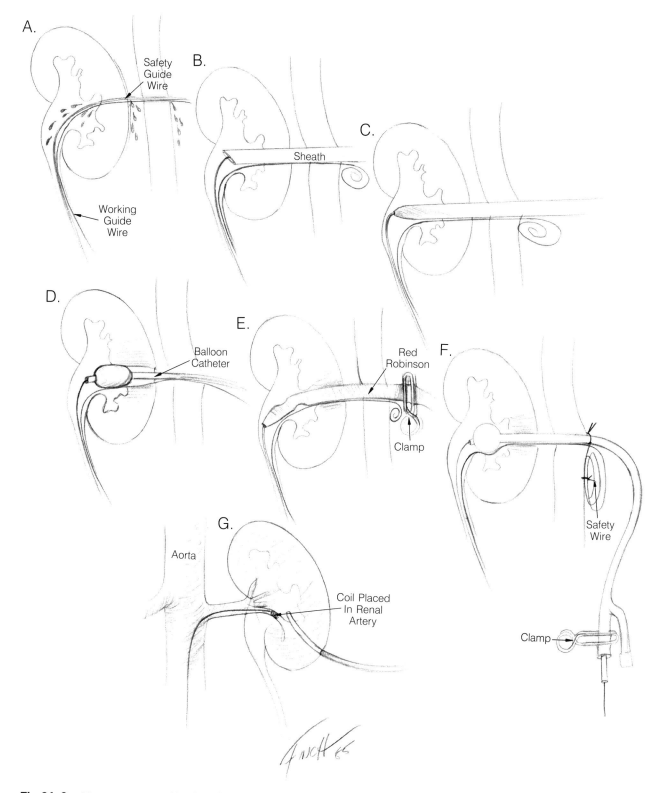

Fig 24–2. Maneuvers to stop bleeding. **A,** bleeding will usually be brisk after dilation if there is no tamponade. **B,** Amplatz sheath is excellent for temporary tamponade while performing endoscopic maneuvers. **C,** fascial dilators are also useful for temporary tamponade when bleeding becomes brisk and continued manipulation ill advised. For more permanent tamponade, a nephrostomy balloon catheter **(D)** can be placed and the balloon filled with 2 to 5 cc. For smaller tracts, an angioplasty balloon may be useful. If bleeding persists, the tube can be clamped **(E and F)** and/or placed on mild traction. Rarely, renal angiography and percutaneous embolization are required **(G)**.

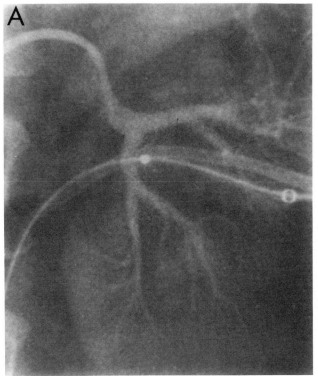

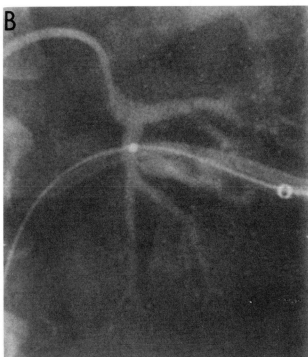

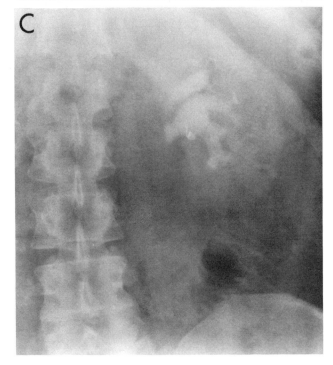

Fig 24–3. **A,** left renal angiogram in patient with brisk persistent bleeding during percutaneous nephrostomy tract dilation to 14 F. Angioplasty balloon tamponade used for 12 hours. No arterial extravasation with balloon inflated. **B,** angioplasty balloon deflated showing tertiary renal artery extravasation. **C,** Gianterio coil in place and all tubes removed (this patient had a lower calyceal stone that was removed percutaneously eight weeks later).

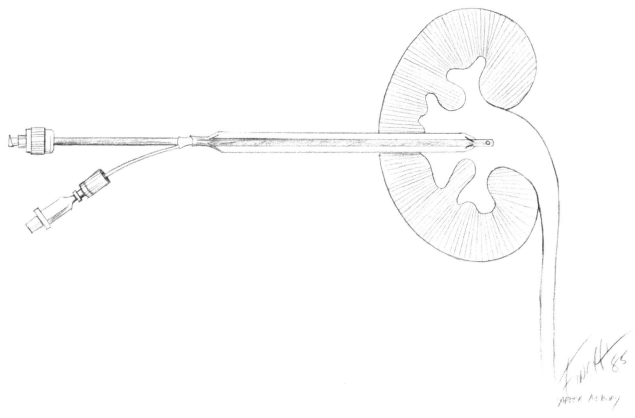

Fig 24–4. The Kaye catheter. This catheter allows nephrostomy tube drainage (14 F) and additional tamponade by a balloon (15 cm; 12 mm; inflation pressure, 2.5 atmospheres).

Fig 24–5. X-ray film showing marked extravasation of radiographic contrast medium during percutaneous nephrostomy tract dilation.

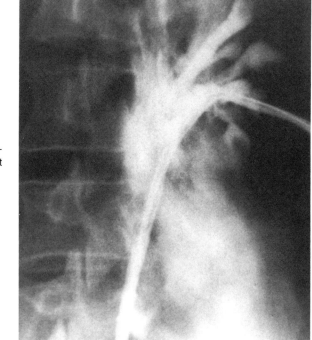

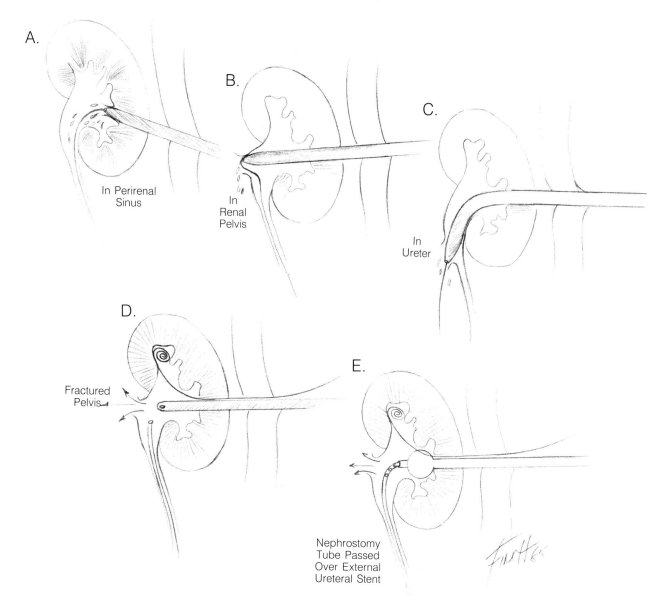

Fig 24–6.   Major sites of renal collecting system perforation in the perirenal sinus **(A)**, renal pelvis **(B)**, and ureter **(C)**. Major extravasation is best managed by terminating the procedure and placing a nephrostomy and ureteral catheter for drainage **(E)**. Alternatively, a multihold ureteral stent catheter can be passed through the nephrostomy tube for multidirectional drainage into the bladder and out the flank.

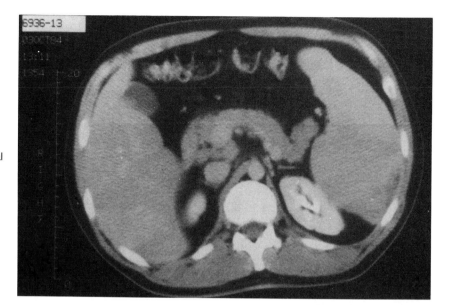

Fig 24–7. Computed axial tomographic scan of patient with splenomegaly. Note the posterior lateral position of the spleen relative to the superior pole of the left kidney.

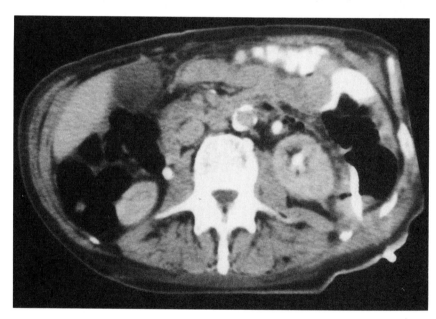

Fig 24–8. Computed axial tomographic scan of patient. Note the posterolateral position of air-filled left colon relative to kidney.

ORGAN PERFORATION

Despite the relative posterior position of nephrostomy tracts, the variability of individual anatomy allows the potential for perforation of other organs. These include the spleen, colon, lung, duodenum, liver, and gallbladder. The technique for transpleural percutaneous nephrostomy is discussed elsewhere (see Chapter 16). Conditions that predispose to splenomegaly or the finding of an enlarged spleen on physical examination should alert the physician to the relative possibil-

ity of a posterolateral position of the spleen. This can be confirmed by computed tomography (Fig 24–7) and is most relevant to the upper and middle poles of the kidney. On the right, similar situations exist for the liver. However, the ascending and descending colon are probably the most vulnerable organs. Studies have determined that in a significant number of people the colon can be normally positioned posteriorly, to the parallel alignment with the horizontal plane drawn to the posterior edge of the kidney. In most of these cases (13%), the position is posterolateral (Fig 24–8) but

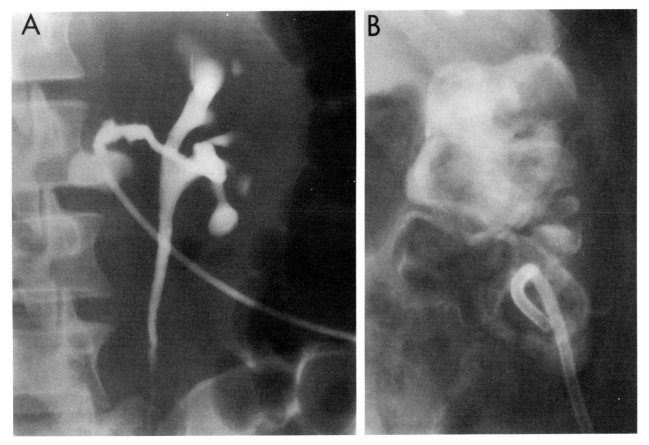

Fig 24–9. A, early-phase nephrogram of patient with colonic fistula. **B,** later nephrogram with nephrostomy tube withdrawn from kidney showing dye extravasation into colon. With conservative management (see text) the fistula and nephrostomy tracts healed without further complications.

in some (0.6%) it is truly retrorenal. These posterior positions are seen most frequently in patients with renal fusion abnormalities (e.g., horseshoe kidneys) and in older women, since as a group they have less perirenal fat than men. In these high-risk groups, it would seem prudent to obtain a computed axial tomographic scan before percutaneous puncture and to be careful to place the puncture especially posteriorly.

The management of a colonic perforation that occurs during percutaneous nephrostomy and dilation has usually been straightforward (Figs 24–9,A and B). Provided that renal parenchyma bleeding has subsided, retrograde drainage of the kidney is instituted and the percutaneous tube is withdrawn sufficiently to remove it from the renal parenchyma, thus allowing drainage of urine, healing of the tract between the kidney and colon, and the prevention of fecal soilage internally. After seven

to ten days, the percutaneous tube is removed altogether and the resultant cutaneous bowel fistula usually closes in several days.

RADIOPAQUE CONTRAST MEDIUM ALLERGY

As in other radiologic procedures, the potential for allergic reaction to radiopaque contrast medium must be judged in the individual patient based on his history. The development of the nephrostomy tract and manipulations in it can cause systemic absorption of radiopaque dye even in mature tracts, and for those patients with history of severe allergic reactions, contrast should not be used. In most of these circumstances, carbon dioxide will give satisfactory delineation. Because of the absorption problem, air should never be used in these circumstances.

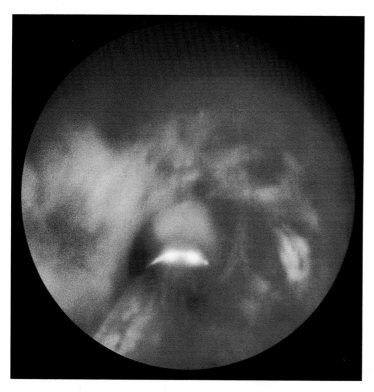

Plate 6. Endoscopic view of ultrasonic lithotripter probe onto stone (yellow) advanced through a narrow infundibulum which would not accomodate the nephroscope.

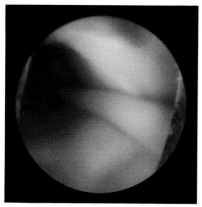

Plate 7. Appearance of mature tract five days after placement of a nephrostomy tube. Note presence of safety catheter.

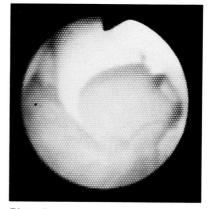

Plate 8. Intrarenal view of sheath inside the kidney photographed through a second nephrostomy tract.

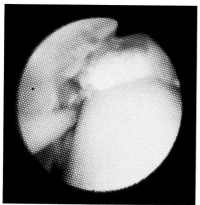

Plate 9. Intrarenal photograph of tip of sheath in the collecting system. Note the safety catheter (red tube) emerging immediately alongside the sheath.

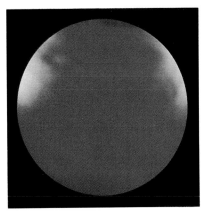

Plate 10. Initial appearance down fresh nephrostomy tract through sheath ("red-out").

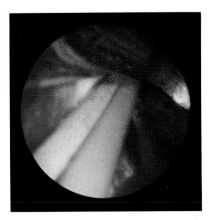

Plate 11. Endoscopic appearance of a guide wire and the safety catheter (red).

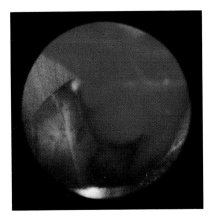

Plate 12. Endoscopic view at the end of the sheath early in a procedure showing clot *(right)* and inflamed hemorrhagic mucosa *(left)*.

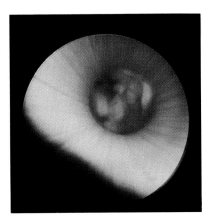

Plate 13. Appearance down the sheath once guide wire has been removed. Note small stones (yellow) in the renal plevis.

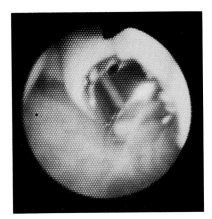

Plate 14. Intrarenal view of sheath in kidney with instrument emerging from it.

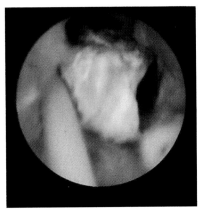

Plate 15. Appearance of stone in renal pelvis adjacent to safety catheter.

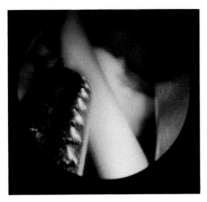

Plate 16. Stone being approached with 7 F grasping forceps.

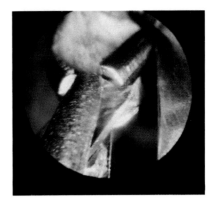

Plate 17. Stone successfully grasped.

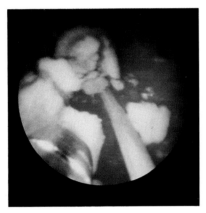

Plate 18. Stone disintegration with ultrasonic lithotripsy. Note tip of ultrasonic probe on left.

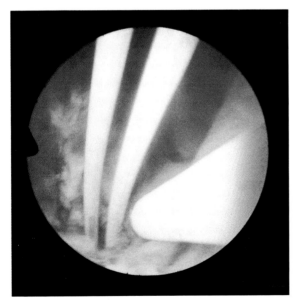

Plate 19. Example of the simple type of ureteropelvic junction obstruction; guide wires can be passed initially.

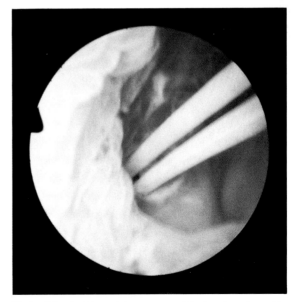

Plate 20. Incision of the ureteropelvic junction alongside the guide wire by electrocautery *(lower left).*

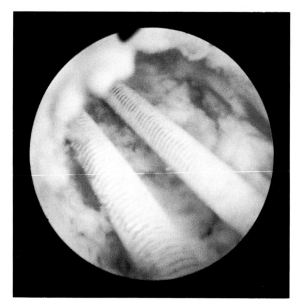

Plate 21. The appearance of the ureteropelvic junction after completion of electrocautery and dilation.

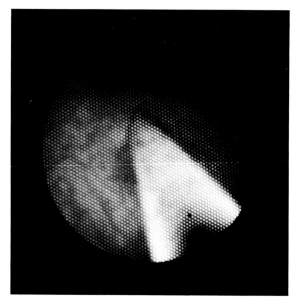

Plate 22. An intrarenal photograph showing a guide wire being passed through the narrow opening of calyceal diverticulum into the diverticulum.

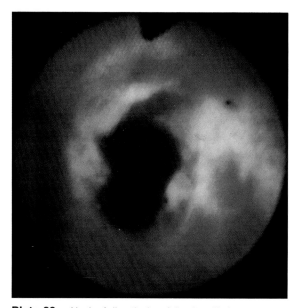

Plate 23. Neck of diverticulum following dilation.

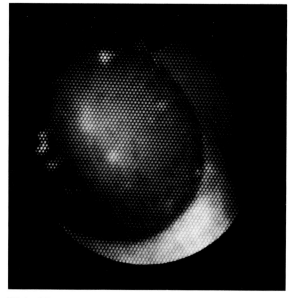

Plate 24. Intrarenal photograph of stone in calyceal diverticulum.

CHAPTER 25

Intrarenal Endosurgical Techniques

John C. Hulbert, M.D., F.R.C.S.

Intrarenal endosurgery encompasses those techniques that are not designed purely for the removal of renal calculi. These involve the management of intrarenal and ureteral strictures, and can also involve conditions intimately related to, but not within, the kidney.

Strictures in the ureter have principally been the realm of fluoroscopic balloon dilation over a guide wire. However, ureteropelvic junction obstruction, infundibular stenosis, and calyceal diverticula are specific anatomical abnormalities that may require endoscopic management aided by intrarenal electrocautery or cold-knife incision.

PRINCIPLES OF INTRARENAL ELECTROSURGERY

The equipment necessary for intrarenal electrosurgery includes the standard endourologic endoscopic instruments. Irrigation solution should be water or glycine; the patient should have an electrode plate placed on the lower limb or buttock so that electrical contact can be improved with electrode jelly; the plate should be connected to an electrocautery power source with adjustable cutting and coagulation currents, which must be grounded. A small 3 F electrode is most suitable for intrarenal cutting (Fig 25–1).

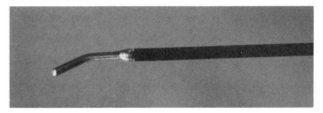

Fig 25–1. Electrode (Grunwald) of 3 F caliber used for endoscopic cutting.

MANAGEMENT OF URETEROPELVIC JUNCTION OBSTRUCTION

Ureteropelvic junction obstruction can be caused primarily by a defect in peristaltic conduction or extrinsic vascular obstruction or secondarily as a result of fibrosis and cicatrization following open pyeloplasty or pyelolithotomy. It is to the latter group that our attentions have been focused.

Cicatrization may complicate pyeloplasty or pyelolithotomy as a result of urinary leak, infection, or ischemia at the site of the anastomosis in the renal pelvis. The resultant fibrosis may result in obstruction and hydronephrosis. Open surgical procedures can be difficult because of this scarring and may even result in nephrectomy. Percutaneous techniques have enabled another less-invasive approach.

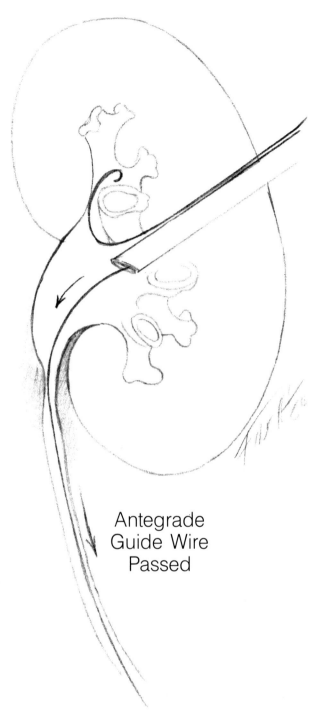

**Antegrade
Guide Wire
Passed**

Fig 25–2. Strictures of the ureteropelvic junction are best approached through the middle- or upper-pole calyx.

Strictures Through Which a Guide Wire May be Passed

These strictures represent the most simple type. The optimal site for percutaneous access is through a middle- or upper-pole calyx, and, after placement of the sheath, a guide wire is passed down the ureter either by means of fluoroscopy (aided often by a Cobra catheter) or endoscopically, with placement of the wire under direct vision (Fig 25–2 and Plate 19). With a wire in place, balloon dilation can be performed. However, it has been our practice and belief that greater success will result if the stenosed segment is cut alone or in combination with balloon dilation (Fig 25–3 and Plate 20). Incision should be performed with exquisite care with a low cutting current, literally dividing the obstruction fiber by fiber; the aim is to develop a full-thickness narrow cut of the entire stricture, and the presence of the guide wire greatly aids orientation when cutting through the ureteropelvic junction. In practice, in the heavily scarred stricture such elegance may not be possible. Final dilation after cutting is useful and may aid in stent placement (Fig 25–4 and Plate 21). A stent should be placed across the ureteropelvic junction for a period of six to eight weeks.

Management of the Obstructed Ureteropelvic Junction Through Which a Guide Wire Will Not Pass But Which Does Retain Patency with the Lower Ureter

If a guide wire cannot be passed through the ureteropelvic junction, other techniques must be employed. The placement of a retrograde catheter beneath the ureteropelvic junction is crucial if patency is to be determined. If contrast will pass into the renal pelvis from the ureteral catheter, one can, of course, determine that there is communication. Attempts can be made to pass the guide wire up from below through a ureteral catheter; if this wire will not pass through the ureteropelvic junction then it should be removed through the ureteral catheter and methylene blue should be infused through the retrograde catheter while the operator is looking through the nephroscope at the area of the ureteropelvic junction. A

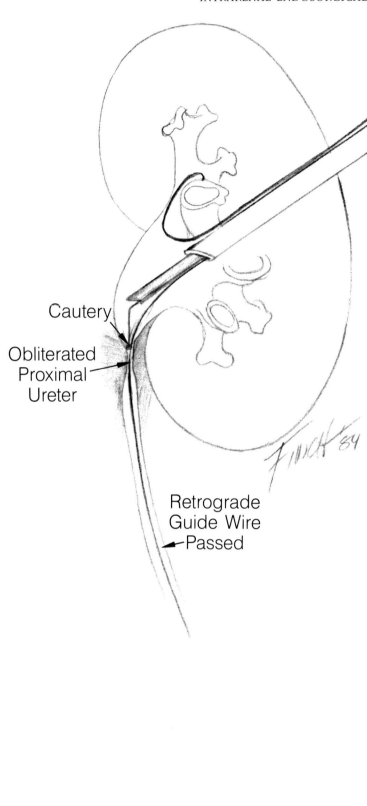

Cautery

Obliterated
Proximal
Ureter

Retrograde
Guide Wire
Passed

Fig 25–3. The most straightforward type of obstruction is that through which a guide wire can be passed and an incision made alongside the guide wire.

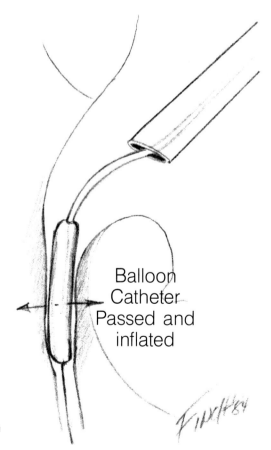

Balloon
Catheter
Passed and
inflated

Fig 25–4. Following incision of the ureteropelvic junction, balloon dilation is a useful adjunct.

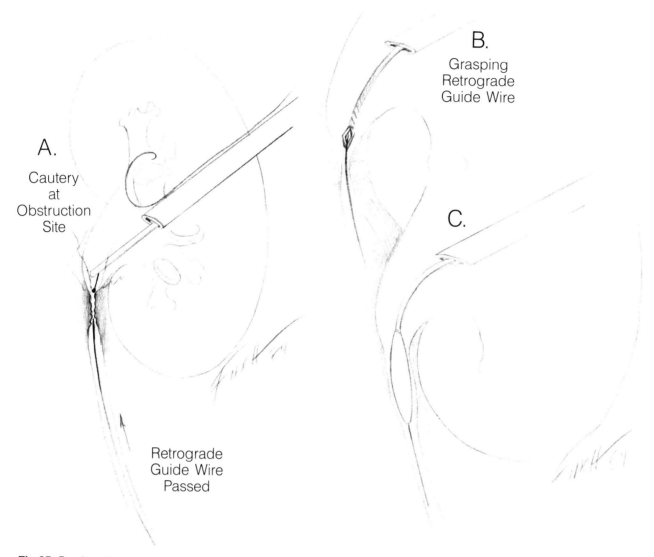

Fig 25–5. **A,** a short, patent ureteropelvic junction through which a guide wire will not pass can be managed by the retrograde infusion of methylene blue and then retrograde pressure with a guide wire while the operator very gently cuts down upon it. **B,** once the wire is seen it can be grasped and pulled through the sheath, thus reestablishing continuity. **C,** incision and balloon dilation can then be performed.

jet of methylene blue may then be seen issuing into the renal pelvis and the spot can be noted carefully by the operator while a guide wire is pushed up through the ureteral catheter until it is adjacent to the stricture. The operator may then carefully cut down on the ureteropelvic junction until the guide wire is seen (Fig 25–5,A). Once the wire has been seen, it can be grasped and pulled through so that continuity is established (Fig 25–5,B) and then dilatation and/or further cutting can take place as previously described (Fig 25–5,C). Of course, stenting is essential after this procedure for a number of weeks.

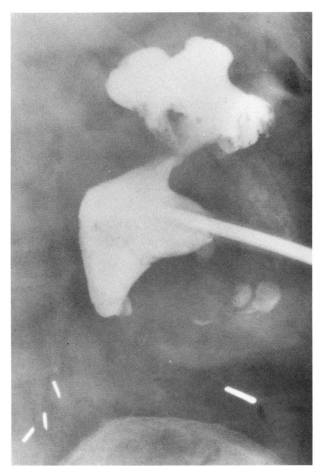

Fig 25–6. Nephrostogram showing a severe ureteropelvic junction obstruction secondary to cicatrization.

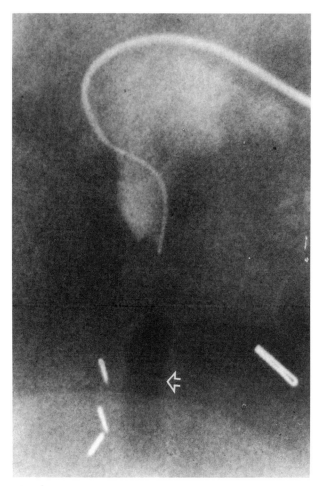

Fig 25–7. Same example of ureteral obliteration as Fig 25–6: contrast in the renal pelvis, and carbon dioxide in the lower ureter *(open arrow)* illustrates the complete loss of ureteral continuity.

Management of the Totally Obliterated Ureteropelvic Junction

In cases of severe fibrosis of the ureteropelvic junction there may be total obliteration of a section of the ureter so that continuity is not possible with wire or contrast (Fig 25–6). In this situation we employ the technique of electrolysis.

After percutaneous access to the kidney has been established, the lower ureter is then filled with contrast or carbon dioxide at the same time as contrast is infused into the collecting system from above, to assess the length of the obliterated segment (Fig 25–7). To cross this obliterated segment, we employ a very fine wire that can be passed through a flexible nephroscope protected by an insulating catheter (Fig 25–8); under very careful combined visual and fluoroscopic control this wire, with the aid of a cutting current, can be guided down through the stricture into the lower part of the ureter. Once the wire has entered the ureter, the protecting catheter can be passed over this wire, crossing the stricture (Fig 25–9). This

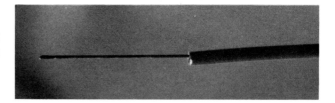

Fig 25–8. Technique of electrolysis. A fine wire is passed through an insulating catheter through which it can be moved easily in and out.

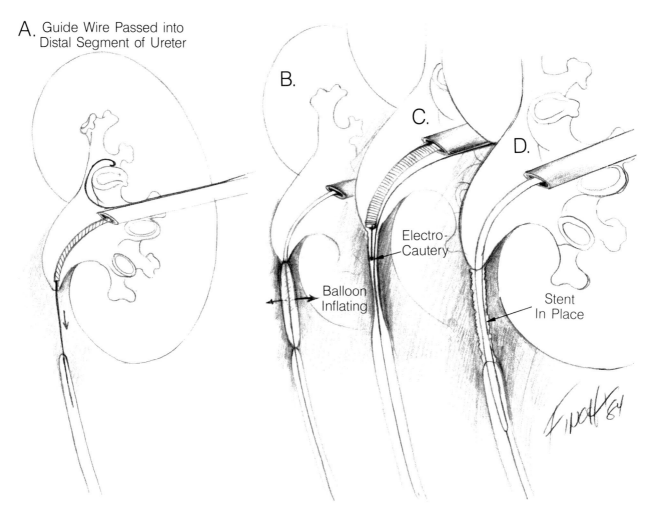

Fig 25–9. **A,** electrolysis: this involves the very careful passage of a cutting wire under both visual and fluoroscopic control directly through the stricture to reestablish continuity. **B,** once continuity is reestablished balloon dilation can take place. **C,** electrocautery can be performed with the aid of the flexible nephroscope. **D,** a stent can be passed through the stricture.

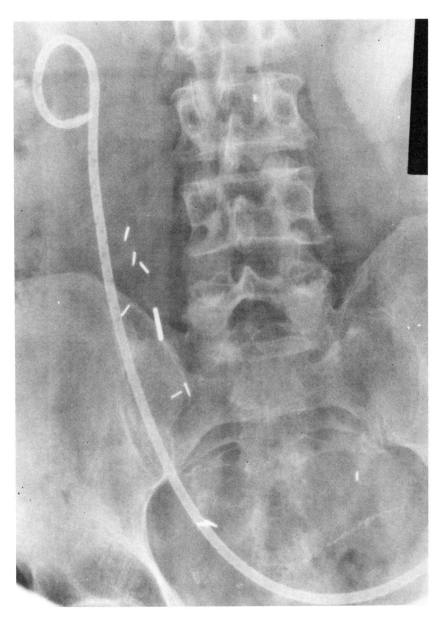

Fig 25–10. Roentgenogram shows a Cope tube in place; this tube is ideal for long-term internal stenting in patients with ileal conduits.

wire is replaced with a routine guide wire passed through the catheter so that communication is re-established. Sequentially, a combination of dilation and cutting is usually performed to open up the ureter sufficiently for stenting (Fig 25–9,C and D). These strictures tend to be much denser than most ureteral strictures and there is a very strong tendency for them to recur; long-term stenting is often necessary (Fig 25–10).

MANAGEMENT OF INFUNDIBULAR STENOSIS

The principles that have been described for the management of different degrees of ureteropelvic junction obstruction can be applied to the management of strictures or obliteration in other parts of the collecting system. Infundibular stenosis can be managed by similar techniques quite success-

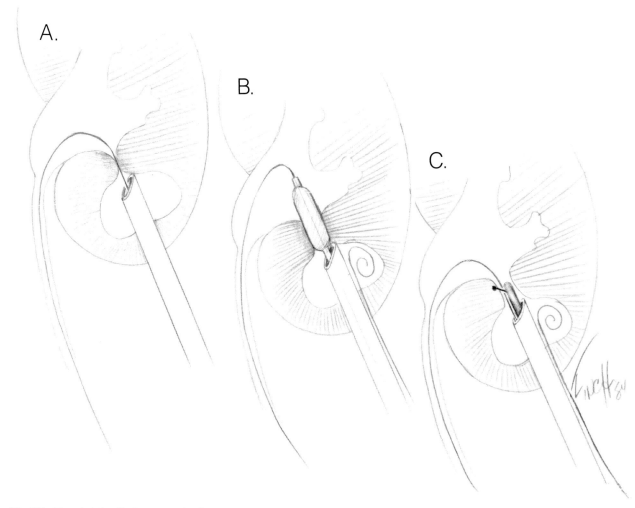

Fig 25–11.   A, infundibulum stenosis: the most simple type–a guide wire can be passed through it. **B,** balloon dilation of a stenosed infundibulum. **C,** incision of the infundibulum may be performed also.

fully; again, it is dependent on the ability to pass a guide wire through the stricture (Fig 25–11,A-C). In many instances in which the infundibulum has been obliterated and stones are trapped in the calyx, electrolysis may be necessary to open the stenosed infundibulum. This can be followed by electrohydraulic lithotripsy. Great care must be taken during this maneuver because of the great proximity of the segmental arteries to the infundibulum (Figs 25–12,A-C and 25–13).

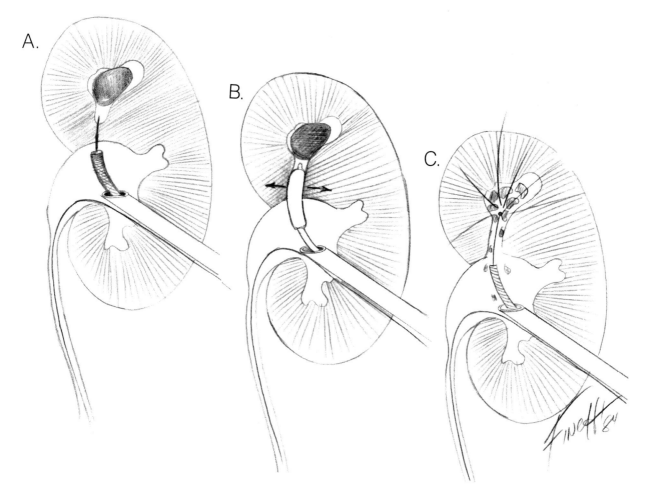

Fig 25–12.   **A,** the completely obliterated infundibulum may be transgressed by electrolysis. **B,** once communication is reestablished, the infundibulum can be dilated or incised. **C,** if a stone is present, it may be reached by either rigid or flexible nephroscopy.

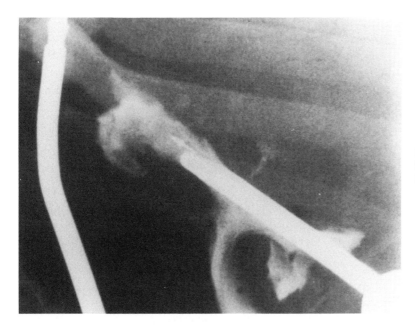

Fig 25–13.   Roentgenogram showing infundibular incision of a stenosed infundibulum by electrocautery with a rigid instrument.

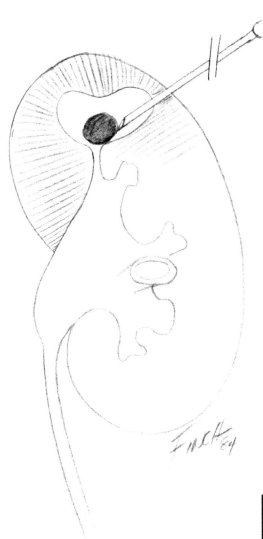

Fig 25–14.   The direct approach to a calyceal diverticula.

Fig 25–15.   Roentgenogram showing direct puncture into the calyceal diverticulum. Note the guide wire coiled in the diverticulum.

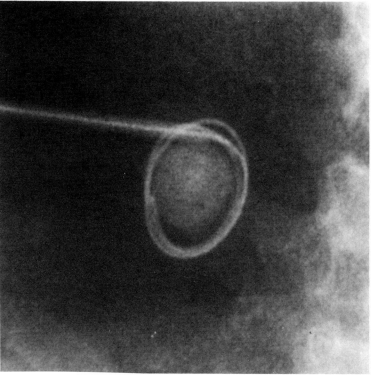

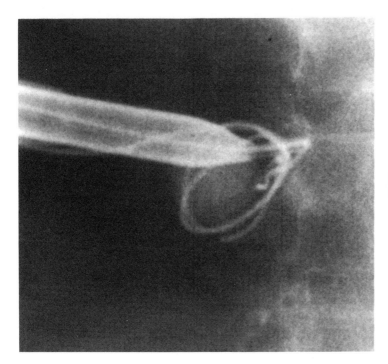

Fig 25–16. Dilation performed with a guide wire in the diverticulum only.

CALYCEAL DIVERTICULA

Calyceal diverticula are found in approximately 0.2% to 0.4% of routine excretory urograms and in most instances are not associated with symptoms and do not require treatment. However, larger diverticula may be complicated by calculus formation and can give rise to symptoms such as pain, recurrent infections, or hematuria. In these instances, the stone should be removed and, if possible, the diverticulum should be obliterated. There are two techniques for dealing with this situation.

Direct Puncture into the Diverticulum

This requires considerable skill, and if the diverticulum is in the upper part of the kidney, puncture above the 12th rib may be necessary (see Chapter 16). Once the diverticulum has been entered a guide wire can be passed in (Figs 25–14 and 25–15). However, it may not pass through the narrow neck of the diverticulum into the main part of the renal pelvis. In this instance, dilation must take place without adequate access having been established to the main part of the collecting system, and will require great care (Fig 25–16). Once a sheath has been inserted into the diverticulum, the stone can be visualized and directly removed (Fig 25–17,A) and then the wire may be passed through the narrow neck of the diverticulum under direct vision if necessary. After dilation of the neck of the diverticulum (Fig 25–17,B) the area should be stented with a suitably sized nephrostomy tube for up to 14 days (Fig 25–17,C). After removal of the tube, the diverticulum will disappear.

Indirect Approach

Diverticula in the upper part of the kidney may be addressed indirectly by puncture into the lower calyx and by approaching the diverticulum with the aid of a flexible nephroscope. A wire is passed through the neck of the diverticulum (Figs 25–18 and 25–19 and Plate 22). The neck of the diverticulum can then be either dilated or incised (Figs 25–20 and 25–21 and Plate 23) to allow the instrument to be inserted inside the diverticulum (Fig 25–22) to remove the stone by either basketing or grasping (Plate 24).

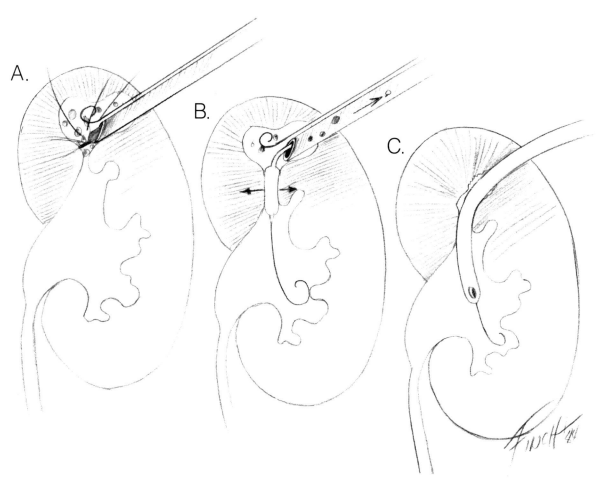

Fig 25–17. **A**, dilation and stone manipulation may have to take place without the wire positioned in the renal pelvis. **B**, dilation of the neck of the diverticulum. **C**, long-term stenting (for 14 days) and the trauma of dilation to the wall of the diverticulum should result in eventual obliteration of the diverticulum.

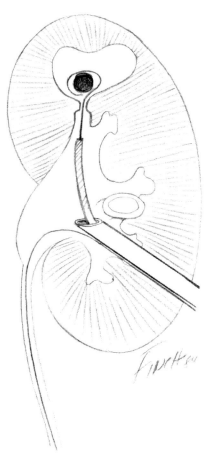

Fig 25–18. The indirect approach to a calyceal diverticulum. Guide wire passed through the narrow opening with the aid of a flexible nephroscope.

Fig 25–19. Roentgenogram showing upper-pole calyceal diverticulum approached indirectly and guide wire passed through narrow communication.

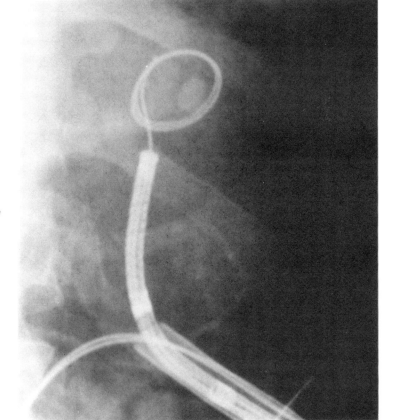

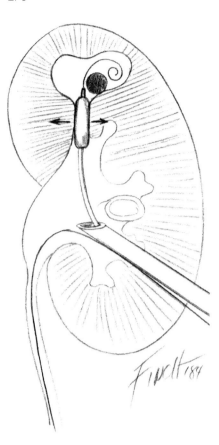

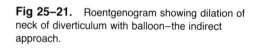

Fig 25–20.   Dilation of the diverticulum.

Fig 25–21.   Roentgenogram showing dilation of neck of diverticulum with balloon–the indirect approach.

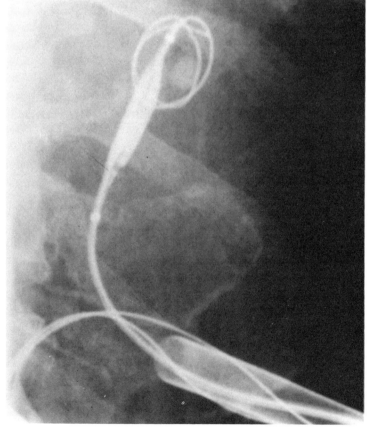

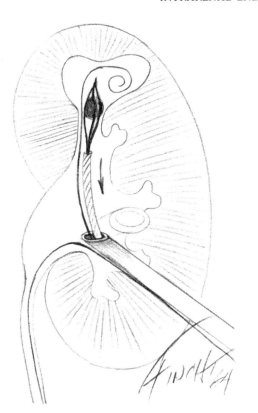

Fig 25–22. Insertion of basket into diverticulum to engage stone.

ENDOCYSTOLYSIS

These techniques can be extended to involve lesions that are not strictures within the collecting system but are intimately related to the kidney. A case is illustrated herein of a patient who had a partial nephrectomy in a solitary kidney and had developed a urinoma that had failed to resolve with both open surgery and an attempt at percutaneous instillation of a sclerosant liquid into the cavity. There was no communication between the cyst cavity and the partially nephrectomized kidney (Fig 25–23,A). Continuity was re-established with the aid of a visually and fluoroscopically guided fine wire and with the aid of a cutting current (Figs 25–23,B and C; 25–24; and 25–25,A), similar to the technique previously described for an obliterated ureteropelvic junction. Once again, both incision and dilation allowed a suitable tract to be established and then fulguration of the wall of the cyst itself encouraged the cyst to collapse around the nephrostomy tube (Fig 25–25,A). Long-term internal stenting allowed the cyst to become completely lysed (Fig 25–25,B and C).

Intrarenal endosurgery is a natural development of the techniques developed for the percutaneous removal of renal and ureteral calculi. Its potential is just beginning. The relationship of this approach to open surgical procedures is still uncertain, particularly in the case of primary ureteropelvic junction obstruction. However, in the poor-risk patient and in the presence of fibrosis, these techniques present a viable alternative to the more established open surgical techniques currently practiced widely.

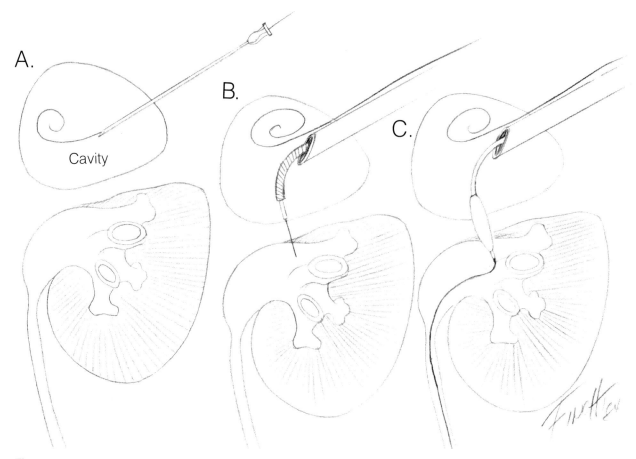

Fig 25–23. **A,** anatomy of endocystolysis case: there is no communication between kidney and cyst. **B,** following dilation of tract into the cyst, communication is established into the collecting system of the kidney by electrolysis. **C,** communication is then dilated and may be incised.

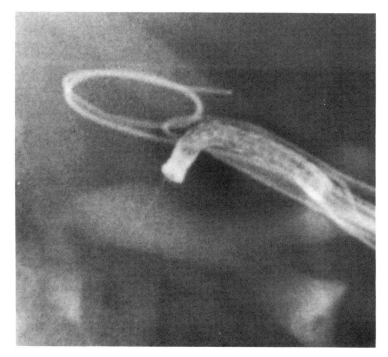

Fig 25–24. Roentgenogram showing establishment of communication between cyst and renal collecting system by electrolysis using flexible endoscopy.

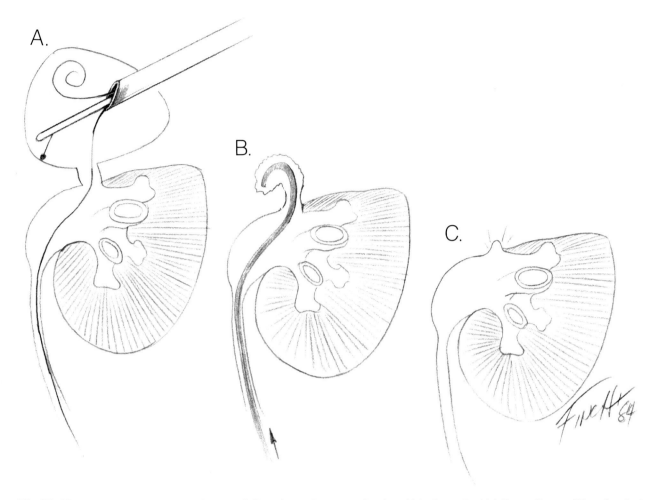

Fig 25–25. **A,** the wall of the cyst is fulgurated. **B,** an internal stent can be placed into the cyst, which then collapses. When the stent is removed the cyst is mostly obliterated. **C,** total disappearance of the cyst.

CHAPTER 26

Endourology of the Ureter: Introduction

Paul H. Lange, M.D.

Endourologic methods are now often used for the diagnosis and treatment of a variety of ureteral lesions, the most common being stones and other causes of obstruction, such as intrinsic or extrinsic tumors or ureteral strictures. Stones are the most common pathologic entities and the indications for intervention are primarily the same as those for open surgical intervention; that is, stones of sufficient size that they cannot or probably will not pass and that cause significant symptoms and obstruction and/or infection. Severely impacted stones formerly were considered a contraindication to endourologic manipulations. However, with increasing success, these stones are now often successfully removed. The location of the stone significantly influences the approach.

Generally, stones in the lower third of the ureter are best approached from below with techniques such as ureterorenoscopy, although this rule is not absolute. (Extracorporeal shock wave lithotripsy is also applicable to some ureteral stones, although these must be located or repositioned in the upper ureter and even there localization of the shock wave is more difficult and success less certain.) The place of endourologic procedures for the correction of anatomical defects such as strictures is being pursued with vigor but their ultimate success rate awaits further experience. Once again, procedures through a percutaneous tract should be avoided in those patients likely to have transitional cell carcinomatous tumors in the upper collecting system.

CHAPTER 27

Endourology of the Ureter: Anatomy

Carol C. Coleman, M.D.

The ureters are paired fibromuscular conduits that are contained in the retroperitoneal space connecting the renal pelvis of each kidney to the urinary bladder. The adult ureter is between 24 and 38 cm in length. There are two segments, abdominal and pelvic, each equal in length.

RELATIONSHIP TO ADJACENT ORGANS

Abdominal Segment

The abdominal segment of the ureters lies in the retroperitoneum on the anterior surface of the psoas major muscle. The right ureter initially is posterior to the descending and transverse portions of the duodenum and the left may be posterior to the tail of the pancreas (Fig 27–1). The upper portions of the ureters are in the perinephric space until about the level of L-5, where they penetrate Gerota's fascia and enter the anterior pararenal space.[1] Five centimeters from the site of origin of the ureters they merge and come into direct contact with the posterior layer of the parietal peritoneum.[2] The ureters are closely attached to the peritoneum. In the case where the kidney is nonrotated or malrotated the proximal few centimeters of the ureter may pass over the lower pole of the kidney, deviating the ureter anteriorly and laterally.[1]

The right ureter is in close proximity but lateral to the inferior vena cava, sympathetic plexus, and vertebral column.[3] The aorta and major aortic lymph node chain are medial to the left ureter. The descending and ascending colon are anterior and lateral to the ureters, the small bowel is anterior and separated from the ureters by a layer of peritoneum.

Each ureter is crossed anteriorly and obliquely by the gonadal vessels between the level of the third and fifth lumbar vertebral bodies. The right ureter is also crossed anteriorly by the right colic and ileocolic vessels and the left ureter anteriorly by the left colic and sigmoid vessels.[4, 5] The abdominal segment of the ureter ends as the ureter crosses the iliac vessels.

Pelvic Segment

The pelvic portion of the ureter is composed of the parietal and intravesical divisions.[5] The parietal division crosses the brim of the pelvis anterior to the bifurcation of the iliac vessels. The right ureter usually crosses the external iliac artery and the left ureter the common iliac artery (Fig 27–2).

Initially, the ureters then generally course laterally following the contour of the pelvic wall before sweeping medially and forward to enter the bladder posteriorly.

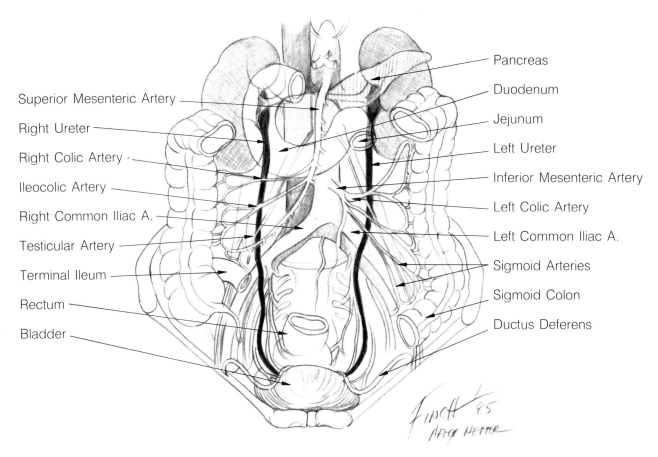

Fig 27–1. Drawing of the relationships of the ureters to adjacent organs and major blood vessels.

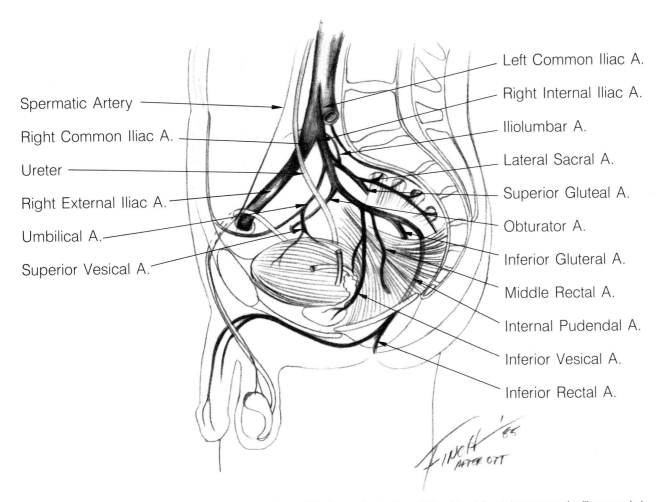

Spermatic Artery

Right Common Iliac A.

Ureter

Right External Iliac A.

Umbilical A.

Superior Vesical A.

Left Common Iliac A.

Right Internal Iliac A.

Iliolumbar A.

Lateral Sacral A.

Superior Gluteal A.

Obturator A.

Inferior Gluteral A.

Middle Rectal A.

Internal Pudendal A.

Inferior Vesical A.

Inferior Rectal A.

Fig 27–2. Artist's drawing of a parasagittal view of the pelvis demonstrating the relationship of the right ureter to the iliac vessels in a male. The right ureter generally crosses the external iliac artery and remains medial to the superior vesical and obturator arteries.

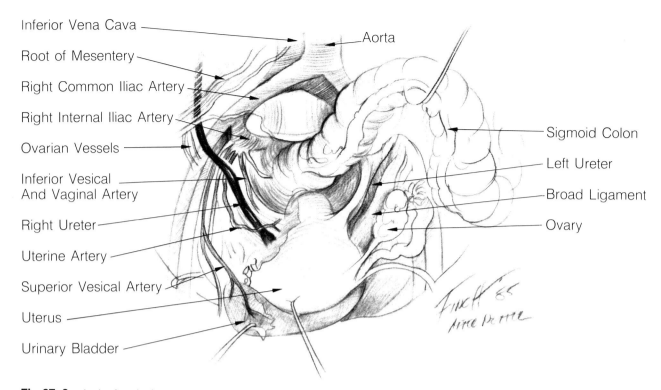

Inferior Vena Cava
Root of Mesentery
Right Common Iliac Artery
Right Internal Iliac Artery
Ovarian Vessels
Inferior Vesical And Vaginal Artery
Right Ureter
Uterine Artery
Superior Vesical Artery
Uterus
Urinary Bladder

Aorta
Sigmoid Colon
Left Ureter
Broad Ligament
Ovary

Fig 27–3. In the female the ureter passes quite close to the ovary, cervix, and fornix of the vagina. The uterine artery crosses the ureter near the ureterovesical junction. It can be seen, therefore, how easy it would be to injure or ligate the ureter during gynecologic surgery.

In the female the ureter has several important relationships. As it descends and turns forward along the lateral wall of the pelvis it is under the parietal peritoneum and behind and below the ovary. Then the ureter courses forward and medially toward the bladder. By doing so the ureter passes close to the cervix of the uterus and lateral fornix of the vagina at a distance of 1 to 2 cm.[5, 6] The uterine artery crosses this segment of the ureter as it passes medially to the uterus from the pelvic wall (Fig 27–3). The proximity of the ureter to these structures makes it vulnerable to ligation or laceration during gynecologic surgery. During oophorectomy the ureter can be injured about 3 to 4 cm above the ureterovesical junction. During hysterectomy when attempting to ligate the uterine artery the gynecologist may accidentally clamp tissue too far laterally and ligate the ureter with the artery. Generally this is about 2 cm above the ureterovesical junction.[1] The close proximity of the ureter to the uterus also makes it quite susceptible to obstruction from cervical and uterine carcinoma. In fact the ureters are quite susceptible to any metastatic gynecologic tumor.

In the male as the ureter reaches the posterolateral aspect of the bladder it is in front of the upper end of the seminal vesicle. The ductus deferens passes anterior and lateral to the termination of the ureter[6] (Fig 27–4).

On the left, the sigmoid colon crosses the ureter and becomes posterior to it.

The terminal portions of the ureters course obliquely through the wall of the bladder for about 0.5 to 1.5 cm. Their internal openings therefore are much closer together than their external penetrations of the bladder wall. This is the most contracted portion of the ureter, being approximately 3 to 4 mm in diameter.

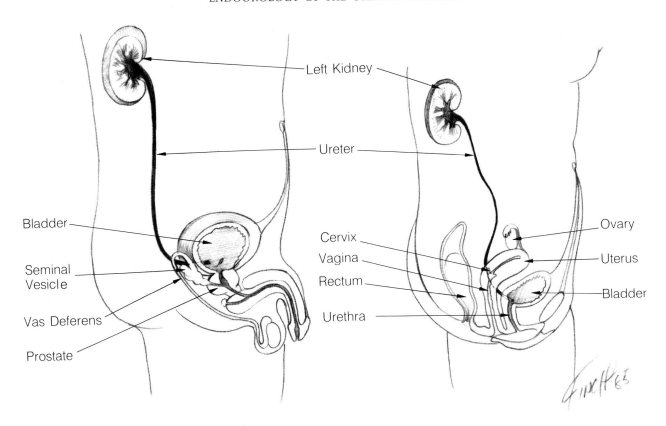

Fig 27–4. Parasagittal views of the ureter of the male and female. In the male the pelvic ureter passes medial to the ductus deferens and anterior to the seminal vesical. In the female the pelvic ureter is in close relationship to the ovary, cervix, and vagina.

RADIOGRAPHIC APPEARANCE

The ureter is adjacent to or courses nearby many important structures throughout its length and is therefore subject to many influences. There are significant variations in the position of the ureter. It is easy to be undone by a normal ureter.

Anteroposterior View

On intravenous pyelograms the entire ureter is often not visualized on one single radiograph because of peristalsis, unless high-dose urography is performed. In this type of examination diuresis may overload the ureters, therefore causing its complete visualization. On immediate postrelease films, the entire ureter may also be demonstrated. Another way to fill the ureters is by placing the patient in the prone position. The upper poles of the kidneys are more posterior than the lower poles; therefore the cranial calyces are more dorsal and hence more dependent and will contain more contrast (contrast is heavier than urine). In the

prone position, these calyces will empty and help fill the ureter. Retrograde ureterograms provide for excellent opacification of the ureter.

At the level of middle to inferior pole of the kidney, the pelvis narrows to form the ureter[5] at a point approximately at the level of the second lumbar vertebra. The abdominal course of the ureter is generally vertical parallel to or passing over the lateral aspects of the transverse processes of the lumbar vertebral bodies. They can be variable in position and are not necessarily identical in their course on both sides. The ureters usually do not cross the pedicles of the first four lumbar vertebral bodies unless a retrocaval ureter is present. As the ureter reaches the L-5 level it becomes more medial, sometimes overlying and coursing medial to the pedicles of L-5 and S-1. The right ureter often approaches the midline, particularly in young adults.[7] Hypertrophy of the psoas muscle can deviate the proximal ureter laterally and the distal abdominal ureter medially. Even in its most lateral course the ureter projects still medially to the sacroiliac joint.

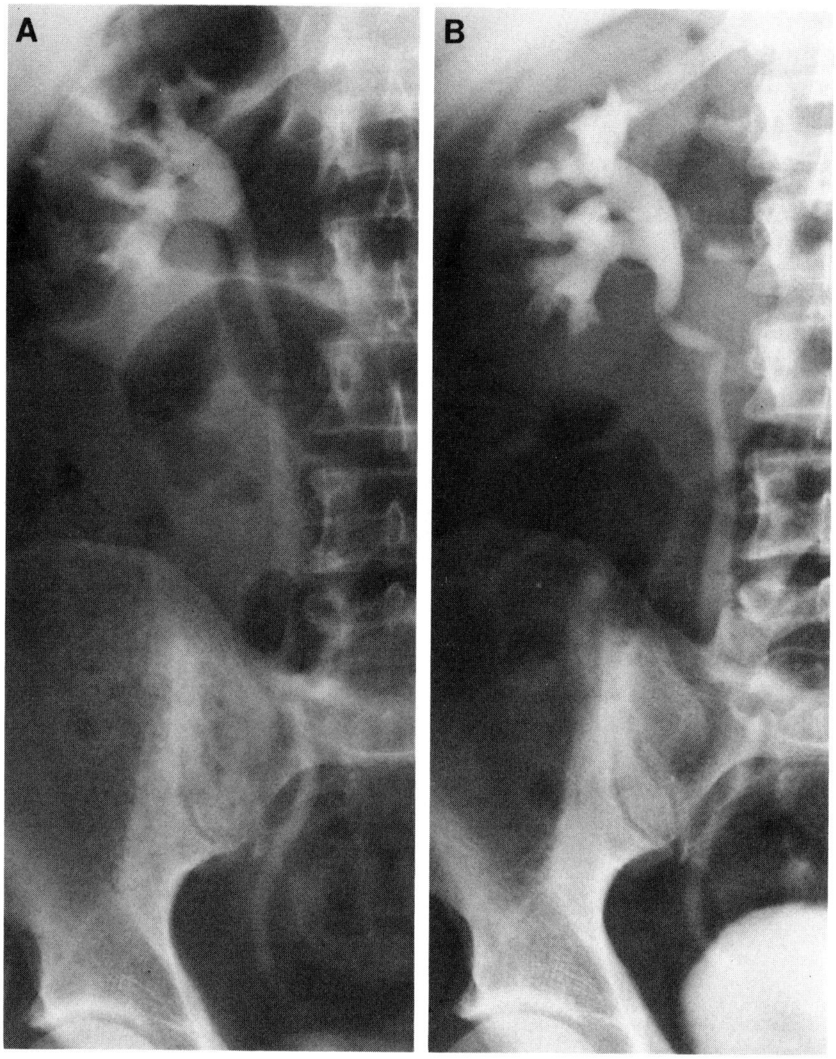

Fig 27–5. Expiration **(A)**, and inspiration **(B)** radiographs from an intravenous urogram. On inspiration the kidney descends. The ureter, being mobile, responds by kinking.

In the proximal ureter kinking may occur for several reasons: (1) Because of the mobility of the kidney and ureter, an inspiratory film will displace the kidney and proximal ureter inferiorly (Fig 27–5). (2) During peristaltic activity the ureter may kink. (3) A well-developed psoas may displace the upper ureter laterally, causing a transverse oblique extrinsic lucent filling defect. The ureter then turns medially with varying degrees of acuteness and descends along the anterior medial surface of the psoas margins. (4) Chronic obstruc-

tion can cause severe kinking, making the passage of a guide wire quite difficult (Fig 27–6).

In the midureter the gonadal vessels cross and often indent the ureters anteriorly at the level of L-3-5[7] (Fig 27–7). Sometimes the contrast material is held up at this point and the ureter above may even be dilated, although this usually does not cause obstruction. In some women the ovarian vein crosses the ureter vertically at S-1 and again at L-4.[1]

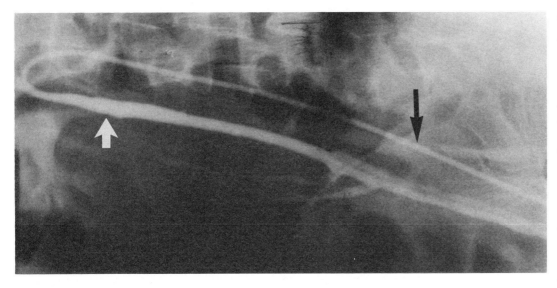

Fig 27–7. Right spermatic venogram performed prior to spermatic vein embolization for varicoceles in male infertility. The right spermatic vein crosses the ureter at the L2-3 level (*white arrow*). The catheter traversing the right iliac vein is crossed by the ureter medial to the sacroiliac joint at the S-1 level (*black arrow*). If using mechanical devices such as coils for embolization, it is better not to place them where the vein crosses the ureter or iliac arteries in case of erosion or perforation by the coil.

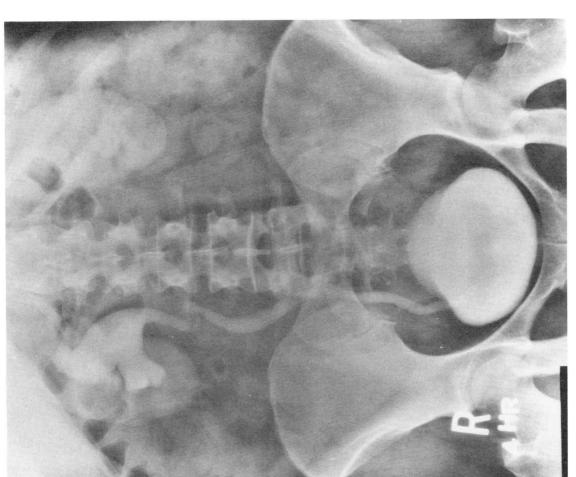

Fig 27–6. An intravenous pyelogram demonstrating a kinked ureter from chronic obstruction. Ureters that have chronic distal obstructions from stones, tumors, or benign strictures dilate and elongate and may often cause severe kinking.

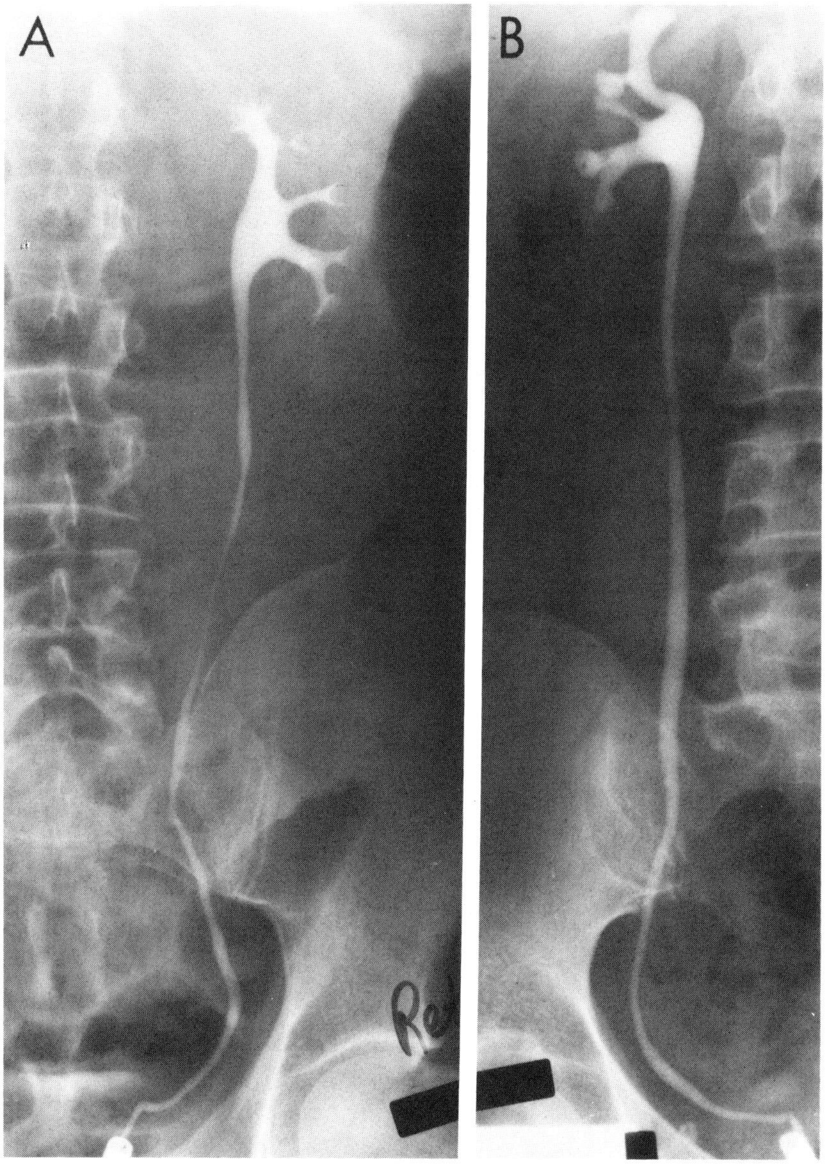

Fig 27–8. Normal lateral course of the pelvic ureters **(A and B). A,** the ureter courses lateral to the psoas muscle before crossing at L4-5, a normal variant. **B,** the distal abdominal ureter is positioned lateral to the L-5 pedicle giving the entire abdominal ureter a straight course.

In the pelvis the ureter may be deviated anteriorly and medially as it crosses the iliac artery. The ureter then usually courses laterally and posteriorly following the contour of the lateral wall of the bony pelvis.[8] It then returns toward the midline medially and anteriorly to enter the trigone of the bladder (Fig 27–8). The ureterovesical junction approximates a line joining the two ischial spines. However there are significant variations. In women there may be straightening or medial deviation of the pelvic portion of the right ureter.[7] This may be why the right ureter is obstructed more frequently than the left in cervical carcinoma.[1] In these women the uterus is more often tilted to the left.[7] In some of both sexes the ureters are medially located to the pelvic inlet even medial to the pedicles of L-5 (Fig 27–9). Also in both sexes the ureters may sweep only slightly lateral in the pelvis[1] (Fig 27–10).

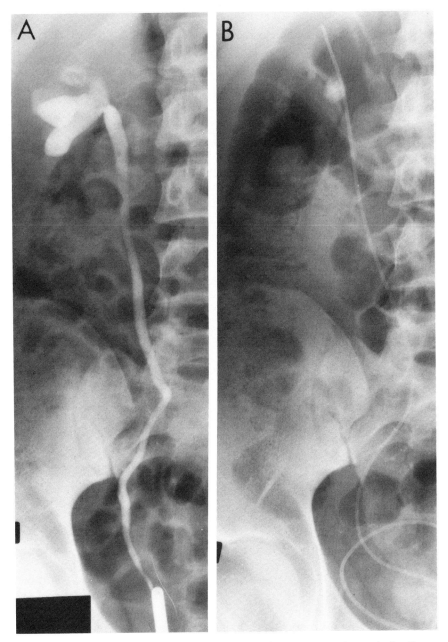

Fig 27–9. Patient with a pelvic stone. **A,** retrograde ureterogram demonstrating the ureter medial to the pedicle of L-5. **B,** the ureteral catheter also clearly identifies the course of the ureter.

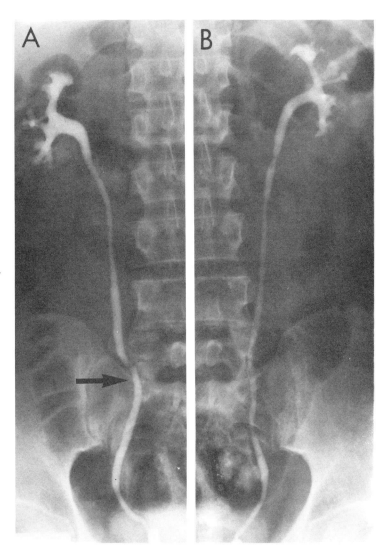

Fig 27–10. Retrograde ureterograms **(A and B)** from a patient whose pelvic ureters sweep only slightly laterally. Note the medial deviation *(arrow)* of the ureter secondary to the iliac vessels in **A.**

There are three normal areas of caliber narrowing of the ureter: (1) uppermost at the ureteropelvic junction; (2) at the transition from the abdominal to the pelvic ureter at the crossing of the iliac arteries, especially in older persons with atheromatous vessels; and (3) lowermost at the uretero- vesical junction. The intramural course of the ureter is the most narrow part of the duct (Fig 27–11). In these segments ureteral calculi may be commonly lodged. There may be mild dilatations between these normal constrictions giving the ureter a spindle shape[5] (Fig 27–12).

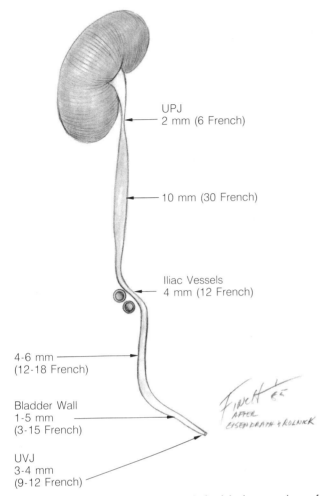

UPJ
2 mm (6 French)

10 mm (30 French)

Iliac Vessels
4 mm (12 French)

4-6 mm
(12-18 French)

Bladder Wall
1-5 mm
(3-15 French)

UVJ
3-4 mm
(9-12 French)

Fig 27–11. There are three natural physiologic narrowings of the ureter. The first at the ureteropelvic junction, the second at the iliac vessels, and the third at the ureterovesical junction.

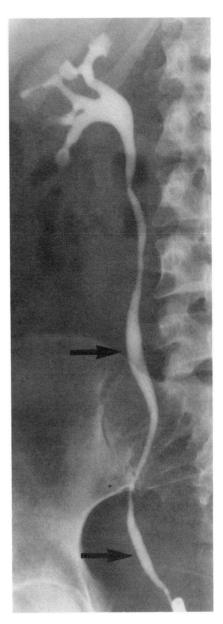

Fig 27–12. So-called spindle ureter. The ureter is mildly dilated above the ureterovesical junction and iliac vessels *(arrows)* where there are normal physiologic constrictions of the ureter.

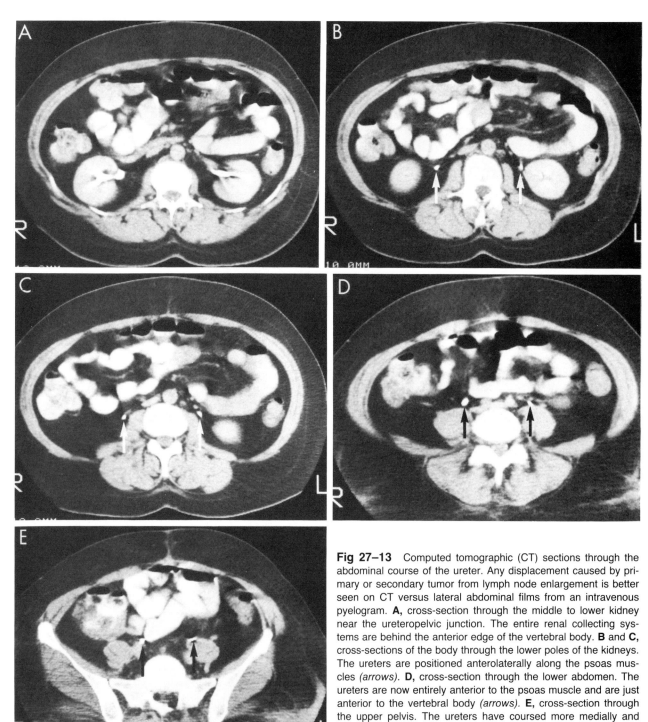

Fig 27–13 Computed tomographic (CT) sections through the abdominal course of the ureter. Any displacement caused by primary or secondary tumor from lymph node enlargement is better seen on CT versus lateral abdominal films from an intravenous pyelogram. **A,** cross-section through the middle to lower kidney near the ureteropelvic junction. The entire renal collecting systems are behind the anterior edge of the vertebral body. **B** and **C,** cross-sections of the body through the lower poles of the kidneys. The ureters are positioned anterolaterally along the psoas muscles *(arrows)*. **D,** cross-section through the lower abdomen. The ureters are now entirely anterior to the psoas muscle and are just anterior to the vertebral body *(arrows)*. **E,** cross-section through the upper pelvis. The ureters have coursed more medially and more anteriorly *(arrows),* corresponding to the typical findings seen on a lateral view from an intravenous pyelogram.

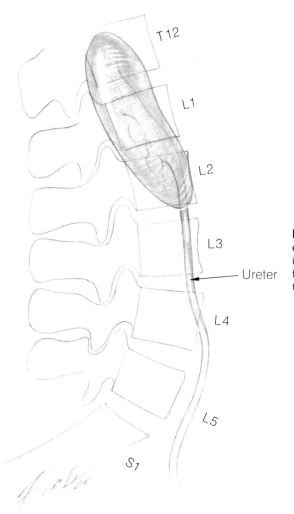

Fig 27–14. Drawing of the position of the ureter seen on lateral view from an intravenous pyelogram. At its origin the ureter is behind the anterior edge of the vertebral body. By L-4 it is in front of the vertebral body and at L-5 lies anteriorly one fourth of the width of the vertebral body.

Lateral View

In the past, lateral views of the kidneys and ureters used to be commonly utilized to diagnose displacement. Nowadays this has been replaced with computed tomography (Fig 27–13). The standard film was taken as a cross-table lateral view, so that no false anterior displacement of the kidney or ureter would occur because of the mobility of the kidney and ureter as seen on the decubitus lateral view.

When the kidney is in its normal lumbar position, the normal renal collecting system should not project beyond the anteriormost portion of the spine.[8] The ureter is initially behind the anterior margin of the vertebral bodies and projects over the anterior margin at about the level of L-4. At the L-5 level the ureter lies approximately one fourth of the width of the vertebral body anterior to the vertebral body[1] (Fig 27–14).

If the kidney is lower than usual it will follow the anterior margin of the psoas muscle and may lie in a more anterior position than normal.

Blood Supply

The blood supply to the ureter has multiple origins (Plate 25). The pelviureteral artery is a major vessel to the renal pelvis and proximal ureter. It is a branch from the anterior division of the main renal artery. The second major source is the gonadal artery, which gives branches to the midureter.[2] The lower ureter is supplied primarily by branches of the superior and inferior vesical arteries (branches of the internal iliac artery). The other more minor blood supply comes from direct small segmental branches from the aorta, lumbar arteries, or iliac arteries.

REFERENCES

1. Friedland G., Filly R., Goris M.L., et al.: Anatomy, in Friedland G., et al.*Uroradiology: An Integrated Approach.* New York, Churchill Livingstone, 1983, pp. 11-153.
2. Bosniak M.A., Siegelman S.S., Evans J.A.: Tumors of the ureter, in Hodes P.J. (ed.): *The Adrenal, Retroperitoneum and Lower Urinary Tract, An Atlas of Tumor Radiology.* Chicago, Year Book Medical Publishers Inc., 1976, pp. 337-437.
3. Cohen J.D., Persky L.: Ureteral stones. *Urol. Clin. North Am.* 10:699-708, 1983.
4. Woodburne R.T.: The abdomen, in *Essentials of Human Anatomy.* New York, Oxford University Press, 1969, pp. 359-459.
5. McVay C.: Abdominal cavity and contents, in *Surgical Anatomy,* ed. 6. Philadelphia, W.B. Saunders Co., 1984, pp. 585-777.
6. Woodburne R.T.: The pelvis, in *Essentials of Human Anatomy.* New York, Oxford University Press, 1969, pp. 474-515.
7. Lich R. Jr., Howerton L.W., Amin M.: Anatomy and surgical approach to the urogenital tract in the male, in *Campbell's Urology,* ed. 4. Philadelphia, W.B. Saunders Co., 1978, pp. 3-33.
8. Pollack H.M.: Intravenous urography, in *Radiologic Examination of the Urinary Tract.* Hagerstown, Md, Harper & Row, 1971, pp. 11-86.

CHAPTER 28

Endourology of the Ureter: Stone Removal by Fluoroscopic Techniques

David W. Hunter, M.D.

Percutaneous removal of ureteral stones was originally done almost entirely with fluoroscopic methods. As endoscopic techniques were added to the armamentarium, results began to improve. Experience with all of the methods led to further improvements in results and with the addition and refinement of the fluoroscopic technique of retrograde flushing, the present success rate of close to 100% was achieved. The retrograde flushing technique is described in Chapter 17.

In our experience removal of stones in the upper ureter is one of the most difficult procedures. Whereas stones in the lower ureter are usually easily removed by baskets (particularly under direct vision through a retrograde ureterorenoscope), stones in the upper ureter require different techniques. Commonly, stones are pushed into the mucosa if instruments are passed; therefore, the first technique to be used is flushing of the stone by injecting contrast medium or carbon dioxide through the ureteral catheter, which is positioned immediately beneath the stone. If this fails, mechanical means have to be attempted.

As a stone lodges in the ureter it rapidly develops a pocket of granulation tissue, which surrounds it and makes it inaccessible to the instruments used for percutaneous removal. Some fluoroscopic techniques are therefore used to dis-lodge stones so that they can be removed by other fluoroscopic or endoscopic means. The most commonly used of these methods is prying a stone loose with the tip of a catheter. A wall-seeking, torque-control catheter such as a Cobra (Cordis, Miami, Fla.) is used. The catheter is advanced over a guide wire (Fig 28–1,A) until the catheter tip is positioned adjacent to the stone. The tip is rotated and moved up and down against the edge of the stone (Fig 28–1,B) in an attempt to free the stone from the pocket of granulation tissue. Once free, it can be basketed or grasped. A coiled guide wire or a two-wire snare can occasionally achieve a similar result.

Another method is to use a balloon catheter to pull a ureteral stone back toward the renal pelvis where it can be more easily grasped. Usually a small catheter such as a Fogarty is passed through a larger catheter so that the balloon is below the stone (Fig 28–1,C).

The balloon is inflated and the catheter withdrawn, hopefully pulling the stone toward the pelvis (Fig 28–2).

Another similar method that has met with limited success in special circumstances is to advance the blunt, cutoff end of a 14 to 20 F Red Robinson catheter over a guide wire to a point immediately adjacent to the stone. Suction is applied with a 60-cc catheter-tip syringe (Fig 28–3) and the stone

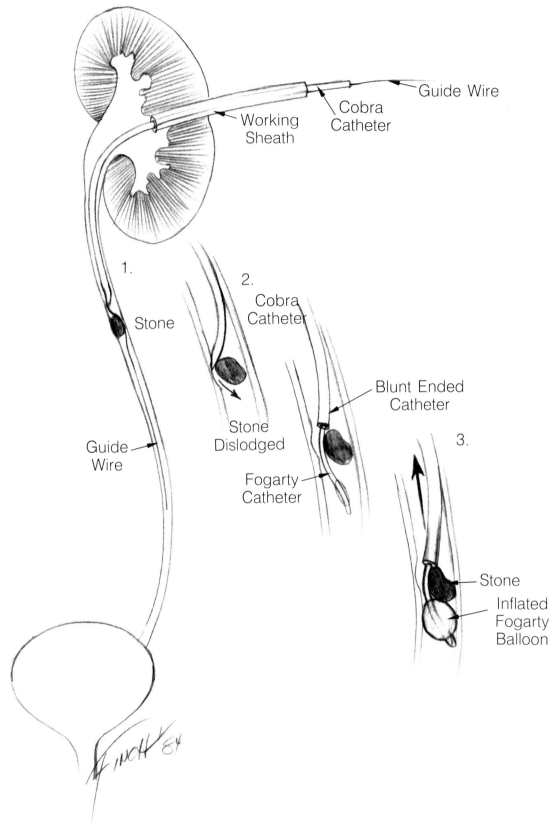

Fig 28–1. **A,** catheter is advanced over guide wire until tip is adjacent to stone. **B,** tip is rotated and moved up and down against the edge of the stone, to free it from the pocket of granulation tissue. **C,** alternatively, balloon catheter is used to pull stone back toward renal pelvis, where it can be more easily grasped.

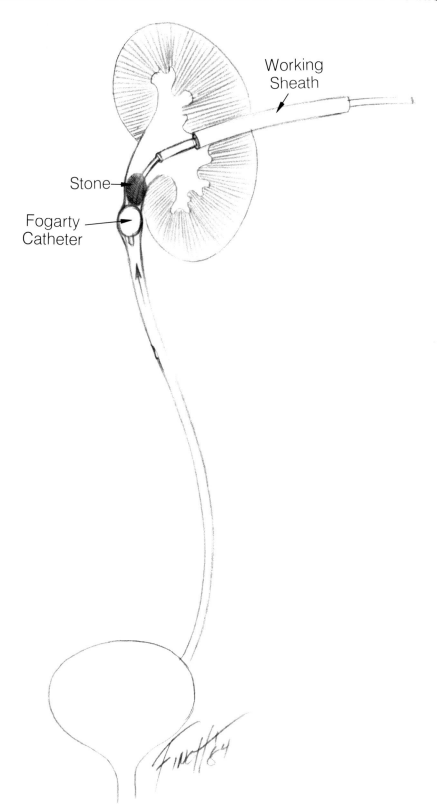

Working
Sheath

Stone—

Fogarty —
Catheter

Fig 28–2. Inflated Fogarty catheter balloon is
used to pull stone toward renal pelvis.

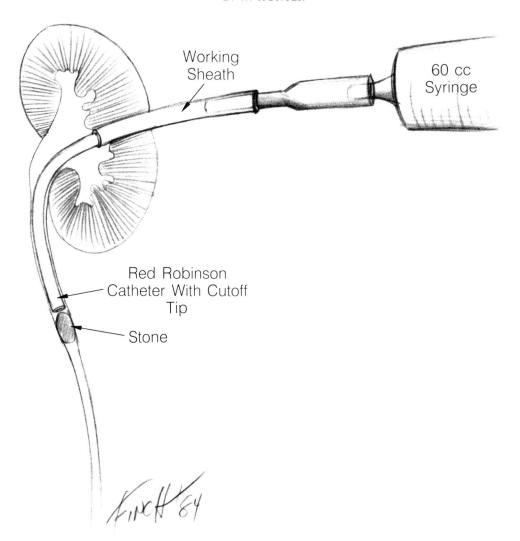

Fig 28–3. Using suction from 60-cc catheter-tip syringe, stone and catheter are slowly withdrawn toward renal pelvis.

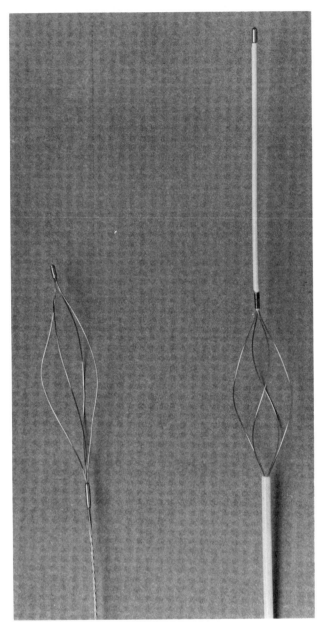

Fig 28–4. Wire baskets used for stone removal.

and catheter are slowly withdrawn toward the renal pelvis. In one instance, the stone was so securely held that it was possible to remove it with this technique.

Other fluoroscopic techniques are used in an attempt to not only dislodge, but to completely remove ureteral stones. By far, the most common method is basketing. The baskets that have met with the greatest success have been one with four straight wires and one with three or four curved wires (Fig 28–4). The straight wire basket allows the stone to enter the basket more easily and has been more successful in dislodging stones that are partially imbedded in the ureteral wall. Curved wire baskets, although they do open more fully in the narrow ureter, have been slightly less successful in engaging the stone. However, once the stone is engaged in such a basket it will never escape.

We always prefer to use baskets with a large, soft "nose" (Fig 28–5) so that if the basket is pulled too far back it can be readvanced to the level of the stone without having to worry about inadvertently injuring the ureter. Injury to the ureter near the stone rapidly results in edema, which makes stone removal almost impossible.

Whenever we attempt to basket a ureteral stone, we place the safety catheter and wire not in the ureter, as is usually done, but somewhere in the collecting system (Fig 28–6,A). Even just a guide wire in the ureter past the stone severely hinders basketing efforts. The entire basketing procedure is carried out as gently as possible to minimize ureteral trauma and edema.

Following tract dilation and working sheath placement a torque-control catheter is used to advance a soft, floppy-tipped wire past the stone (see Fig 28–1). A 9 F nontapered catheter is advanced over the guide wire to a position just above the stone (Fig 28–6,B). In some cases, the catheter goes past the stone without resistance. This position is desirable, since it allows the basket to be

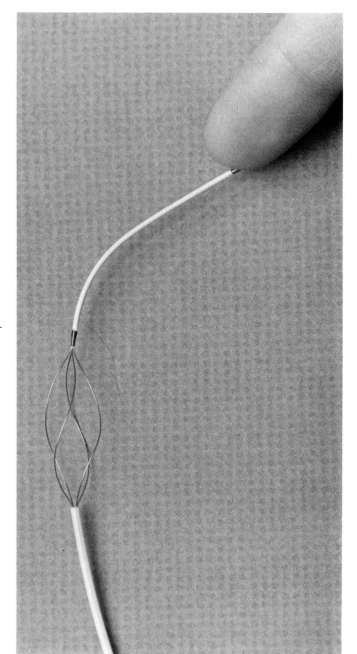

Fig 28–5. Basket with large, soft "nose" to prevent inadvertent injury to the ureter.

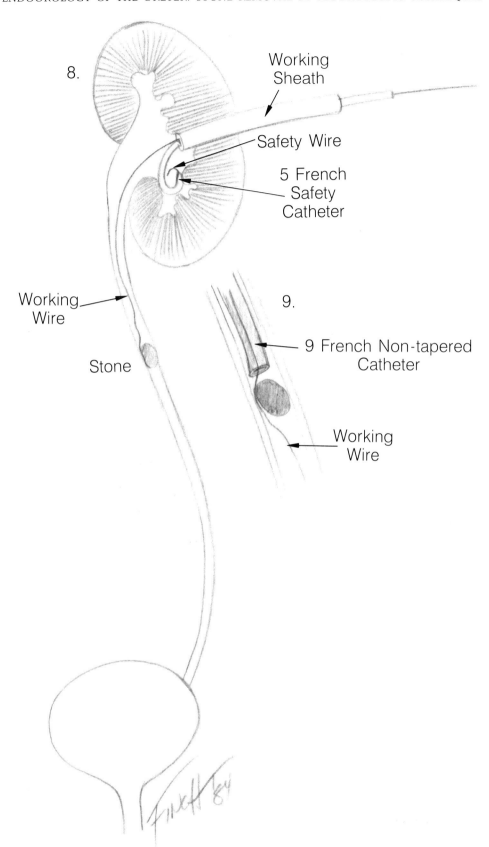

8.

Working
Sheath

Safety Wire

5 French
Safety
Catheter

Working
Wire

Stone

9.

9 French Non-tapered
Catheter

Working
Wire

Fig 28–6. **A,** during basketing, safety wire and catheter remain in collecting system; after dilation of tract and placement of working sheath, a torque-control catheter is used to advance a soft, floppy-tipped wire past the stone. **B,** 9 F nontapered catheter is advanced over guide wire to a position just above the stone.

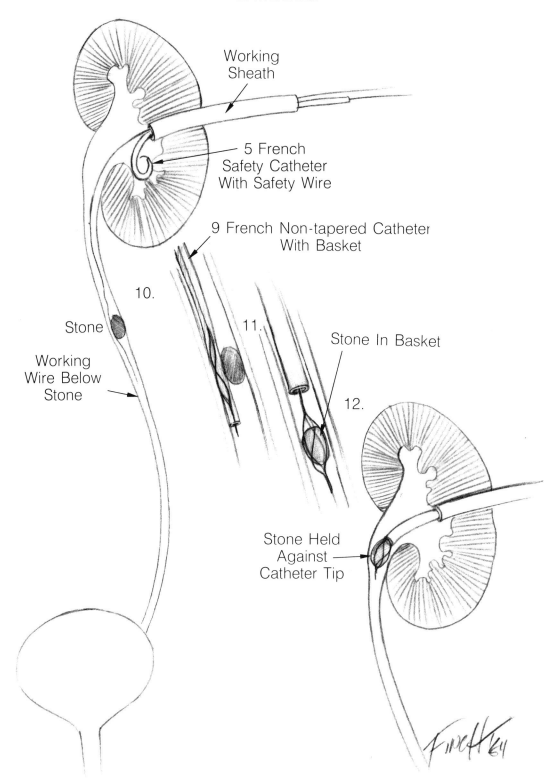

Working
Sheath

5 French
Safety Catheter
With Safety Wire

9 French Non-tapered Catheter
With Basket

10.

Stone

Working
Wire Below
Stone

11.

Stone In Basket

12.

Stone Held
Against
Catheter Tip

Fig 28–7. **A,** catheter advances past stone, allowing basket to be placed at level of stone. **B,** basket is passed through catheter until it can be opened at level of stone. **C,** stone is engaged in basket, and basket and catheter are slowly withdrawn as a unit.

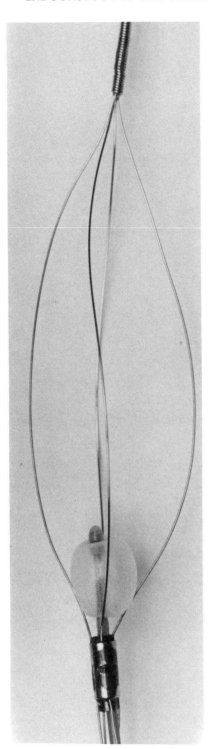

Fig 28–8. Basket with balloon.

placed at the level of the stone (Fig 28–7,A), but it is not necessary or even preferable to do this since there is always the risk that the catheter will further push the stone into the wall and prevent its removal. The basket is passed through the 9 F catheter until it can be opened at the level of the stone (Fig 28–7,B). Once the basket is opened, jerky up-and-down movements and spinning motions, first in one direction and then the other, are used to try to coax the stone into the basket. Once the stone appears to be in the basket, the basket is held still while it is gently closed by advancing either its own catheter or the 9 F introducing catheter toward the stone. With the stone engaged, the basket and catheter are slowly withdrawn as a unit (Fig 28–7,C).

Next to dislodging the stone from its mucosal pocket, the most difficult problem has been to get the basket open in the ureter. Several baskets have been designed to try to overcome this problem, including baskets with balloons (Fig 28–8) and a through-and-through basket, which can be opened by pushing on the basket from both sides (Fig 28–9). Neither effort has been very successful. Dilating the ureter above and below the stone with a balloon prior to basketing has also been tried without much success. Choosing a basket with stiffer wires, or using one of the curved wire baskets that spring open with greater force, and using shaking and twisting movements have been the only reasonably successful ways to combat this problem. A more definitive solution is lacking.

Another fluoroscopic method used to remove ureteral stones is with any of several graspers (Fig 28–10) placed through an introducing catheter. Unlike the introducing catheter used with a basket, the catheter used with a grasper must have a steerable tip like a Burhenne, or a gently curved tip so that the grasper can be accurately directed at the stone (Fig 28–11). When using any grasper in the ureter under fluoroscopic control, a C-arm or some other way of seeing the grasper and stone in more than one projection is critical. Before the "jaws" of the grasper are even opened, we always check to be sure that the grasper is immediately adjacent to the stone. Without such precautions there is an unacceptably high risk of mucosal injury and ureteral perforation.

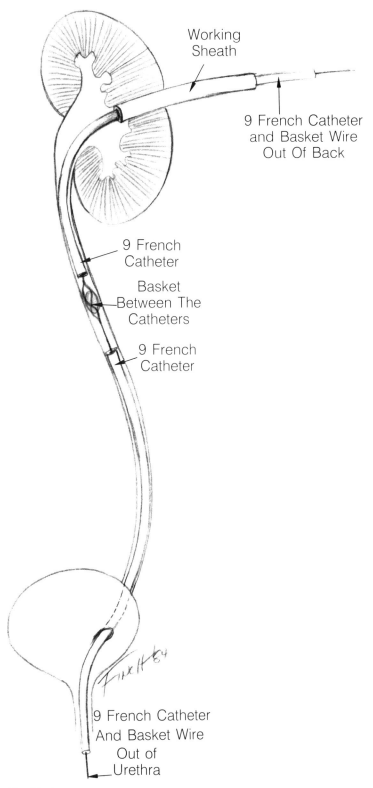

Working
Sheath

9 French Catheter
and Basket Wire
Out Of Back

9 French
Catheter

Basket
Between The
Catheters

9 French
Catheter

9 French Catheter
And Basket Wire
Out of
Urethra

Fig 28–9. Through-and-through stone basket, which can be opened by pushing from both sides.

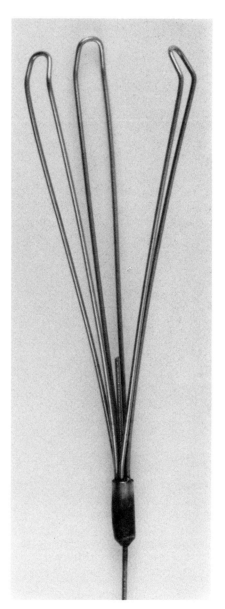

Fig 28–10. Stone grasper.

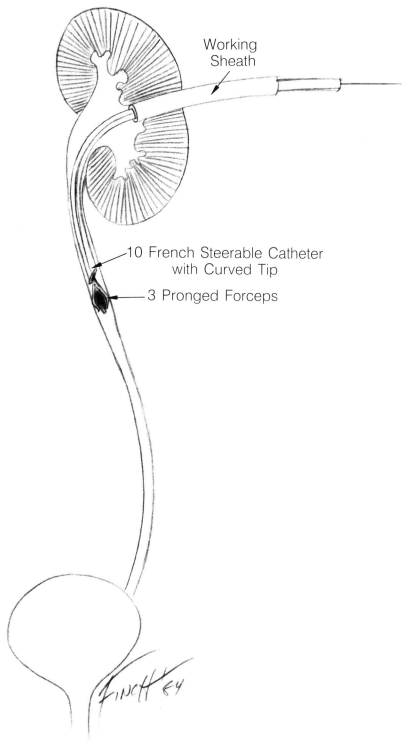

Fig 28–11. Steerable catheter with three-pronged stone graspers, shown securing ureteral stone.

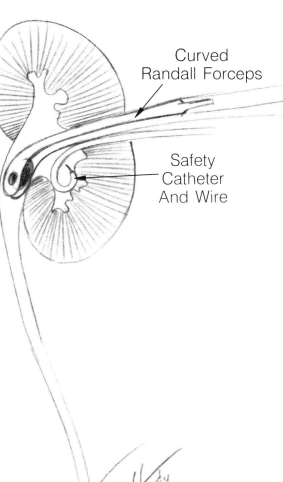

Curved
Randall Forceps

Safety
Catheter
And Wire

Fig 28–12. Curved Randall forceps, which can be used for stones in the ureter near the ureteropelvic junction.

For stones in the ureter near the ureteropelvic junction, a Randall forceps can be used (Fig 28–12). We use the grooved Randall forceps, which can be advanced over a guide wire to the stone. Similar precautions to those used with the graspers, including the use of two or more fluoroscopic planes for position verification, are required when using the Randall forceps. If the Randall forceps will not open easily or adequately in the ureter, they should never be forced open, because it is quite easy to overdistend and rupture the ureter.

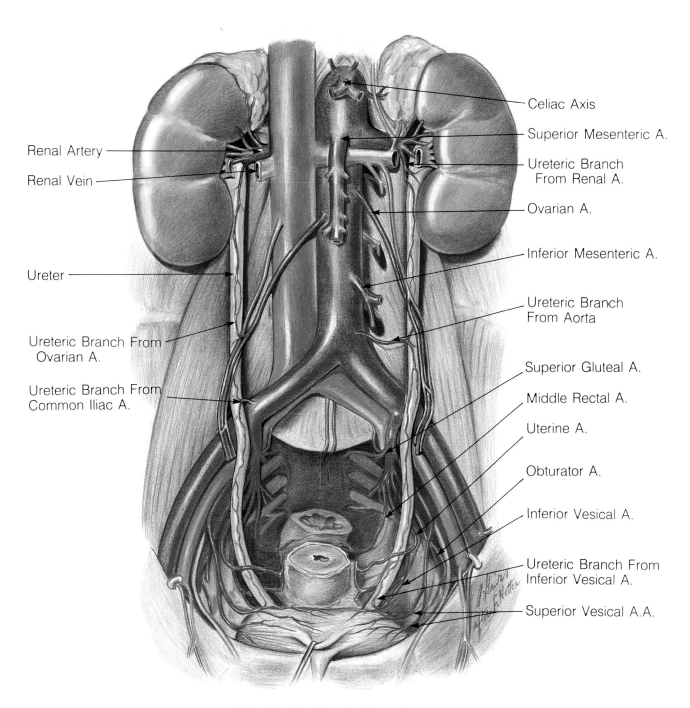

Renal Artery

Renal Vein

Ureter

Ureteric Branch From
Ovarian A.

Ureteric Branch From
Common Iliac A.

Celiac Axis

Superior Mesenteric A.

Ureteric Branch
From Renal A.

Ovarian A.

Inferior Mesenteric A.

Ureteric Branch
From Aorta

Superior Gluteal A.

Middle Rectal A.

Uterine A.

Obturator A.

Inferior Vesical A.

Ureteric Branch From
Inferior Vesical A.

Superior Vesical A.A.

Plate 25.   Blood supply of the ureter.

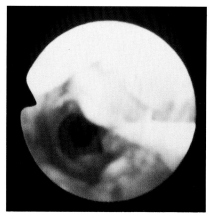

Plate 26. Antegrade view down ureter; note narrow lumen.

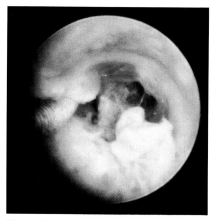

Plate 27. Ureteral calculus impacted in the ureter; note the considerable periureteral edema and the guide wire located adjacent to the stone.

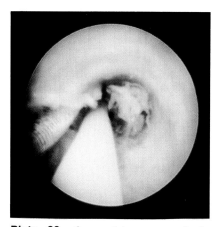

Plate 28. Successful passage of closed stone basket (white catheter) past the stone; note the apparent impaction of the stone within the ureteral wall.

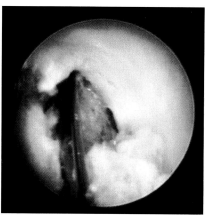

Plate 29. Open basket engaging the stone.

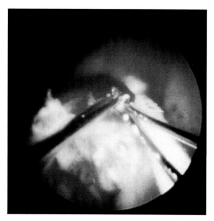

Plate 30. Stone successfully basketed; note the significant trauma to the ureteral mucosa.

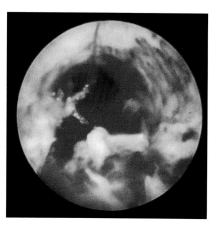

Plate 31. Ureter after successful antegrade stone manipulation; note significant ureteral edema and hemorrhage.

CHAPTER 29

Endourology of the Ureter: Percutaneous Endoscopic Removal of Ureteral Calculi

John C. Hulbert, M.D., F.R.C.S.

When a calculus passes into the ureter, pain is often the presenting symptom. Approximately 80% of ureteral calculi will pass spontaneously; however, stone removal is indicated when the pain is severe and the stone has ceased to move down the ureter, when infection is present, or when the kidney is obstructed by such a calculus. Traditional techniques of removal have been relatively blind retrograde stone manipulation with the aid of a stone basket for those stones below the pelvic brim, and open ureterolithotomy for those above the pelvic brim or those below the pelvic brim that could not be engaged with a retrograde basket. With the development of percutaneous techniques antegrade ureteral stone manipulations were preferred initially, using baskets and fluoroscopy. With the subsequent development of instruments for the visualization of the interior of the collecting system, in particular the flexible fiberoptic nephroscope, it has become apparent that endoscopy aided by fluoroscopy, whenever possible, is preferable to fluoroscopy alone for removal of ureteral stones. Two broad categories of techniques will be discussed in this chapter; first, antegrade endoscopic techniques for the removal of ureteral calculi, and second, retrograde flushing as an aid to the removal of these stones.

ANTEGRADE ENDOSCOPIC TECHNIQUES

Antegrade attempts at stone manipulation depend on the ability to pass instruments down to the stone in order to engage it with either a basket, snare, three- or four-prong grasper, or grasping forceps. The ureter, however, has a narrow lumen (Plate 26), such that it may be impossible for these instruments to open adequately in order to engage the stone; furthermore, an impacted stone can be surrounded by considerable edema. Attempts to pass a wire may result in perforation of the ureter (Fig 29–1) or dissection of the wire under the ureteral mucosa so that tissue is interposed between the stone and the guide wire (Fig 29–2). Even if neither of these complications occurs the lumen of the ureter may not allow the basket to open sufficiently to engage the stone (Fig 29–3). The use of endoscopy may assist in visualizing the stone, as obstruction of the ureter by the stone may have dilated the ureter proximally, facilitating the passage of the flexible nephroscope. It may then be feasible to engage the stone with a grasping forceps or a basket (Figs 29–4 and 29–5). The stone in the ureter, however, may be surrounded by considerable edema (Plate 27) and in order to

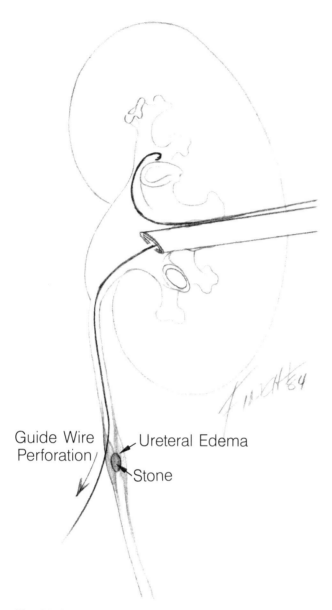

Guide Wire
Perforation

Ureteral Edema

Stone

Fig 29–1. In the presence of periureteral edema around a stone, the potential for ureteral perforation by the guide wire is significant.

basket the stone, the closed basket must be able to pass the stone before being opened (Plate 28). The basket can then be gently opened and attempts can be made to "persuade" the stone to fall into it (Plate 29). Even with appropriate care, significant trauma to the ureter may occur during basketing such that the ureteral epithelium is abraded and edematous (Plates 30 and 31). Attempts to grasp the stone with grasping forceps may also cause similar problems. In fact, ureteral perforation and periureteral extravasation do occur, but the ureter seems to sustain such trauma with remarkably little long-term effect as long as it is stented adequately.

Thus endoscopic and/or fluoroscopic controlled antegrade manipulations in the ureter are very successful, but failures and complications do occur. Consequently we devised the retrograde flushing technique, which has further reduced both the complications and failure rates when applied to calculi in the middle and upper ureter.

RETROGRADE FLUSHING
OF URETERAL CALCULI

By moving the stone up to the renal pelvis by forces from beneath the stone, the risks of perforation and extravasation associated with passage of wires and baskets past the stone are greatly reduced. The technique is surprisingly simple; a retrograde catheter of at least 7 F caliber, without side holes, is positioned carefully about 1 cm beneath the stone in the ureter (Figs 29–6 and 29–7). The percutaneous tract is established, preferably through a middle- or upper-pole calyx and the sheath positioned over the ureteropelvic junction (Figs 29–8 and 29–9). Only when access has been established is flushing attempted; flushing without a percutaneous tract may rupture the calyces. Initial flushing is performed with carbon dioxide and injected through the retrograde catheter by hand (Fig 29–10). If this is not successful, flushing with diluted liquid contrast by means of a pressure-infusion pump at a rate of between 5 to 10 ml/second should move the stone up into the renal pelvis (Fig 29–11). This technique has proved very effective for stones in the middle and upper ureter and even those that have been impacted for four weeks or more. Retrograde flushing for lower ureteral stones, however, is not as successful, and ureterorenoscopy is more appropriate.

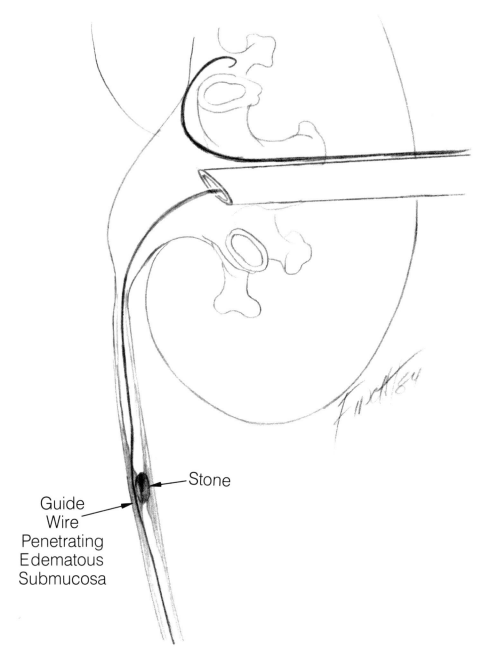

Fig 29–2.   The wire may not perforate the full thickness of the ureter but may, however, dissect beneath the mucosa.

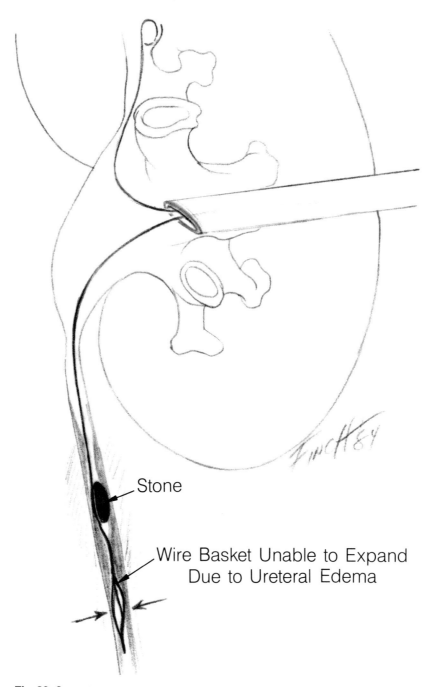

Fig 29–3. Although the basket may be maneuvered beyond the stone, it may not open adequately to engage the stone because of the narrow lumen of the edematous ureter.

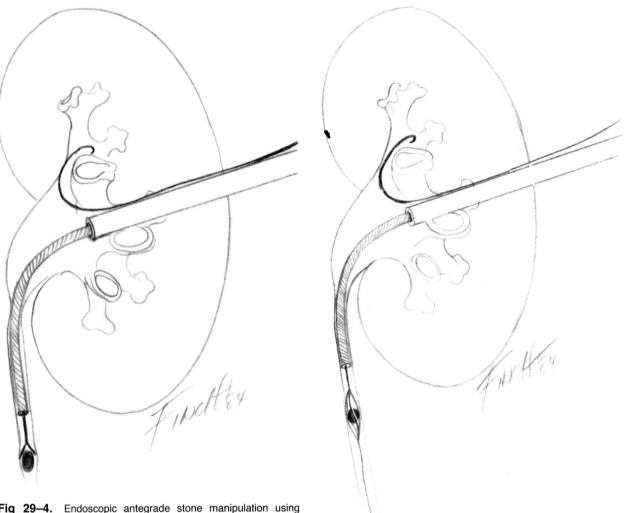

Fig 29–4. Endoscopic antegrade stone manipulation using grasping forceps.

Fig 29–5. Endoscopic antegrade stone manipulation using a stone basket.

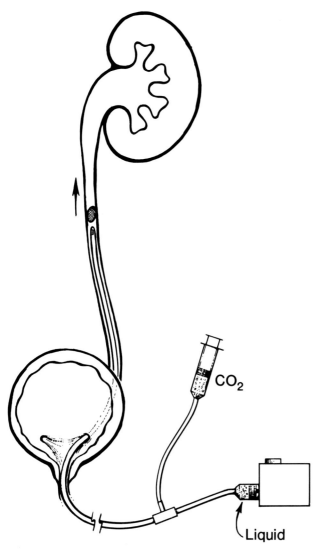

Fig 29–6. Schematic illustration of retrograde flushing technique. (From *J. Urol.* 134:29, 1985. Reproduced by permission.)

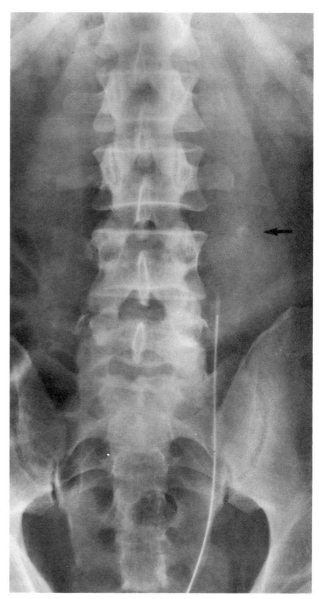

Fig 29–7. Radiological appearance of ureteral catheter beneath stone.

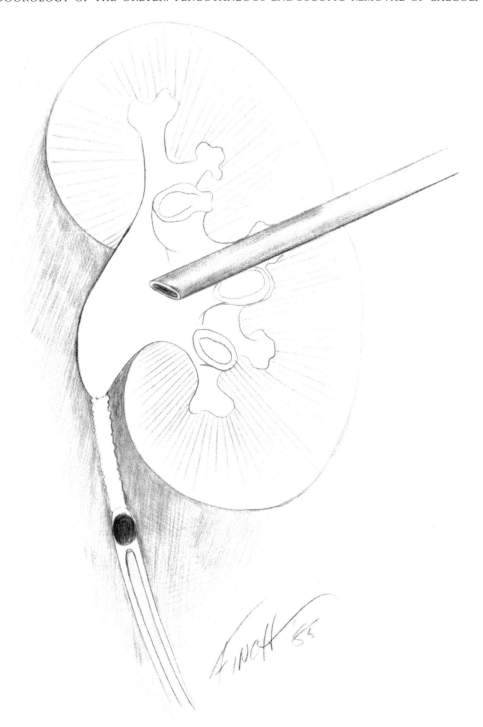

Fig 29–8. Position of sheath at the ureteropelvic junction for retrograde flushing.

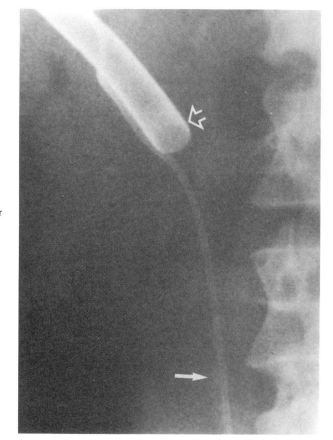

Fig 29–9. Roentgenogram of sheath *(open arrow)* positioned for retrograde flushing *(arrow* marks stone).

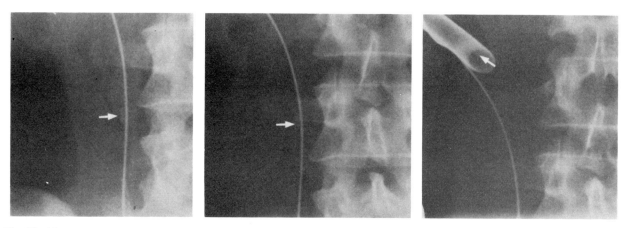

Fig 29–10. Roentgenograms showing flushing with carbon dioxide; note on the righthand frame the presence of carbon dioxide in the collecting system. The stone can be seen moving up (indicated by *arrow*).

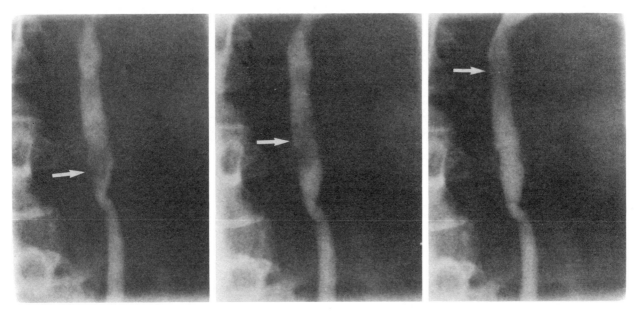

Fig 29–11.   Roentgenogram showing retrograde flushing with liquid contrast; stone *(arrow)* moves easily up the ureter into the renal pelvis. (From *J. Urol.* 134:29, 1985. Reproduced by permission.)

CHAPTER 30

Ureteropyeloscopy for Diagnosis and Treatment

Demetrius H. Bagley, M.D.

Transurethral endoscopy of the upper urinary tract has become possible through ureteropyeloscopy. Ureteropyeloscopic techniques have grown with the development of appropriate instruments.

Lyon et al.[1] reported a technique using pediatric cystoscopes for distal ureteral endoscopy in females. With the development of instruments specifically for ureteroscopy, the reach of the endoscope extended to the pelvic brim in both males and females.[2] Techniques for dilating the ureterovesical junction also advanced with these series. After the longer ureteropyeloscope became available, a rigid instrument could be passed as high as the renal pelvis.[3] The combination of this instrument with a long ultrasonic probe and transducer made possible the fragmentation and removal of calculi throughout the ureter and even in the renal pelvis.[4]

INSTRUMENTS

Ureteropyeloscopes presently include two basic designs, the conventional sheathed instrument and the operating ureteropyeloscope with an offset lens. Each instrument has its own advantages and disadvantages. The design and limitations of each instrument should be considered in selecting one for use in a specific patient with a specific clinical problem.

The conventional sheathed ureteroscope is very similar in design to the standard cystoscope (Fig 30–1). There is a sheath that may or may not have a working channel and will accept different telescopes, usually a forward and a lateral viewing lens. The working channel will accept no larger than a 5 F instrument. This is adequate for passing a basket, biopsy forceps, or electrode. This instrument is limited since it will not accept an ultrasound probe with direct visual control. The telescope must first be removed to allow placement of the ultrasound probe.

The operating ureteropyeloscope with an offset lens is specifically designed to accept an ultrasound probe for fragmentation of a calculus under vision (Fig 30–2). The offset telescope permits placement of the rigid ultrasound probe directly through the straight working channel within the instrument. There is also a small working channel on the side to permit passage of a device to restrain the calculus. This endoscope is also useful for passing larger working instruments, since its channel is approximately 6 F. Thus, a more substantial biopsy or foreign body forceps or electrode can be passed and used under direct vision.

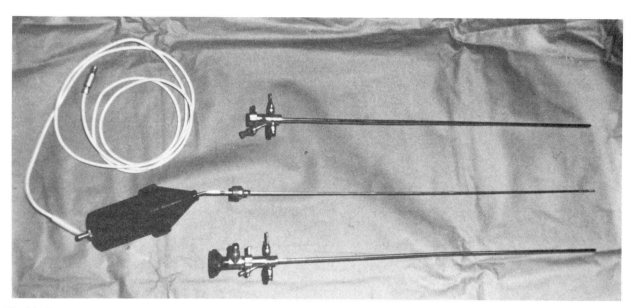

Fig 30–1. The standard sheathed ureteroscope has interchangeable lenses. A forward or lateral viewing lens can be placed into the sheath. There is also a 5 F working channel.

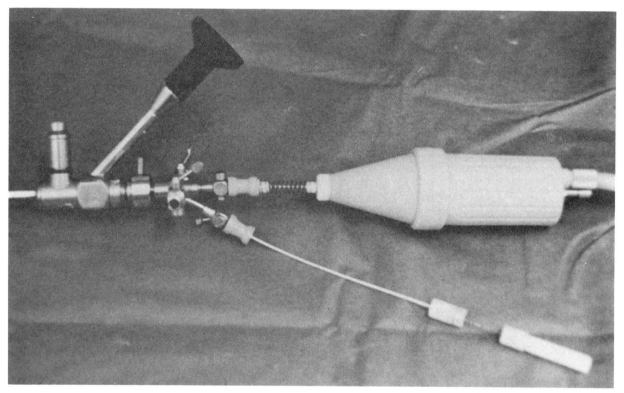

Fig 30–2. The offset lens operating ureteropyeloscope has a straight working channel for the ultrasound probe and a side channel for smaller working instruments, such as a stone basket.

Several of the same factors are significant disadvantages for the operating ureteropyeloscope. The offset lens may be extremely inconvenient for passage of the instrument or for use in certain positions. For example, the position of the calculus determines the optimal position for the tip of the instrument. Thus, if it appears best to place the ultrasound probe at the upper aspect of the calculus, then the instrument must be turned upside down and the urologist must place his head under the instrument to view through the offset lens. The total size of the working channel permits passage of only a small ultrasound probe and a very small basket or balloon for restraining the calculus to be fragmented.

Other designs of ureteropyeloscopes will certainly become available. Early models now exist of an instrument with a flexible offset telescope and another that has a rigid offset telescope that is interchangeable with a standard forward viewing telescope. These instruments will certainly add to the convenience of visual ultrasonic lithotripsy.

TECHNIQUE OF URETEROPYELOSCOPY

The technique for ureteropyeloscopy includes cystoscopy with a retrograde pyelogram performed using a cone-tipped catheter, dilation of the ureterovesical junction, and actual passage of the ureteropyeloscope.

Retrograde Pyelogram

The retrograde pyelogram provides accurate documentation of the entire ureter to the ureterovesical junction and indicates any nondistensible segments within the ureter. For this specific reason, it is more useful than an intravenous urogram, which may also show the ureter. It is impossible to determine from the excretion study whether a narrow area in the ureter is truly nondistensible or just represents a peristaltic contraction.

Dilation of the Ureterovesical Junction

Dilation of the ureterovesical junction, including the intramural ureter, has been an essential step for ureteropyeloscopy. Although the proximal ureter will usually dilate with pressure from the irrigation fluid, in many patients there are nondistensible segments that also require dilation. Several different techniques have been employed for dilating the ureterovesical junction and the proximal ureter.

Unguided Cone-Tipped Metal Bougies

Lyon et al.[1] described the use of cone-tipped metal bougies for dilating the ureterovesical junction for ureteroscopy. Dourmashkin[5] described the use of similar instruments, in the early part of the century, for dilating the ureter to facilitate stone passage. Commercially available cone-tipped metal dilators consist of a cone-shaped metal tip attached to a flexible carrier. The sizes range from 8 to 16 F.

The smallest dilator is passed through the cystoscope and into the appropriate ureteral orifice under direct vision. It can be followed visually as it enters the orifice and should be directed along the expected course of the ureter (Fig 30–3). A definite "give" is felt as the instrument passes through the intramural ureter into the lumen of the distal ureter. Successively larger instruments are similarly passed to dilate the orifice further.

Dilators greater than 12 F must be backloaded into the cystoscope. To position these dilators, the telescope and bridge are removed from the sheath of the cystoscope and the dilator is loaded into the bridge in a retrograde fashion. The assembled unit, consisting of the telescope bridge and dilator, is then reinserted into the sheath of the cystoscope and into the bladder. Under direct vision, the larger dilator can then be passed into the ureter. Again, considerable care should be taken to direct the dilator along the path of the intramural ureter.

Graduated Dilators

Graduated dilators of increasing size can also be used for dilating the intramural ureter. These dilators are passed over a guide wire that has been placed into the appropriate ureter. The smaller dilators, up to 12 F, can be passed through the cystoscope into the ureter under direct vision (Fig 30–4). Larger dilators will not pass through the bridge of the instrument and therefore must be placed into the ureter with radiologic control, preferably fluoroscopy. Care must be taken to pass the dilator into the ureter without coiling within the bladder. This can usually be avoided by using a heavy-duty guide wire or a Lunderquist guide wire to lead the dilator into the orifice.

Olive-Tipped Metal Bougie Dilators

Olive-tipped metal dilators can be passed over a guide wire through a cystoscope into the ureteral orifice. The dilator can be placed under direct vision into the orifice and advanced to dilate the

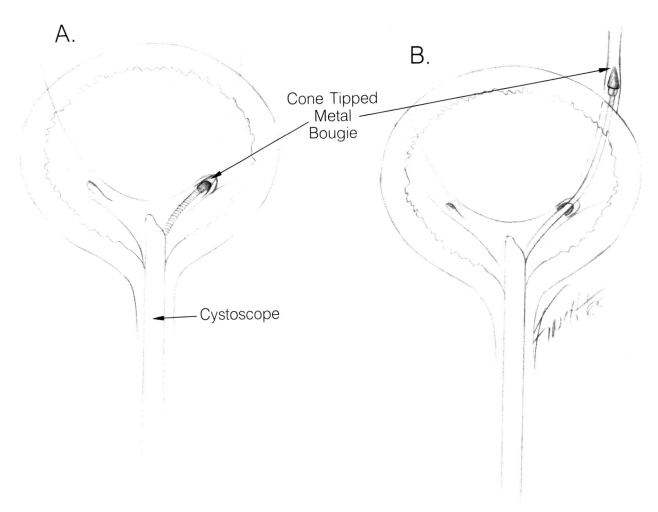

A.

B.

Cone Tipped
Metal
Bougie

Cystoscope

Fig 30–3. **A,** the cone-tipped metal bougie is passed from the cystoscope into the ureteral orifice under vision. **B,** it is directed along the course of the ureteral lumen and passed through the intramural portion of the ureter.

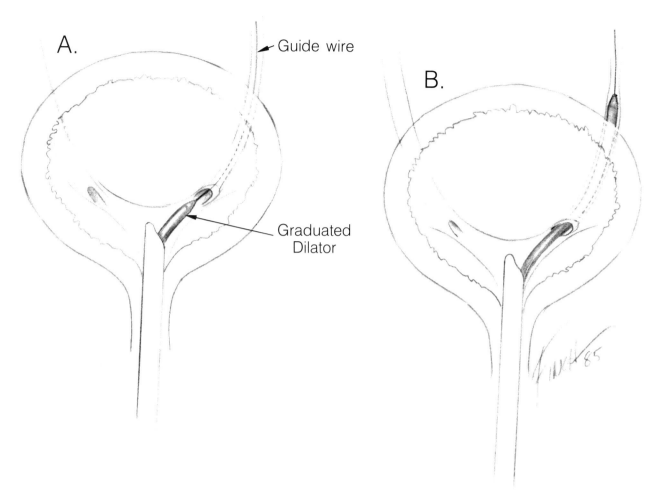

Fig 30–4. **A,** the graduated dilator is passed through the cystoscope over a guide wire into the ureteral orifice. **B,** it is passed through the lumen of the ureter to dilate the intramural portion. Its position can be confirmed fluoroscopically.

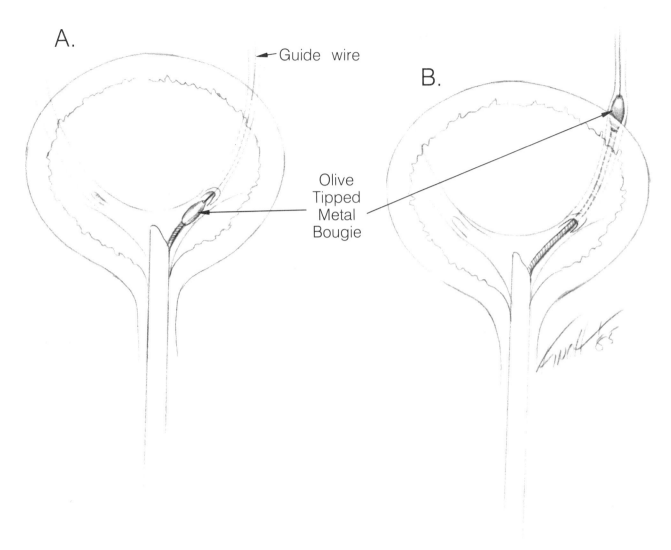

Fig 30–5. **A,** the olive-tipped metal bougies can be passed over a guide wire under direct vision into the ureteral orifice. **B,** it is advanced over the wire through the intramural portion of the ureter and can be advanced more proximally if necessary.

ureterovesical junction (Fig 30–5). Its position can be confirmed fluoroscopically. Successively larger dilators can be placed to the limit that the cystoscope will accept. Larger dilators can then be backloaded into the instrument. In this fashion, the telescope and bridge of the cystoscope are removed, leaving the guide wire in place. The olive-tipped dilator and its carrier are then placed over the guide wire, the combination of which is reassembled into the bridge of the cystoscope or "backloaded." The larger dilator can then be passed under direct vision into the orifice. These dilators afford full dilation of the orifice, excellent radiographic visualization, and reusability.

Balloon Dilating Catheters
Balloon dilating catheters can effectively dilate the ureterovesical junction. The high-pressure balloons, which can withstand pressures up to 17 atmospheres, have been particularly valuable. Older balloons, which were used for transluminal angioplasty and could withstand pressures of only 5 at-

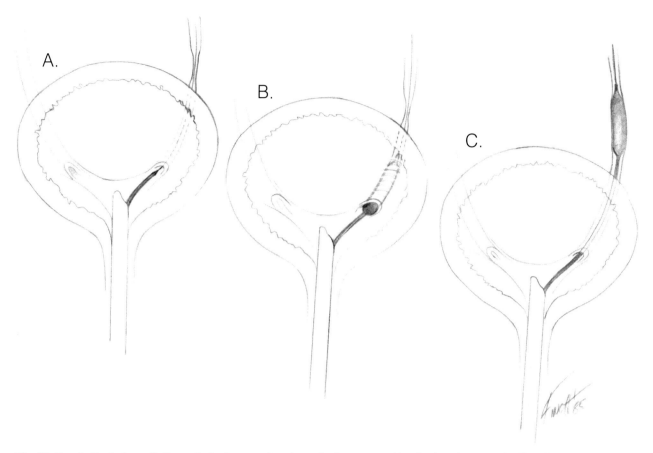

Fig 30–6. **A,** the balloon dilating catheter is passed cystoscopically over a guide wire into the ureteral orifice. **B,** it should be positioned so that the cylindrical portion of the balloon can be seen at the orifice as it is inflated. **C,** the balloon can be deflated, passed more proximally in the ureter, and again inflated to dilate segments of the ureter at any level.

mospheres, have proved less useful and often could not provide full dilation. Catheters are available from 5 to 9 F with balloons 5 or 6 mm in diameter and at least 4 cm in length, which can be passed over a guide wire. Pressures up to 15 to 17 atmospheres have been required for dilation.

After a guide wire is passed into the ureter cystoscopically, the balloon catheter is passed over the dilator through the cystoscope into the orifice (Fig 30–6). The balloon is then positioned so that it can be seen within the bladder and so that the cylindrical portion of the balloon will inflate to dilate the ureteral orifice and the intramural ureter. The balloon is then inflated with a solution containing radiographic contrast media (30% iodine). Balloon catheters can also be positioned to dilate more proximal portions of the ureter.

Inflation of the balloon should be monitored

fluoroscopically to confirm full dilation of the balloon. If there is a persistent "waist," then dilation is not sufficient. If waisting persists after the balloon is inflated, then it should be inflated to a higher pressure. The specific dilating balloons will not overexpand, but will rupture if inflated beyond their pressure capacity. The pressure generated by a hand-held syringe is inversely related to the size of the syringe with the smaller syringes providing a higher pressure. The specific limitations and directions for inflation for each balloon are provided with the manufacturer's specifications.

Catheters with latex balloons such as the Fogarty embolectomy catheter should not be used for dilating the ureter. The latex balloon is elastic and may overexpand in the nonstenotic segment and injure the ureter.

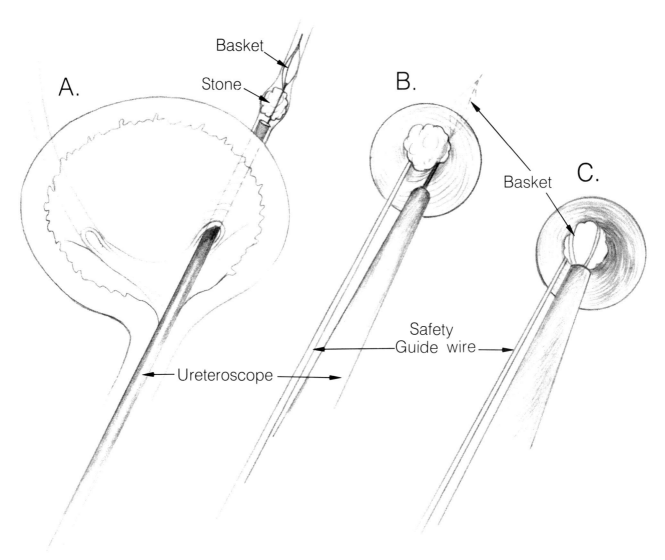

Fig 30–7. **A,** a basket is passed beyond the calculus under direct vision through the ureteroscope. **B,** an appropriate point between the calculus and the ureter can usually be visualized endoscopically. The safety guide wire can be left in place throughout the procedure. **C,** under vision, the basket may be opened at the level of the calculus in an attempt to place the wires around the calculus and engage it within the basket.

TREATMENT OF URINARY CALCULI

Urinary calculi have become a major indication for ureteropyeloscopic procedures. Calculi can be removed intact if they will pass through the ureter under vision or may be fragmented for removal. The ureteropyeloscope can reach throughout the ureter and usually into the renal pelvis as well, but the ease and success of stone retrieval are highest in the distal ureter.

The ureteropyeloscope is placed into the ureter as described previously. The guide wire used for dilating is usually left in place to act as a safety

wire. The instrument is then passed to the level of the calculus, and a stone basket is passed through the instrument beyond the calculus and withdrawn to engage the calculus (Fig 30–7). This maneuver is often difficult, even under direct vision. It may be of value to open the basket at the same level as the calculus and to manipulate it so that the wires are on either side of the calculus. An appropriately sized basket should be used to fit around the calculus. The ureteroscope, basket, and calculus are then withdrawn from the ureter as the operator keeps the calculus in the basket under vision. It should move freely within the lumen of the ureter. If the calculus is firmly impacted within the ureter or does not move freely as the instrument is withdrawn, then it should be fragmented for removal.

Ultrasonic Ureterolithotripsy

Ultrasonic ureterolithotripsy has proved to be an effective and safe technique for fragmenting and removing ureteral calculi that are too large to retrieve intact from the ureter. In general, two techniques have been developed for fragmenting calculi within the ureter with an ultrasound probe. Each provides accurate control and each has its own specific advantages and indications as well as disadvantages. These are: (1) the tactile or auditory technique, and (2) the direct visual technique.

Tactile Ultrasonic Ureterolithotripsy

The conventional sheath ureteropyeloscope with interchangeable lenses is used for this procedure. The instrument is passed to the level of the calculus as described above. The calculus is then engaged in a basket that can be passed through the 5 F working channel (Fig 30–8). The calculus can be drawn down the ureter with a basket as far as possible until the size of the lumen precludes further withdrawal. The calculus is then positioned at the tip of the ureteropyeloscope so that nothing but the calculus can be seen with the forward viewing telescope. The calculus and basket are then held in that position as the telescope is removed. A rubber gasket fitting is placed into the end of the ureteropyeloscope through which the ultrasound probe is introduced. The probe is passed to the tip of the sheath until it contacts the calculus. It is quite easy to feel the probe touch the calculus with both of the operator's hands as the stone is held within the basket and the probe is advanced. As irrigation is continued, the probe is activated and fragments are aspirated with suction. As the probe is activated in contact with the calculus, there is a distinctive sound that changes as the probe passes the calculus. Positioning can be confirmed fluoroscopically but this does not provide as fine a resolution as tactile and auditory monitoring.

After the probe has disintegrated the calculus or has fragmented a portion of it to form a groove through which the probe can pass, resistance is no longer felt with the probe and pressure is no longer felt against the calculus within the basket. The probe is then removed and the telescope replaced to visualize the calculus and reposition it at the tip of the ureteroscope. The entire procedure is then repeated. Fragmentation is continued until the entire calculus has been removed or the calculus is sufficiently small to be extracted from the ureter.

Visual Ultrasonic Ureterolithotripsy

By using the operating ureteropyeloscope with the offset ocular lens, a rigid ultrasound probe can be introduced into the ureter under direct vision (see Fig 30–2). The ureteropyeloscope is passed in the usual way to the level of the calculus. If the calculus is firmly lodged within the ureter, particularly within the distal ureter, the ultrasound probe may be introduced immediately and applied to the calculus and activated (Fig 30–9,A). If the calculus is moving freely, then it should be engaged in a basket or the proximal ureter should be obstructed to prevent proximal migration of fragments (Figs 30–9,B and C). Placing a basket to engage the calculus offers the greatest security and control of the calculus. After it has been placed within the basket, the ultrasound probe is introduced and the calculus fragmented under vision. If the calculus is too large to fit into a basket, then the basket or a balloon catheter can be placed beyond the calculus into the proximal ureter to prevent migration of fragments. The basket offers some advantage over a balloon since the calculus can sometimes be engaged in the basket as it is fragmented and thus be securely restrained for fragmentation or removal. It is difficult to obstruct the entire ureter and prevent proximal migration of fragments with a balloon catheter alone.

Although the probes that fit through the offset lens ureteropyeloscopes are quite small, fragments can usually be aspirated through the lumen. Obstruction with a fragment of calculus is not unusual and can be avoided by irrigating rather than aspirating through the lumen of the probe. Although pieces of the calculus are not removed, fragmentation is often achieved more quickly.

Postoperative Management

Following removal of the calculus, an open-ended ureteral catheter, diversionary catheter, or double-pigtail stent is placed over the safety guide wire within the ureter, which is subsequently removed. Catheter drainage is maintained for 24 to 72 hours while a stent allows early discharge of the patient and can be removed several days later at the patient's convenience. Mild lower abdominal discomfort may be seen after ureteroscopy but severe pain is distinctly unusual. Mild hematuria is expected.

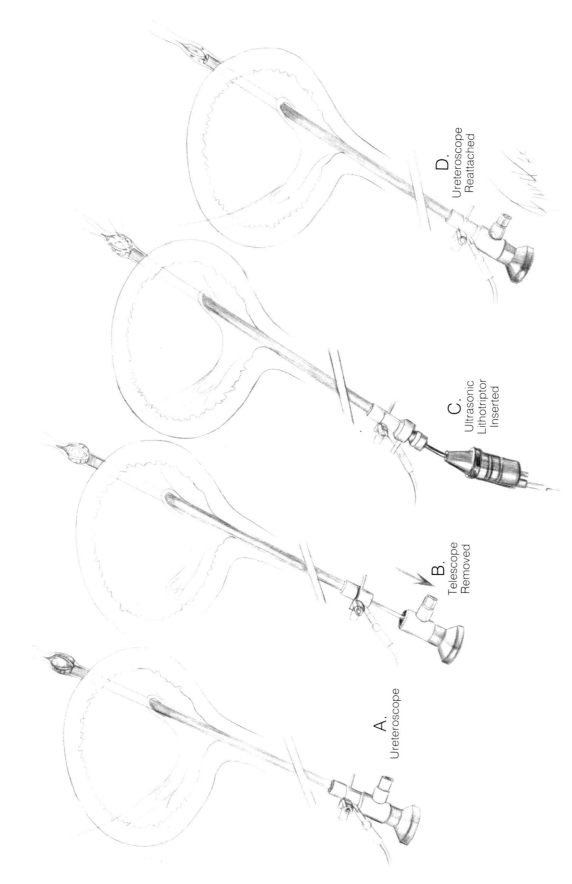

Fig 30—8. **A,** calculi can be fragmented with the ultrasonic lithotriptor utilizing the nonvisual or tactile technique. The calculus is engaged in a basket under vision and drawn to the tip of the ureteroscope. **B,** as the calculus is held in position, the telescope is removed from the ureteroscope. **C,** the ultrasound probe is passed through the sheath to contact the calculus and, as irrigation continues, used to fragment the calculus. The force of the probe against the calculus can be felt by the urologist holding the calculus and the probe. **D,** as a calculus is fragmented, the probe will pass the calculus and resistance is no longer felt. The calculus should then be repositioned under vision.

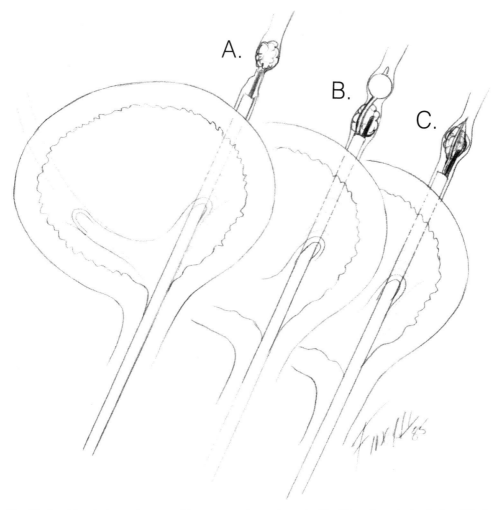

Fig 30–9. Visual ultrasonic ureterolithotomy can be performed with: **(A)** an impacted calculus; **(B)** after obstruction of the ureter proximal to the calculus, or **(C)** with the calculus engaged in a stone basket.

DIAGNOSIS AND TREATMENT OF UROTHELIAL TUMORS

Urothelial tumors have been diagnosed and in some cases treated ureteropyeloscopically.[6] Observation and biopsy under vision have proved most useful for ureteral and renal pelvic filling defects. Resection of urothelial tumors in a fashion similar to that employed for bladder tumors has been employed in several patients but awaits longer series and follow-up before establishing its role in the routine treatment of such lesions.

Biopsy

When ureteropyeloscopy is being performed for diagnostic purposes, particular care should be taken in placing a guide wire and dilating the ureter. Every effort should be made to avoid traumatizing a filling defect or suspicious area being investigated. The ureteropyeloscope can be passed to the area of interest using the usual techniques. Urothelial lesions of the ureter and renal pelvis possess the same morphologic characteristics as those within the bladder. However, they can also

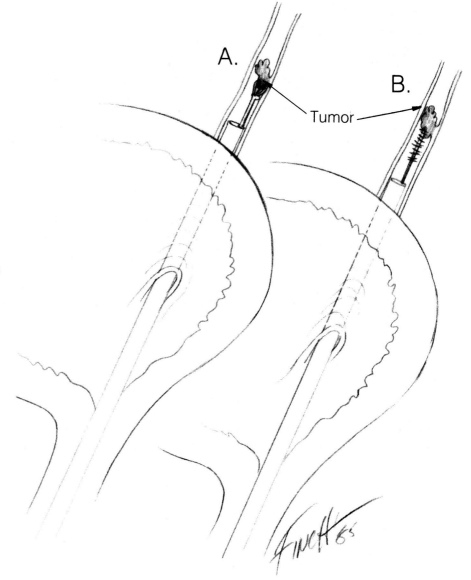

Fig 30–10. Ureteral neoplasms can be biopsied with **(A)** a cold cupped forceps, or **(B)** a brush under direct vision.

be confused with inflammatory lesions and the diagnosis should always be confirmed with biopsy. As the lesion is visualized, a 5 F biopsy forceps can be passed through the ureteropyeloscope to sample the lesion directly (Fig 30–10,A). A brush can also be passed under direct vision to obtain tissue from the lesion (Fig 30–10,B). A small tumor can be fulgurated with an electrode as similar lesions are in the bladder.

Larger tumors can be resected with the ureteropyeloscopic resectoscope. This instrument is passed to the level of the lesion in the same fashion as the diagnostic or operating ureteropyeloscopes. Resection is performed by extending the loop to the tumor and then withdrawing it into the sheath before cutting (Fig 30–11). Thus, the wall of the ureter is not damaged by the cutting loop. It may be a slow procedure since the resectoscope has a relatively small lumen and the resected bits of tumor must be irrigated from the field. An indwelling ureteral catheter should be left in place for at least 24 to 48 hours after resecting within the ureter.

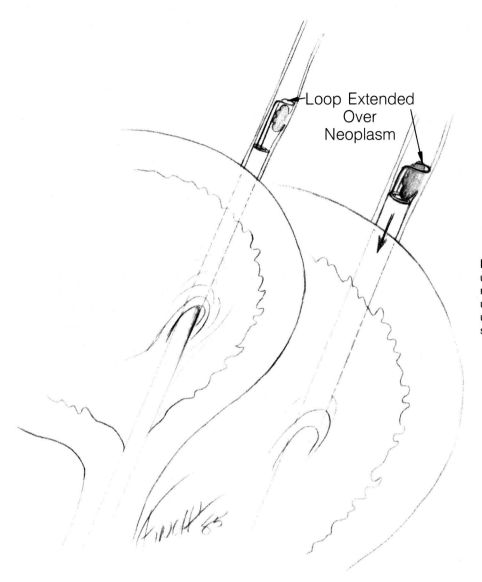

Loop Extended
Over
Neoplasm

Fig 30–11. The resecting ureteropyeloscope can be used for removal of neoplasms within the ureter. The loop is extended and used to draw the lesion into the sheath before cutting.

FLEXIBLE URETEROPYELOSCOPY

Ureteropyeloscopy was first performed in a planned fashion with flexible instruments.[7, 8] The technical limitations prevented widespread application of these techniques. Although development of rigid instruments and techniques for their use have far surpassed the employment of flexible instruments, the latter are being increasingly appreciated for their unique features. Flexible instruments can pass tortuosities within the ureter and enter lateral portions of the intrarenal collecting system that are inaccessible to rigid instruments. The major difficulties with these instruments have been in introducing them into the ureteral orifice, providing irrigation, and having a channel adequate for useful working instruments.

Introducing the Flexible Ureteropyeloscope

Flexible ureteropyeloscopes can be passed through the bladder into the ureteral orifice in several ways. Each technique must direct the instrument into the orifice and prevent it from buckling and coiling within the bladder. Variations of the guide tube techniques are most widely applicable. This technique generally includes placing a tubular instrument from the urethra through the bladder and into the ureter through which the flexible instrument can be passed. A cystoscope can be employed as a guide tube by positioning the sheath adjacent to the ureteral orifice and then maintaining it in that position as the flexible instrument is passed through the sheath into the orifice. It is usually easier to pass a flexible Teflon tube over a graduated dilator into the orifice[9] (Fig

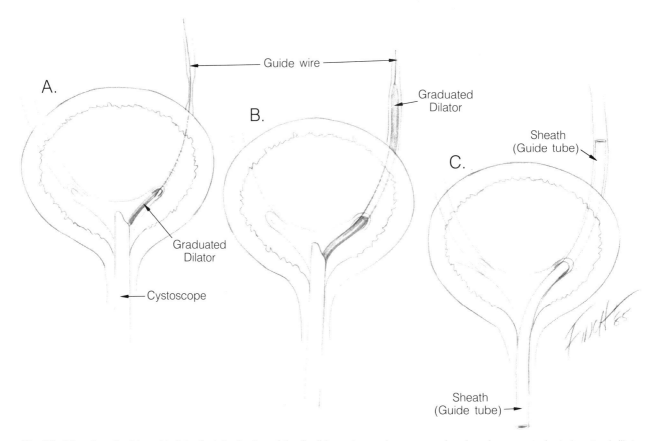

Fig 30–12. **A,** a flexible guide tube for introduction of the flexible ureteropyeloscope can be placed over a graduated ureteral dilator. A guide wire is first placed into the ureter under cystoscopic visualization. **B,** the ureter is dilated with the graduated dilators under visual and fluoroscopic control. **C,** a sheath of selected size is passed over the dilator, which is subsequently removed, leaving the guide tube extending from the urethral meatus into the ureter.

30–12). After the dilator has been removed, a flexible endoscope can be passed through the lumen into the ureter. The sheath of the rigid ureteropyeloscope can also function as a guide tube[10] (Fig 30–13). After the conventional ureteropyeloscope has been passed into the ureter, the rigid telescope can be removed and a flexible instrument (2.7-mm Olympus ureteropyeloscope) can be passed through the sheath and used as a flexible deflectable telescope. This combination benefits from the best features of each instrument. The rigid sheath provides passage through the bladder and allows for irrigation and placement of a working instrument while the flexible instrument can be maneuvered into otherwise inaccessible intraluminal locations.

Instruments with a working channel adequate to accept a guide wire can be passed over a guide wire and through the bladder into the ureter.[11] The guide wire prevents coiling of the flexible instrument within the bladder.

Irrigation

Irrigation can be provided through the working or irrigation channel in instruments that have that feature. For the other small instruments, irrigation can be provided through the working sheath or the sheath of the rigid ureteropyeloscope. A small ureteral catheter can often be inserted alongside the flexible endoscope to provide irrigation at the proximal portion of the urinary tract near the tip of the ureteropyeloscope.

Working Instruments

Only the flexible ureteropyeloscopes with a working channel greater than 1 mm will accept any working instrument. The 3.6-mm Olympus ureteropyeloscope has a 1.2-mm working channel that will accept simple instruments such as a snare or grasper if the instrument itself is used as the sheath. The newer 3 F instruments can also be passed through this channel. To perform any tasks

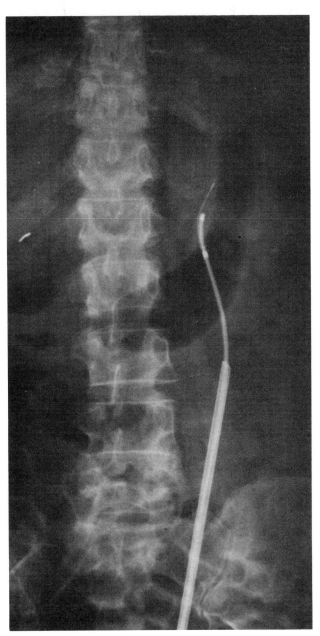

Fig 30–13. The small (2.7-mm) flexible ureteroscope has been passed through a rigid ureteropyeloscope sheath to function as a flexible telescope. Irrigation and a working channel are provided by the rigid sheath.

under vision with the other instruments, the auxiliary working instrument must be passed alongside the endoscope. Although this necessitates separate manipulation of each instrument, the task can be performed under direct vision and affords much greater accuracy than that provided by fluoroscopic control.

REFERENCES

1. Lyon E.S., Kyker J.S., Schoenberg H.W.: Transurethral ureteroscopy in women: A ready addition to urologic armamentarium. *J. Urol.* **119:**35, 1978.
2. Lyon E.S., Banno J.J., Schoenberg H.W.: Transurethral ureteroscopy in men using juvenile cystoscopy equipment. *J. Urol.* **122:**152, 1979.
3. Perez-Castro Ellendt E., Martinez-Pineiro J.A.: Transurethral ureteroscopy—a current urological procedure. *Arch. Esp. Urol.* **33:**445, 1980.
4. Huffman J.L., Bagley D.H., Schoenberg H.W., et al.: Transurethral removal of large ureteral and renal pelvic calculi using ureteroscopic ultrasonic lithotripsy. *J. Urol.* **130:**31, 1983.
5. Dourmashkin R.L.: Cystoscopic treatment of stones in the ureter with special reference to large calculi: Based on the study of 1,550 cases. *J. Urol.* **54:**245, 1945.
6. Huffman J.L., Morse M.J., Bagley D.H., et al.: Endoscopic diagnosis and treatment of upper tract urothelial tumors—a preliminary report. *Cancer* **55:**1422–1428, 1985.
7. Marshall V.F.: Fiberoptics in urology. *J. Urol.* **91:**110, 1964.
8. Takagi T., Go T., Takayasu H., et al.: Fiberoptic pyeloureteroscope. *Surgery* **70:**661, 1971.
9. Takayasu H., Aso Y.: Recent development for pyeloureteroscopy: Guide tube method for its introduction into the ureter. *J. Urol.* **112:**176, 1974.
10. Bagley D.H., Huffman J.L., Lyon E.S.: Combined rigid and flexible ureteropyeloscopy. *J. Urol.* **130:**243, 1983.
11. Bagley D.H., Huffman J.L., Lyon E.S.: Flexible fiberoptic ureteropyeloscopy, in Bagley D.H., Huffman J.L., Lyon E.S. (eds.) *Urologic Endoscopy: A Manual and Atlas.* Boston, Little, Brown & Co., 1985, pp. 207–217.

CHAPTER 31

Endourologic Procedures Relating to Extracorporeal Shock Wave Lithotripsy

Joseph W. Segura, M.D.

Extracorporeal shock wave lithotripsy (ESWL) has become more and more important as a primary method of renal stone removal. While the relative roles of ESWL and endourology in stone removal remain to be demarcated, it seems apparent that ESWL will be the procedure of choice for some 70% to 80% of renal stones, especially smaller stones. Its noninvasive nature and ability to convert stones into tiny pieces, which may then pass down the ureter and into the bladder with relative ease, seem to be distinct advantages.

Despite its usefulness, ESWL cannot itself deal with all renal calculi. Further endourologic procedures are often necessary to optimize the effectiveness of ESWL or deal with some complication ESWL has generated. In the first 300 ESWL patients treated at Mayo, 126 had some preoperative endourologic procedure (Table 31–1) and 10% had some postoperative procedure. The majority of the preoperative ancillary treatments were indicated to optimize the visualization of the stone, and the majority of the posttreatment procedures were directed toward problems related to obstruction from the stony fragments. Also, staghorn calculi were treated in a prospective manner with a combined planned treatment of percutaneous ultrasonic lithotripsy with subsequent ESWL.

INDICATIONS FOR ENDOUROLOGIC PROCEDURES

Visualization

A major limitation of currently available shock wave lithotripsy equipment is in its intraoperative fluoroscopy. While fluoroscopy is essential to the operation of the unit, as the stones become smaller or less calcified, fluoroscopic visualization becomes less and less certain, to the point that it may very well be impossible to find the stone for which lithotripsy is indicated. In such circumstances, it has been our practice to pass a ureteral catheter prior to the shock wave treatment. This considerably facilitates finding the stone, or at least in outlining the collecting system to outline the calyx, infundibulum, or where the stone should be. Contrast may be injected at will and irrigated out, if necessary, at will. I have found this clearly superior to the use of intravenous (IV) contrast medium. While IV contrast medium will eventually collect in the kidney, the degree of concentration varies with the patient's state of hydration and the concentration and visualization may be in no sense timely.

TABLE 31–1.—Type of Preoperative Endourologic Procedure in First 126/300 Patients Who Had ESWL

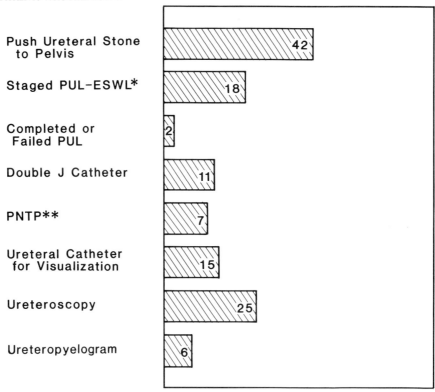

*Percutaneous Ultrasonic Lithotripsy

**Percutaneous Nephrostomy Tube Placement

We usually remove ureteral catheters at the end of the procedure as they no longer serve a useful purpose, and if left in will only prevent the pieces from passing down the ureter. In the case of uric acid stones, the retrograde catheter is left in for an extra 24 hours so that the status of the stone may be evaluated with retrograde injection of contrast medium the next day.

Ureteral Stones

Most ureteral stones that do not pass are 5 mm in diameter or greater, and most are usually less than 1 cm in diameter, as larger stones usually will not fall down into the ureter. Extracorporeal shock wave lithotripsy is useful in treating these stones, especially those in the upper ureter. When the stone is located in the ureter, it is usually visible readily on one but not both of the two monitors. On the second monitor, the stone will overlay the spinal column and it will usually be impossible to find it. Furthermore, ureteral stones often become fixed to the ureteral wall. Even if the stone is broken up by the shocks, the pieces

may remain in place, fixed by the ureteral mucosa that has grown around the stone.

For these reasons it is desirable that the stone be pushed back into the renal pelvis, if possible, to where breakage occurs much more reliably and where visualization is possible without the concern of overlying bony structures. We usually attempt to pass a retrograde catheter immediately prior to the procedure and attempt to push or irrigate the stone back up in the renal pelvis. Our success rate in doing this is approximately 50%. A much higher success rate could be achieved if a percutaneous nephrostomy tube were previously inserted and the techniques described by Hulbert et al.[1] employed. Because we can usually break the stone up successfully in the ureter, the extra effort that this method requires does not seem justified in this circumstance.

In some clinical situations, the anatomy of the ureter may be such that the stone may be expeditiously removed by a ureteroscopic technique. Certainly, if the ureter below the stone is of adequate caliber and particularly if the stone is rather large, it may be that transureteral ultrasonic lith-

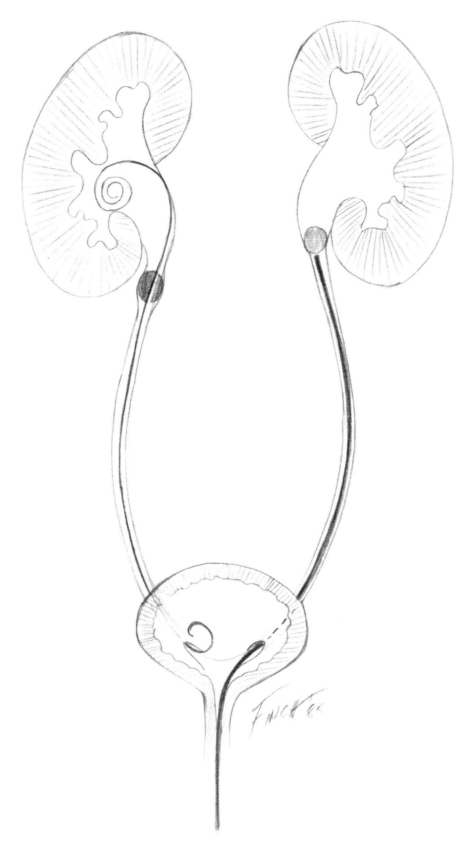

Fig 31–1.　Illustration depicting several uses of ureteral catheters prior to extracorporeal shock wave lithotripsy (ESWL). The stone in the upper third of the left ureter may be destroyed in situ with shock wave lithotripsy. Localizing it with ESWL fluoroscopes will be much simpler if the catheter is left indwelling below the stone or if the stone is pushed to the renal pelvis. On the right side, a double-J stent has been placed as a temporizing device because of acute colic. In this situation the double-J should remain in until the stone is broken up by ESWL, and then the catheter immediately removed.

otripsy might be more expeditious and quicker than shock wave lithotripsy.

If we have been unable to move the stone with a catheter or by irrigation, the ureteral catheter is left in place with its tip just distal to the stone and it is then tied around the Foley catheter. This will mark the position of the stone on the fluoroscopic monitors. The catheter usually is obvious, and with the catheter in position, it is possible to localize the stone on both monitors. Should it still be difficult to see, injection of contrast medium through the ureteral catheter will elucidate the position of the stone (Fig 31–1).

Despite seemingly adequate disruption of the stone at the time of the ESWL, 24 to 48 hours may pass without any passage of fragments. If passage is still unsatisfactory, it has been our practice to attempt to dislodge the fragments with a catheter or to employ ureteroscopy to remove the stones. Such direct treatment avoids the uncertainty associated with a second ESWL treatment and ensures that on dismissal from the hospital the patient's clinical problem has been solved.

Ureteral Obstruction

Patients who have obstructive stones in the ureter or ureteropelvic junction and have elevated temperatures and associated urinary tract infections should not undergo shock wave lithotripsy until the acute infection is controlled and the condition stabilized. In many cases, this will mean insertion of a percutaneous nephrostomy tube and, perhaps, a retrograde catheter to achieve proximal drainage. Once a percutaneous nephrostomy tube has been placed, defervescence will occur and ESWL may be performed as an elective procedure. Should it have been necessary to insert a percutaneous nephrostomy tube, the surgeon should consider whether the situation might be managed by performing a percutaneous stone removal instead of ESWL.

STAGED PERCUTANEOUS ULTRASONIC LITHOTRIPSY-ESWL

While ESWL has undeniable advantages for smaller stones, the advantages begin to blur as the size of the stone increases. Multiple treatments may be necessary and ancillary treatments may become important. It has been obvious that the treatment of infected stones of large volume (staghorn calculi and partial staghorns) present difficult problems that may not be best managed by ESWL alone.

Owing to the size of these stones, large volumes of stony fragments will be formed after fragmentation from ESWL. The quantity of stone will exceed the capacity of the ureter to pass the fragments in a timely fashion and an obstructive uropathy will ensue. Because these are infected fragments, a pyonephrosis will result, and the patient will develop signs of localized infection with pain, fever, and chills. Second, while a single ESWL treatment may break up all of the infected stone, it is very likely that multiple treatments will be necessary, thus prolonging the time period in which the patient will be at risk for sepsis and ureteral obstruction.

The problem may be obviated by combining the virtues of ultrasonic lithotripsy, with which large volumes of stone are readily removable from areas readily accessible, and the virtues of ESWL, with which small volumes of stone can be effectively removed, especially in places that are not readily accessible. All except the smallest struvite stones are thus managed in a stepwise fashion. The patients received 24 to 48 hours of the appropriate intravenous antibiotic—usually gentamicin, but occasionally ampicillin as well, for susceptible bacteria. A percutaneous nephrostomy tube is placed and percutaneous ultrasonic lithotripsy performed. If the patient's anatomy is such that all of the material can be removed, the procedure is then terminated and no shock wave procedure performed.

The role of shock wave lithotripsy when the initial percutaneous procedure has not cleaned out the stone is essentially to replace the percutaneous manipulations and secondary procedures that would have been done to completely clean out the kidney (Fig 31–2). In other words, instead of using the flexible nephroscope or a second nephrostomy tract to remove a calyceal stone or fragment not directly accessible from the original access site, the shock wave machine would be used. We have routinely administered 1,000 to 2,000 shocks for such purposes two days after percutaneous ultrasonic lithotripsy without apparent ill effect. Most of the newly pulverized stone will exit through the preexisting nephrostomy tube placed at the time of percutaneous lithotripsy. When the remaining infected stone appears to have been reduced to a level at which obstruction seems unlikely, a nephrostomy tube may be removed. Occasionally, we have manipulated fragments through the percutaneous tract prior to removal of the nephrostomy tube.

The biggest disadvantage of this procedure is the uncertainty concerning the final result. When

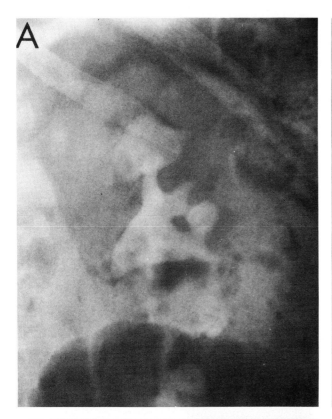

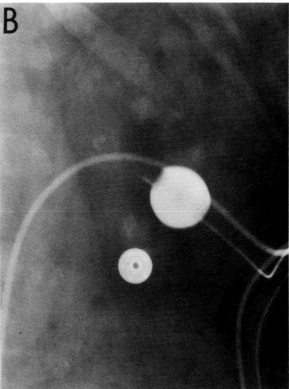

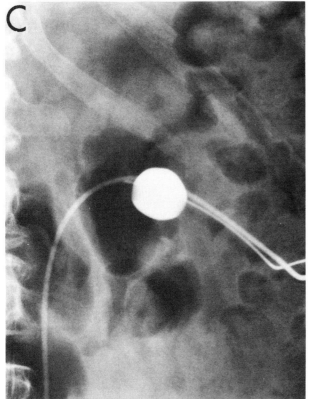

Fig 31–2. A, staghorn calculus in left kidney. **B,** this postprocedure roentgenogram of the kidney illustrates the material remaining after the percutaneous ultrasonic lithotripsy. This material was treated with 1,500 shocks at 20 kV with extracorporeal shock wave lithotripsy. **C,** all of the material in the kidney has passed out of the nephrostomy tube, except for a small amount of material on the lower-pole calyx. This may be removed via percutaneous methods or the stent and the nephrostomy tube removed and the patient may pass material in the months to come.

the patient is dismissed from the hospital, it is still not known whether he will ultimately be stone-free or not. At the present time, there are insufficient data to establish whether this combined treatment is equal to or superior to treatment with percutaneous methods alone or even open surgery. The problem is made more acute and underlined by the fact that 9% to 25% of shock wave cases will have residual fragments. Any residual fragment after treatment of infected stone represents a partial failure.

Post-ESWL Ureteral Obstruction

Ten percent or more of ESWL patients may require some post–shock wave procedure because of obstructing fragments in the ureter. Treatment may be required because of pain, fever, or other symptoms of obstruction. While such obstruction may be from one or two small stones than were insufficiently fragmented, more often the problem is from a column of stones collecting in the lower ureter. This is called a "Steinstrasse" or stone street (Fig 31–3). Such a collection of stones is more likely to occur with larger stones when the ureter is suddenly presented with more stones than can be passed over reasonable time.

In our opinion, these Steinstrasse should be aggressively managed. A preferred approach is to remove these fragments by the ureteroscope. Cystoscopic inspection of the ureteral meatus will reveal the swelling and edema typical of a meatus from which stones have passed or are about to pass. It is usually impossible to pass a guide wire or basket up past these stones, but because the stones have the effect of dilating the ureter, I have always found it possible to introduce a ureteroscope through the ureteral meatus without dilation up to the base of the column of stones. It may then be possible to implant a guide wire catheter and, under vision with the ureteroscope, start to knock the stones loose. The small bits of stone will gradually be knocked loose until a "keystone" is reached, and then the whole column seems to fall through at once.

A more rapid and efficient method is to use the ultrasonic probe to aspirate the pieces that have already been broken up. The preferred probe is that which has a lumen adequate to aspirate small pieces. The solid probes are probes that have no lumen or whose lumen is so small that aspiration of pieces is impossible and will not be effective. These probes are best used if the stone has not been previously broken up and represent no advantage in this circumstance. Once the lower ureter is clear of stones, I usually leave one or two ureteral catheters in place for 24 to 48 hours.

If ureteroscopy is not practical or possible, and if pain or sepsis is present, a percutaneous nephrostomy tube should be placed. This is particularly true if the stone is infected. If a percutaneous nephrostomy tube is not done prior to ESWL, sudden sepsis may develop. The tube should be placed as soon as possible after the temperature spike to prevent the development of pyonephrosis. On two occasions we delayed the placement of the nephrostomy tube for 24 and 48 hours past initial temperature spike and were greeted by what was essentially pus in the obstructed system.

Post-ESWL Percutaneous Lithotripsy

Extracorporeal shock wave lithotripsy may fail. Occasionally, the stone either does not break up or does not break up into pieces small enough that they can reasonably be expected to pass. While this is most likely to occur with cystine stones, calcium oxalate monohydrate stone will occasionally behave in such a manner. While repeated ESWL treatments are always possible after initial failure, the certainty of treatment by a percutaneous method would seem to make this preferable to the uncertainty of repeated shock wave lithotripsy treatments.

Bilateral ESWL

There is no reason not to treat both sides at a single time under the same anesthetic when bilateral stones are present. The chief risk to be considered under this circumstance is ensuing bilateral ureteral obstruction from simultaneous passage of fragments. We have tried to restrict bilateral treatments only to those cases in which the stone burden on one side was small enough that obstruction seemed unlikely. If the surgeon guesses wrong, a percutaneous nephrostomy tube or retrograde catheter should be inserted, if and when anuria is present and if it persists beyond a few hours.

REFERENCE

1. Hulbert J.C., Reddy P.K., Lange P.H., et al.: Percutaneous management of ureteral calculi facilitated by means of retrograde flushing with carbon dioxide or dilute radiopaque dye. *J. Urol.* 134:29–32, 1985.

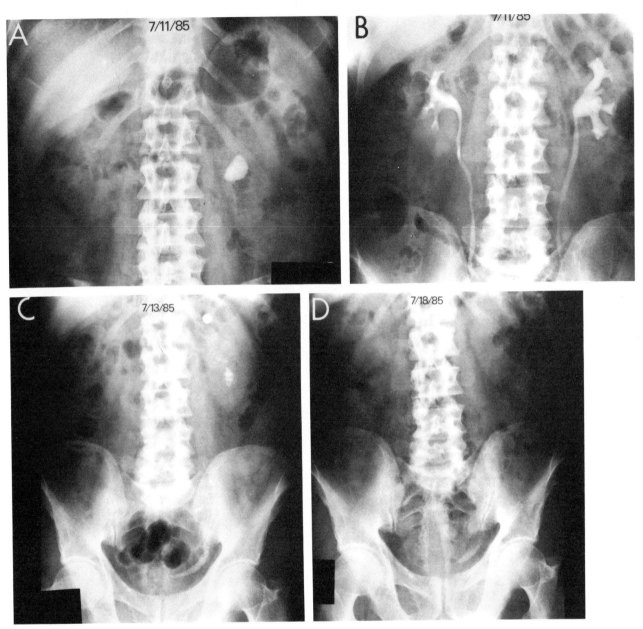

Fig 31–3.   **A,** a substantial renal pelvic stone. **B,** the collecting system is otherwise normal with a normal ureter. **C,** roentgenogram of kidney, ureter, and bladder after extracorporeal shock wave lithotripsy: note the "Steinstrasse" in the left lower ureter. A considerable amount of material is present and unpassed material is also still present in the pelvis and in the lower pole of the kidney. This material in the lower ureter was removed with the ureteroscope. **D,** all of the material in the left kidney is now present in the lower ureter. This material passed spontaneously without further manipulation.

Subject Index